Praise for *The Wisdom of Healing*

"I hope this understandable book will be read open-mindedly not only by those who are sick and those who do not want to become sick, but by those who manage health care organizations."
George Freeman Solomon, M.D.,
Professor Emeritus of Psychiatry and
Biobehavioral Sciences, U.C.L.A.

"Dr. Simon distills the vast wisdom of healing from the ancient Ayurvedic system of India and places it at the fingertips of the modern Western reader. His book is one of the most important additions to the literature of Ayurveda in modern times and should be read by all who are interested in this profound subject."
Dr. David Frawley,
author of *Ayurveda and the Mind*

"Ayurveda encompasses the healing of the body, mind, and consciousness of each individual in his or her day-to-day life and in daily relationships. As a practical text for self-healing, Dr. David Simon's book guides both the professional and the layman through his integral approach and his own wonderful journey toward total healing."
Vasant Lad, B.A.M.S., M.A.Sc.,
author of *The Doctor's Book of Ayurvedic Home Remedies*

THE WISDOM OF HEALING

The
WISDOM
~ *of* ~
HEALING

*A Natural Mind Body Program
for Optimal Wellness*

DAVID SIMON, M.D.

Foreword by Deepak Chopra, M.D.

THREE RIVERS PRESS • NEW YORK

Copyright © 1997 by David Simon, M.D.

Introduction copyright © 1997 by Deepak Chopra, M.D.

Published by Three Rivers Press, a division of Crown Publishers, Inc.,
201 East 50th Street, New York, New York 10022.
Member of the Crown Publishing Group.

Originally published in hardcover by Harmony Books,
a division of Crown Publishers, Inc., in 1997.

Random House, Inc. New York, Toronto, London, Sydney, Auckland
www.randomhouse.com

THREE RIVERS PRESS and colophon are trademarks of
Crown Publishers, Inc.

Printed in the United States of America

Design by June Bennett-Tantillo

Library of Congress Cataloging-in-Publication Data
Simon, David, M.D.
The wisdom of healing : a natural mind body program
for optimal wellness / by David Simon.
p.   cm.
Includes bibliographical references (p. 313)
1. Medicine, Ayurvedic.   2. Holistic medicine.   3. Health.
I. Title.
R605.S565   1997
615.5'3—dc21   97-9296   CIP

ISBN 0-609-80214-3

Contents

Illustrations

Foreword

DEEPAK CHOPRA

In the world of forms and phenomena, change is the only constant. In life, change proceeds in the direction of evolution—how more can be accomplished with less energy expenditure. Human evolution has moved through several epochs over the past several million years, from the hunter-gatherer stage to the Agricultural Age, on to the Industrial Age and now, the Information Age. Each age has had its own worldview—its own paradigm—which defines the expectations and limitations of the people living in the period. I believe that the transition from the Industrial Age to the Information Age has again resulted in a transformation of our worldview. We are beginning to see, thanks to information technology, a paradigm shift from a material worldview to a consciousness-based worldview. We are beginning to understand that what exists at the essential core of matter is information and energy. I hope and believe that the Information Age is going to be the stepping-off point for the Age of Consciousness. What is consciousness, if not information and energy that has become alive with self-referral? In other words, consciousness is information that responds to feedback, which is also information. Through this self-referral loop, consciousness influences its own expression in more abstract and unpredictable ways, and in this process, consciousness becomes intelligence.

This underlying nonmaterial basis for existence is already taken for granted in the information technologies of our civilization—fax machines, cellular phones, satellite television transmissions, and the Internet. These tools of our age demonstrate the basic premise of our time, which is that the essential nature of the material world is not material; that the essential stuff of the universe is "nonstuff"; that the atom, which is the basic unit of matter, is not a solid entity, but a hierarchy of states of information and energy in a huge void.

This profound and valuable knowledge has been missing from our biological sciences. Our current health-care system needs to integrate this understanding of consciousness in order for it to evolve to the next phase. Our current therapeutic interventions in medicine are based upon a mechanistic view of life that views the human body as a physical machine with consciousness as the epiphenomenon. Although modern medicine has made great advances, saving millions of lives through sophisticated technology and pharmaceuticals, it has come at a high price. Modern medicine has not evolved sufficiently to deal with the underlying causes of disease in our society. There is a need, therefore, for a system of health care that is truly holistic.

This book by Dr. David Simon offers a new vision of health care that embraces the best of East and West. It brings together the insights of ancient healing wisdom with what we know about the workings of nature through the window of science. Wisdom requires knowledge and experience and this book provides the keys to both.

I have known David for more than ten years and have worked closely with him for the past five. Together, he and I have developed courses that have trained thousands of physicians, nurses, and other health professionals in the principles and practice of mind body medicine. As a result of these courses, we have certified hundreds of health-care providers to teach "The Magic of Healing," which is being taught to thousands of people all across the world. In my opinion, Dr. David Simon is the most qualified person to translate the ideas and concepts that I have been exploring and writing about for the past ten years into practical programs that anyone—health-care professions and the general public—can access.

There has been a need for this book for many years. Dr. Simon has painstakingly researched every statement made in this book and diligently gathered the scientific evidence that documents the benefits of the techniques of mind body medicine that he explores in each chapter. I believe *The Wisdom of Healing* will become a classic of great value to both the general public and health-care professionals. Along with *Perfect Health,* it is a valuable companion for those wishing to understand and apply holistic concepts of health to real-life challenges.

David, a remarkably talented physician, is the medical director of The Chopra Center for Well Being in La Jolla, California, and has been responsible for creating a number of health-care programs with me that are based upon a holistic perspective of the human being: "Magical Beginnings, Enchanted Lives," a course for pregnant mothers; "The Healing Heart Program," for people facing heart disease; and "Return to Wholeness," for people confronting cancer. These programs are being embraced by health-care organizations and providers around the world. *The Wisdom of Healing,* by David Simon, takes us a giant step closer to bringing the principles and practices of integrated mind body medicine fully into the mainstream of society and health care; I am privileged to be associated with him at The Chopra Center for Well Being and in all the work we do together on behalf of that larger goal.

Acknowledgments

This book has provided me a precious opportunity to recount my personal healing journey. Along my path, countless guides have shared their love and wisdom with me—to these souls I am deeply grateful.

I wish to express special gratitude:

To the wonderful team of dedicated people who have made The Chopra Center for Well Being a spiritual intensive care unit;

To my extended family at Infinite Possibilities International for their commitment to an enlightened world;

To my dear friends and colleagues, Jude Aluce, Margo Anand, Donna Anton, Brent BecVar, Bruce BecVar, Brian BecVar, Bija Bennett, Rama Birch, Ginna Bragg, Ray Chambers, Mallika Chopra, Rita Chopra, Heidi Clark, Diane Cook, Manjari Ehrlichman, William Elkus, Rebecca Flynn, David Frawley, Annie Frensdorff, Jeremy Geffen, Tom Gegax, Becky Hanson, Carol Hyde, Jan Kinder, Paul Johnson, Sunil Joshi, Vasant Lad, Karen Martin, Mary Maskell, Sarah McLean, Paige Megna, Chuck Meier, Catherine Miller, Vidya McNeill, Muriel Nellis, Richard Perl, Candace Pert, Carolyn Rangel, Tom Rautenberg, Marcia Ross, Adriana Silva, Sylvia Sepielli, Deepak Singh, Geeta Singh, Ira Strongin, Clara Toro, Francis Warner, and

Barbara Wheeler for their unwavering dedication to our shared vision of healing the world;

To my adored tribe of infinite possibilities co-dreamers, Stephen Bickel, Arielle Ford, Debbie Ford, Danielle Dorman, Roger Gabriel, Nan Johnson, Adriana Nienow, Gayle Rose, and Kimberly Wise;

To Mitch Sisskind and Peter Guzzardi for their resolute pursuit of excellence;

To Deepak for his inspiration, wisdom, and vision;

To my divine parents, Myron and Lee Shirley, for their boundless nurturing and for instilling in me the values of service and integrity;

To my beloved Howard, Dana, and Samantha for their constant love and support;

To my dear Lori, Bruce, Judy, and Al for their loving acceptance and caring;

To my cherished son, Max, for his extraordinary courage and spirit;

And, to my darling, Pam, for her unconditional love and acceptance.

Introduction

Twenty-First-Century
Health Care

"Something we were withholding made us weak,
Until we found it was ourselves."

Robert Frost

In ancient India, the doctor wore his money bag on his belt. As he made his rounds through the village, he visited each home. If every member of the family was healthy, the head of the household placed a coin in the doctor's bag. If, however, someone in the home had fallen ill, the doctor was held responsible for not providing the necessary knowledge to the patient. The cost of herbs, special foods, or specific therapeutic treatments was paid for by the doctor. Thus was born the first health maintenance organization (HMO).

We are in the midst of a health revolution. With modern medical technology we can penetrate the genetic code to reveal the broken molecule that underlies an inherited illness, we can see changes in the brain's metabolic activity that underlie thoughts and intentions, we can focus gamma rays to carve out a brain tumor without cutting the skin. Yet more than one in three Americans seeks out unconventional health care for illnesses ranging from chronic pain to cancer. There is a perplexing disparity between the amazing medical miracles we have available to us and the growing dissatisfaction with our modern health-care system.

Since entering medical school almost twenty-five years ago, I have felt discontent with our prevailing approach to health and disease. My expectations upon entering medical school were great, but

I found my training disappointing. I wanted and expected to be taught the sacred principles of health. Instead, I learned about *interesting* aspects of disease. I expected to learn from professors of medicine who were models of humility and compassion, and instead I saw them revered mainly for their problem-solving skills, as if healing were a branch of mechanical engineering. At times I was deeply demoralized that the notion of human beings as fully conscious, spiritually aware creations had been totally lost from the medical model of life and health.

Over the last few years, however, I have been encouraged by the new awareness of health issues that is growing in our society. Increasingly, people are expecting their health-care providers to be more than master disease technicians. The concept of doctor as teacher is returning.

What do we really want from our healers? We want the best acute treatment available when needed. If a child develops a high fever and an earache at two in the morning, we want instant access to a competent physician and an effective antibiotic. If we are in a serious automobile accident, we want to have state-of-the-art X-ray equipment available to diagnose our broken bones and expert orthopedic doctors to set them straight. We want our providers to show compassion, whether we are suffering with cancer or an annoying muscle spasm. We want our doctors to practice what they preach, radiating health in their own lives. We want to be taught what we can do to avoid illness and the ravages of aging. And we want it all to be inexpensive and easy!

These are tall orders, and thus far we have had to accept compromises. We have paid an emotional price for the high-technology medicine of our time, sacrificing humane caring for efficiency. And we are paying an ever-increasing financial price as well. It is reassuring that our highly skilled surgeons can clean out or bypass blocked blood vessels to the heart, or transplant an organ, but now we are finding that there is often not enough money in the bank to provide these treatments. As a result, a vast transformation is underway in the way we look at health and health care.

One effort to change our approach to health is the rise of managed care. Although the theory behind health maintenance organizations (HMOs) is to provide incentives to doctors and hospitals to keep people healthy, there is growing concern that the effort to save money sometimes leads to withholding appropriate care. Although it will require a fundamental shift in the way both patients and physicians think about health care, I am convinced that an answer to these problems is now available. To put it succinctly, the solution lies in providing people with the means and the information they need to make lifestyle changes that will diminish the need for expensive medical care. Rather than rationing our limited resources, we can reduce the need for those resources by empowering human beings to lead healthier lives.

This doesn't mean encouraging people to abandon medical care for alternative providers. Although I believe there is great potential value to acupuncture, massage, homeopathy, nutritional counseling, and other alternative approaches, I don't think an alternative health-care system is going to solve all our problems. Throughout my exploration of healing technologies since my premed days, I have been struck by the fact that, in every system of health care, some people get better and some do not. The problem lies at the heart of almost every therapeutic approach in every tradition, from every historical period, and from every area of the globe: No matter where we look, the patient is always the passive recipient of the healer's efforts. To use a metaphor from our own part of the world, the doctor always pitches and the patient always catches.

I am suggesting that it is time for the patient to step up to bat. I have witnessed chiropractors who adjust spinal subluxations, homeopaths who choose the correct tincture, acupuncturists who place needles into blocked meridians, and herbalists who treat symptoms with specific botanical preparations. Although these alternative approaches to illness have demonstrable value, they do not represent a real shift in the doctor-patient relationship. While most natural-medicine traditions emphasize disease prevention through healthy life choices, the day-to-day practice of these healing arts often fails to make *knowledge* about health an important component. For the most part, the patient remains the passive recipient, relinquishing authority to an all-knowing healer.

I vividly remember my experience with an herbalist who was offering consultations at the rate of thirty people an hour. I waited along with one hundred others until I was ushered into the small office of the medicine man. Without asking me any questions, he felt my pulse for about twenty seconds. He whispered that I had "too many thoughts" and dictated a prescription to his assistant. I was escorted to the next room, where several bags of herbal tablets were filled for me. I paid about twenty-five dollars for the herbs—there was no charge for the visit—and I was sent on my way.

The most fascinating thing to me about this experience was listening to the other patients describe their own brief visits. Reactions like "He seemed able to thoroughly read me," or "I felt better just by his touch," impressed me because the most common complaint I was hearing about medical doctors was that they weren't spending enough time with their patients. In some subtle yet profound way, and in just a few minutes, these people felt that a need had been met. It seemed to me that a spiritual connection had been made between patient and healer and that this experience had a powerful effect.

Although I understand the potent benefits of a visit with a medicine man, I doubt that this type of consultation will find widespread acceptance in the West. Increasingly, Westerners ask to be respected partners in their health care and I don't believe my patients would be fully satisfied with a healing encounter without knowledge of how to sustain and expand the experience. However, the feeling of being accepted, understood, and acknowledged as a fellow human being must be an integral part of every exchange with a doctor. My vision of health care for the next millennium values the best of Western scientific medicine while embracing the essence of the great healing traditions. Acknowledging the integral link between healing and spirit, we also need to empower people with the knowledge and practical approaches to improve their own health.

To accomplish this, we need to make the experience of health care relevant to patients' emotional lives. A visit with a healer/doctor ought to be inspirational and even spiritual on occasion. Here the ancient healing traditions have much to offer, for in their definitions of health they include not just body and mind, but spirit also. This is vitally important, because genuine good health means more than having normal laboratory studies. It's a dynamic state of *well-being* in every sense. It's joy in the gift of living a human life.

In this book, I want to share with you my experiences of the healer's art as it has been understood around the world. In the ancient wisdom traditions of India, Tibet, and China I have found both profound philosophical concepts and practical techniques for combining concepts of body, mind, and spirit into a comprehensive definition of health. Throughout my medical career I have worked to integrate the theory and practice of these ancient health sciences into my medical practice in the West.

My first exposure to an Ayurvedic physician left a lasting impression on me. A gentle, humble *vaidya* (doctor of Ayurveda) had been visiting the United States for just a few weeks and intuitively seemed to understand the deeper needs of Westerners. His demeanor radiated compassion and I was surprised at how often his polite exploration of the issues underlying a person's problem elicited tears. His kind-hearted nature encouraged trust, which allowed those seeking his counsel to gain a deeper understanding of the source and meaning of their concerns. With his simple explanations and encouragement, the steps to recovery seemed readily attainable.

Each patient was given basic advice about diet, exercise, and daily routine. A few Ayurvedic herbs were usually prescribed along with information on when and how to take them. He encouraged people to begin a daily spiritual practice and often suggested they spend time alone in nature.

The information he provided was at once simple and profound, but the most powerful aspect of his therapy was his own presence. Although he was seeing several patients each hour, there was a timelessness about him that made each person feel his only concern was for his or her well being. More than an expert on health, he seemed to be a living representative of a healthy person, balanced in body, mind, and spirit. In this man, I saw the possibility that a physician could be more than a technical master of pathology—a doctor could guide his patients to health through his actions, words, and being.

For the past four years I have had the privilege and opportunity of devoting my full time to the development of The Chopra Center for Well Being. This program is unique in its mission of integrating holistic concepts and practices into a mainstream health-care system. We are finding growing acceptance of these holistic principles as complementary, not alternative, to standard medical care. Patients are no longer acquiescing to a passive role in their recovery processes, but are actively seeking every possible means to activate their internal healing systems. It has been my experience that a combination of mind body approaches and best-quality, appropriately administered medical care provides the optimal opportunity for healing. And when there is not an effective standard medical approach to a problem, mind body medicine offers hope and options at minimal cost with often surprising results.

Beyond "A Pill for Every Ill"

This new view of health seeks to expand, not overthrow, the prevailing paradigm. Contemporary health science sees the human body as a physical machine that has inexplicably learned to manufacture thoughts. But if we think of the human body that way, as a flesh-and-bone thought-manufacturing machine, then we are viewing consciousness as a side effect of matter. Feelings, desires, instincts, falling in love, being moved by poetry or music—all are understood as by-products of biochemistry. Moreover, just as emotions are seen as by-products of molecules, so are sickness and health.

Science has attempted to understand the mechanics of disease in the hope that by disrupting those mechanics, disease can be eradicated. Thus, if we can learn how bacteria multiply, we can presumably use antibiotics to interfere with that process and before long there won't be any more infections. If we know how cancer cells replicate their DNA, we can interfere with that process too, and then we won't have cancer anymore. If we know how cholesterol is manufactured in the liver, we can intervene in the process of cholesterol development, and heart disease will soon follow cancer into the dustbin of history.

While this model of the body has been extremely useful in acute intervention, has saved many lives, and has made great improvements in the general state of public health, it has only partly fulfilled our intentions. For example, the mechanical or materialistic model has not significantly affected morbidity and mortality from chronic disease in society at large, nor has it influenced the age-adjusted mortality from illness. It has very effectively succeeded in getting rid of certain epidemics, but other epidemics have appeared in their place. We no longer have polio, smallpox, and malaria, but we do have cardiovascular disease, stroke, cancer, degenerative disorders, AIDS, drug addiction, and alcoholism.

It is now also clear that treating illness with a purely mechanistic approach very frequently sows the seeds of illness for the future. It has been estimated that over 1.5 million people develop hospital-acquired infections each year in the United States, and many thousands die from antibiotic-resistant bacteria.[1] The cost of caring for these iatrogenic, or treatment-related, infections is estimated to reach to three billion dollars per year.[2,3] More than one-half of all antimicrobial drugs may be prescribed inappropriately.[4] This has created a situation in which problems that recently were considered easily treated, such as common staph or strep infections, are now resistant to antibiotics and are striking with lethal force in immuno-compromised patients.

Since 1928, when Alexander Fleming's observation of a mold that contaminated his bacterial cultures led to the discovery of penicillin, we have proceeded under the assumption that there is a "pill for every ill." Recent studies have shown that between fifty and eighty percent of the adult population in the United States and England swallows a medically prescribed chemical every twenty-four to thirty-six hours.[5,6] Over one-third of patients in a university hospital may be suffering from iatrogenic diseases.[7] If a study of hospital-acquired injuries from New York is typical of the United States, 180,000 people die each year of iatrogenic injury, the equivalent of three jumbo-jet crashes every two days.[8] It is known that the number one cause of drug addiction in the world is not street drugs, but medical prescriptions legally prescribed by physicians. And, despite our presumption that the standard practice of Western medicine is scientifically based, studies suggest that less than half of medical interventions are supported by solid scientific evidence.[9,10]

The materialist model of the body focuses on disease mechanisms rather than the basic life functions of the human mind body system. These life functions are simply what we do every day, eating, breathing, digesting, metabolizing, and eliminating. Mind body medicine emphasizes the crucial influence of consciousness on each and every one of these processes. If they are effortless and spontaneous, there is health; and conversely, the origins of disease can be found in a disruption of the spontaneity and effortlessness with which the life functions occur.

What "Holistic" Really Means

The recognition of consciousness or spirit as a central factor in the etiology of an illness is the fundamental distinction between the healing traditions of the East and conventional Western health care.

Although I've found much that is valuable in all the healing traditions, what ultimately attracted me to the Ayurvedic medicine of India was its all-inclusiveness, its willingness to put the welfare of the patient above any doctrinal or ideological imperatives. Simply put, Ayurveda advocates whatever restores or strenghtens the health of the patient and whatever retards or eliminates the process of disease.

One of the first patients I saw at The Chopra Center was a delightful man who worked as a massage therapist at the Esalen Institute in northern California. For several years he had been troubled by a tingling sensation in his face, and as someone who was thoroughly at ease with alternative approaches to health care he had sought help from chiropractors, acupuncturists, and homeopaths. Each doctor had prescribed a course of treatment that provided temporary relief, but his symptoms invariably returned.

This patient now came to us hoping to try an Ayurvedic approach—but as I listened to his story, I became increasingly concerned that he might have a rare brain tumor. After providing his history and allowing me to examine him, he asked me for my thoughts as an Ayurvedic physician. I replied that I fully supported the use of natural approaches when appropriate, but in this instance I recommended a brain MRI scan as soon as possible. Although the massage therapist was understandably dismayed, he agreed to the study because he trusted me as a holistically oriented doctor. In fact, the scan did show a small tumor on his hearing nerve, which was successfully removed neurosurgically without any complications.

To me, this was a successful application of mind body medicine. There is a saying that runs, "If the only tool you own is a hammer, everything looks like a nail," and all too often this is true of health care. For medical doctors, the hammer is a prescription pad; for chiropractors, it is a spinal adjustment; for acupuncturists, it is a needle; for homeopaths, a miasmic tincture. My concept of truly holistic health care is ensuring that the correct tool is available for the task at hand, and using that tool, whatever it may be. And very often—but not always, as illustrated by the case described above—the most powerful tool is not anything on the outside, but rather the healing powers of the patient's own body, mind, and spirit.

It is encouraging to note that the World Health Organization has defined health as not merely the absence of disease, but as a state of physical, mental, and emotional well being.[11] It is now time to add a fourth element: spiritual well being. We could even go further and redefine health as a higher state of consciousness—a state in which we open ourselves to entirely new categories of creativity and vitality, including the ability to influence biological processes through the power of our own awareness.

Information and Energy

The idea that something as subtle as our attention can influence something as concrete as our physical body may at first be difficult to accept. Yet, our whole concept of what is "real" is changing today. Our technology—fax machines, cordless phones, computers, and television—is based on a new understanding of reality. All these technologies have evolved from one paradoxical idea: that the essential nature of the physical world is that it is *not ultimately physical;* that the atom, for example, which is the basic unit of matter, can also be seen as a *network of information and energy.*

A flower, for example, is made up of information and energy. The *energy* is the raw electromagnetic, gravitational, and atomic forces that allow the flower to be perceived by our senses; the color, shape, texture, and fragrance are the specific packages of *information* that are available to our consciousness. Consciousness is also information and energy, but it is more than that. Consciousness is alive—it is *living* information and energy. We can refer to it as intelligence, although the intelligence manifested by a flower is in many respects different from that of an animal or human being.

Ayurveda teaches that intelligence is information and energy that is self-referral. Self-referral means the ability to learn through experience to reinterpret and influence one's choices. When, through our intelligence, we make different choices, we change the energy and information that enters our mind and body and by so doing, we transform who we are.

The human body is really a river of intelligence. And like a river that is always changing despite the appearance that it is the same, our human bodies are undergoing continuous transformation. We replace almost all the atoms in our body each year. From reconstituting our stomach lining every week to the calcium and phosphate in our bones every few months, our physical structure is in constant and dynamic exchange with the world around us.

This may not be the way we are used to perceiving our bodies, but sensory experience is often unreliable. Our senses tell us that the earth is flat, yet we know that it is round. Sensory experience informs me the earth is the center of the universe, yet I know that it is just a tiny speck of matter in a remote corner of the galaxy. If we could see the human body as it truly is, rather than through the filter of human sensory experience, we would see it as a field of energy and information.

If we conceive of our bodies as fixed physical structures, it makes sense to intervene with surgery to remove broken parts or add medications to alter the body's chemistry. If, however, we begin to grasp the nature of a human life as a magnificent network of intelligence, entirely new possibilities for healing can be considered. From this perspective, we can influence health through our choices and interpretations: through the food we ingest, the emotions we experience, the sensory input we are exposed to, the daily patterns and rhythms of our lives. We can re-create ourselves by changing the quality of our experiences.

The Roots of Mind Body Medicine

Although these concepts may have been discredited in some circles as being "New Age," the roots of mind body medicine are in time-honored healing traditions from around the world. As I learned in medical anthropology classes in college, as long as human beings have existed, we have sought means to offset the suffering caused by injury, illness, and aging. In prehistoric times extended families came together into clans and tribes, enabling the emergence of specialized roles, of which the medicine man was among the earliest. Traditional healers had to begin by resolving their own health issues, through which they gained firsthand experience about sickness and recovery. The knowledge of how to utilize nature's gifts to heal was passed down from generation to generation, eventually becoming systematized in the great ancient healing traditions.

Medical historians recognize a number of major traditional health systems whose roots go back thousands of years. The medical science of ancient Greece is identified with Hippocrates, who was born about 450 B.C. He considered health to be a natural state that could be lost through forsaking a balanced lifestyle. Hippocrates emphasized moderation as the road to a sound mind and body and resolutely preached the need to be in harmony with nature. Although many medical students recite the Hippocratic oath at the time of graduation, the basic principles of Greek medicine that integrated body, mind, and spirit have been relegated to footnote status in today's medical schools.

The major healing traditions of the East are intimately interwoven, sharing many common principles and therapeutic interventions. Tibetan medicine's origins go back approximately twenty-five hundred years to the time of the Buddha. Medicine provided an opportunity for Buddhist monks to practice compassion, help relieve suffering, and convert the comforted to their spiritual path. The classical Tibetan medical treatise, *Tantra of Secret Instruction on the Eight Branches, the Essence of the Elixir of Immortality,* is commonly known as *The Four Tantras.* Magnificent pictorial texts that depict a detailed Tibetan understanding of anatomy, physiology, and embryology expound the origin, diagnosis, and treatment of disease. Virtuous conduct, a healthy diet, and regular daily and seasonal routines are promoted for a long and healthy life. If you fall ill, Tibetan medicine includes a vast herbal pharmacopoeia. Although under severe threat from Chinese occupation, Tibetan medicine is still widely practiced in its native land and has spread to Nepal, India, and recently to the West. Tibetan medicine is a rich and elegant healing system that deserves the attention of healers around the world.

Traditional Chinese Medicine (TCM) became familiar to Americans after President Richard Nixon's visit to China in 1972. Although most widely known for acupuncture, TCM includes an extensive herbal pharmacy. The earliest known oriental medical text, *The Yellow Emperor's Classic of Internal Medicine,* dates back as far as 2600 B.C. Westerners were exposed to acupuncture in the seventeenth century when Jesuit missionaries to China returned with amazing accounts of doctors curing patients by placing needles in their skin. Oriental medical doctors hypothesize that life energy, called chi, flows throughout the body within specific pathways, or meridians. This vital force circulates as a result of opposite forces, known as yin and yang, that are continuously seeking a dynamic balance. Illness results when the life force is obstructed or when the polar principles become imbalanced. Traditional Chinese Medical practitioners have gained considerable credibility in the West and are now commonly members of pain-treatment teams. Although Western scientists may have difficulty with the concept of chi traveling through invisible channels, there is a growing body of evidence supporting the role of TCM in the treatment of neuromuscular and arthritic pain, post-surgical pain, menstrual cramps, nausea from chemotherapy, and drug addiction.[12-16]

Ayurveda, which means "science of life" in Sanskrit, may be as ancient as humankind. Although its precise origins have been lost in the mists of history, one thing can be said with certainty about this comprehensive, philosophical, eminently practical system of health science: *Ayurveda is very old.* The Rig Veda, a collection of more than one thousand poetic hymns that includes many of the central concepts of Ayurveda, was composed between 1200 and 900 B.C. Thus, the Ayurvedic system was already centuries old during the time of Charaka, the most celebrated of the ancient physicians of India, who lived around 700 B.C.

In his book known as the Samhita, which is the principle source for our knowledge of his thinking, Charaka described a gathering of the most learned men of India who came together in the foothills of the Himalayas to discuss the problem of disease. They agreed that disease was spreading misery and death and was standing in the way of humanity's achieving spiritual enlightenment, the true purpose of existence. In the Charaka Samhita, the sages elected a delegate to call upon the celestial being known as Indra, who then revealed the *science of life* to the great sage, Bhardwaja. In this way the principles of Ayurveda are described as coming to mankind directly from the gods. From the very beginning Ayurveda was intended to serve spiritual as well as physical purposes.

For anyone reading the Samhita and other ancient Ayurvedic texts today, many of the books' ideas seem amazingly sophisticated and up-to-date. The Charaka Samhita, for example, includes a carefully formulated classification of diseases and their treatments, as well as sections on anatomy and embryology, nutrition, and herbology. In all, Ayurveda's understanding of human health is every bit as comprehensive as the healing systems of ancient Greece and China, though these have, until recently, received far more attention from Western historians.

It would be wrong, however, to imagine that there was rivalry or competition between the health sciences of the various ancient civilizations. Early physicians were eager to learn from one another, and the extensive trade routes of the ancient world made it surprisingly easy for them to do so. Ayurvedic texts had probably been translated into Greek by the time of Hippocrates, who would have been familiar with the work of Indian physicians. The expansion of medical knowledge that occurred during the Han dynasty in China (circa 200 B.C.) must also have been influenced by the earlier developments in India.

It's unfortunate that the ancient world's willingness to share and accept medical knowledge from various cultures did not extend into more recent times. During the medieval period Ayurvedic medicine began to be forcibly replaced by alternative systems imposed by the ruling classes, and its decline accelerated after the conquest of India by Moslem invaders in the twelfth and thirteenth centuries. Later, beginning in the eighteenth century, Ayurveda was almost completely suppressed by India's British rulers. Tragically, one conqueror after another has seen Ayurvedic learning as a threat to his political control, rather than as a resource for linking the Indian nation with its proud heritage and for bettering the health of its people.

When India gained independence from Britain in 1947, the way was opened for a revival of Ayurveda's long-suppressed tradition. It is only very recently, however, that the science of life has at last begun to receive the interest that it deserves, not only in India but around the world. Western medicine is now beginning to acknowledge that we must treat the person as well as the disease, that we must recognize the underlying causes of ill health and try to address them even before symptoms appear, and that good nutrition, appropriate exercise, emotional well being, and spiritual fulfillment are as important to human health as drugs or surgery. These principles, of course, were well understood by even the earliest Ayurvedic physicians. While it's regrettable that their insights have been cast aside for many hundreds of years, it's also heartening to see how the situation is beginning to change for the better. Through *The Wisdom of Healing,* I hope to accelerate this change by offering detailed knowledge of Ayurvedic medicine to an audience of both laypeople and health-care practitioners. Moreover, by integrating Ayurvedic insights with the most advanced concepts of Western science, I hope to at last make possible the physical, emotional, and spiritual well being that was the highest purpose of Charaka and the ancient sages of India.

The new model for health offered in this book embraces the best of the objective, scientific interventions of Western medicine with the subjective, holistic approaches of the ancient healing traditions. It empowers and honors the inherent healing power within us all, acknowledging the imperishable linkage between body, mind, and spirit. Health is then understood as the return of the memory of wholeness. Healing is a lifelong process of unfolding, without clear beginnings and with no anticipated end. For me, coming to understand this has been a journey of discovery, and in these pages I hope you will find the fruits of that journey.

PART ONE

CONSCIOUSNESS:
THE RAW MATERIAL
OF THE UNIVERSE

The ideas that structure mind body medicine are both old and new. They are derived from the profound insights of physicists and molecular biologists whose work was done in this century, or even in just the past few years—but they are also grounded in a Vedic conception of the universe that is thousands of years old. Breakthroughs of twentieth-century science such as relativity theory and quantum mechanics were anticipated in surprising detail by the ancient seers of India. My purpose in Part I of The Wisdom of Healing *is to show how these ideas from widely separated times and places form a new vision of health, of life, and even of matter itself. Vedic philosophy in general, and in particular the science of health known as Ayurveda, sees human life as an inseparable part of a continuum that extends outward to include the most distant galaxies of the universe and inward to the faintest energy traces of subatomic particles.*

The model of an endlessly flowing reality in which elements blend and turn back upon themselves like ocean waves is a vision that contemporary physicists share with ancient poets and philosophers—but it stands in contrast to the materialistic, mechanistic conception that forms the basis of Western health care. While I do not for a moment deny the enormous achievements of the prevailing mechanistic approach, it is equally obvious that many fundamental health problems remain unsolved, and in recent years serious new problems have appeared for which medical science as yet has no answer. I believe a consciousness-based understanding of human health can transcend the limits of mechanistic thinking. By presenting this vision of a consciousness-created reality, I hope to offer a new instrument for healing at a time when there is a very clear need for it.

I

Healing the Healer

*"Science cannot solve the ultimate mystery of Nature . . .
because in the last analysis we ourselves are part of the mystery
we are trying to solve."*

Max Planck

I am six years old and running a 104°F fever. It seems I have inadvertently loaned my body to a community of viruses that has seized the opportunity to expand its population rapidly. Even watching My Little Margie *on television does not appease the aching in my muscles. My mother is particularly concerned because the St. Joseph's Aspirin for Children that she has been pumping into me every four hours has had a minimal effect on my alternating fevers and chills.*

I notice that Mom is frantically cleaning up the house because the doctor is coming. Dr. Benjamin Stein, noted suburban pediatrician, is making a house call and my mother wants the Simon household to mirror the antisepsis of Northshore Memorial Hospital. My father has called several times today to see how I am feeling and has come home an hour early from work to be here when Dr. Stein arrives. Mom has just completed the finishing touches on my bed, puffing up the pillows and pulling the bedcovers tight across my chest, when the front doorbell rings, announcing the arrival of the doctor.

Looking into my ears, he remarks that there are no potatoes growing in my acoustic canals and, tapping on my knees, reassures all in attendance that I am still alive and kicking. After a few minutes of tender probing, poking, looking, and listening, he declares with authority that I have "a bug that is going around." It requires no antibiotics (no shot!) and the doctor promises my much-relieved parents that I'll be better in a couple of days. He scribbles a prescription for some cough syrup and tells my mother to call him toward the end of the week.

Dr. Stein departs and within hours my fever breaks, the toxic invaders seem to vanish from my body, my parents breathe a sigh of relief, and the red-breasted robins resume their song outside my window.

This is one of my earliest memories of healing. Although it happened decades ago in a Midwestern suburb, the visit from Dr. Stein has much in common with encounters that have taken place between patients and doctors for hundreds of years in all parts of the world. For centuries a physician's words, gestures, and simple nostrums were the only available responses to illness, but despite his limited ability to affect the disease process directly the doctor was honored, appreciated, even loved. And his patients often recovered.

At least in the emotions that are evoked, the typical encounter between doctor and patient is largely unchanged today. Seeing a physician is always a fundamentally regressive experience for a sick person. It's as if you're once again a little boy who has tried and failed to button your coat by yourself, or a toddling one-year-old girl who can't walk across the room without help. You call for help—not because you want to, but because you must.

For most people, then, a meeting with a doctor is colored by powerful feelings of hope and fear. This is as true for an Eskimo fisherman meeting with his tribal shaman as it is for a Manhattan businessman visiting his cardiologist. Every patient naturally hopes that his or her problem isn't serious or that it can be resolved easily. This hope often translates into a deeply held faith on the part of the patient, a trust that the doctor possesses special knowledge that allows him to make a sick person feel better, to cure illness, and to prolong life when life is threatened. The patient's faith, in turn, gives the physician extraordinary authority. One sometimes hears it said of a doctor, occasionally with bitterness but just as often with awe, "He thinks he's God!" A joke that most second-year medical students learn captures this sentiment.

A recently departed gentleman standing in line at the pearly gates became irritated when a young, bearded, long-haired fellow in a white coat, swing-

ing a stethoscope, walked past the waiting line right into heaven. When the man complained to the sentry angel that it wasn't fair that the chap was allowed to bypass the waiting line just because he was a doctor, the angel dismissed his protest, saying, "That wasn't a doctor, that was God. Sometimes he just likes to play doctor."

For the most part, the physician's authority and even much of his healing power has always derived from the patient's hope and belief that the doctor can make things right. But healing is only one of the hopes that a patient focuses on a physician. For many people, particularly as they get older, the doctor may be the only person who offers a caring relationship. Aging in America almost always includes isolation, death comes to be feared as the ultimate solitary experience, and the doctor can be the last person who stands between the patient and that self-locking door. Often the doctor is not just a surrogate parent, but a whole surrogate family—someone who provides attention, affection, and appreciation. When people become unhappy and frustrated, it's often because they're emotionally deprived, and that alone can give rise to physical illness with all its consequences.

From the doctor's point of view, hope and fear are also the central emotions of an encounter with a patient, though of course the doctor cannot disclose these feelings. Again, this has remained unchanged for hundreds of years—but now some new, important elements have been added to the equation. With the unprecedented advances in scientific medicine in the last thirty years, there has been an erosion of what might be called the ceremonial, or perhaps even the theatrical, sides of medicine. I mean *theatrical* in the most elevated sense: not as falsification, but as a performance in which the doctor provides a kind of catharsis for the patient's needs, just as can happen in an encounter with great art of any kind.

In his very thoughtful book entitled *How We Die*, the surgeon and medical historian Sherwin Nuland writes at some length about the place of hope in the doctor-patient relationship.[1] As his title suggests, Nuland's book is concerned principally with cases in which chances of recovery are very remote. Nonetheless, he suggests that there is much to hope for even in so-called hopeless cases. There is much a doctor can hope to accomplish for a patient who is not going to get well, and there is likewise a great deal that such a patient can hope to achieve for himself or herself. Serenity, insight, the sharing of love with family and friends—these are not just sentimental clichés. In a very real sense, they are what life is all about, despite the fact that they can't be detected by an MRI scan.

Unfortunately, in recent years there has been a general hardening on both sides in the relationship between doctor and patient. Many younger patients, for example, are now much more sophisticated about medicine than was true when doctors still made house calls for childhood illnesses. Well-informed about the differences among viruses, bacteria, and parasites, well-read in the popular literature of health and self-help, a new generation of patients is unlikely to accept just any medical advice or prescription. Rather than viewing the doctor as a healer or even a type of clergyman, a new generation of patients today is just as likely to see the healer as a businessman and view him with some of the same skepticism one might bring to an encounter with a salesman or repairman.

The doctor's orientation is also growing more hard-edged. Few doctors routinely visit the homes of sick children anymore—what would be the point? The fevers and chills associated with common childhood infections will go away by themselves, and if the symptoms persist, an office provides a better setting to run the tests that will yield an accurate diagnosis. This shifting of focus and responsibility from intuitive diagnosis to quantified test results has transformed and largely eliminated the "bedside manner" that was historically so important to the doctor's art.

This brings up an important point. I believe that with the unprecedented development of scientific medicine over the past fifty years, the primary focus of doctoring has shifted toward formulating a precise diagnosis and away from providing the comfort and compassion that for so many centuries were the only options. My medical training taught me that reaching a precise diagnosis was what distinguished real doctors from quack healers who provided therapy without knowing what diseases they were treating. I was taught to make use of advanced diagnostic tools to explore living anatomy and physiology, and to accept the dominance of high technology in interactions with patients. I accepted the premise that a temporary inconvenience to the patient was a reasonable price to pay for gaining information that could ultimately be beneficial.

A CAT scanner, for example, functions optimally at a temperature of 65°, and can process one patient every twenty minutes. While watching my patients move through such a scanner, I have sometimes had the impression that people are being served *to* rather than *by* technology, and I've found myself wondering how or if we could humanize the process without losing the critical information the machines provide. But the underlying premise of current medical science is that we must understand the mechanism of disease in greater and greater detail in order to intervene in ways that are more and more precisely targeted, as if healing were analogous to the "smart bombs" and computer-guided missiles of modern warfare. Indeed, many doctors do adopt the role of officers in an army mobilized against disease, and hospitals are in fact organized along quasi-military lines, with chiefs of staff and chains of command.

While this approach has led to unprecedented advances in treatment for a wide range of human afflictions, we have also witnessed the development of a widening gulf between the human experience of medicine and its marvelous technological arsenal.

Today it has become increasingly difficult for doctors to navigate between their traditional roles as healers and their new requirements as master disease diagnosticians and destroyers. To put this in more philosophical terms, instead of viewing the patient as another fellow being, the patient is in danger of becoming an object in the physician's eyes. This not only robs the patient of his essential being, it also cuts off the physician himself from a source of life and love in his work. And as Sigmund Freud, one of the great physicians of our century, rightly suspected, the opposite of love is death. In this sense, the powerful technology of modern medicine can itself be a source of suffering and pathology, both for patient and doctor as each is less nurtured by their interactions.

In light of contemporary medicine's emphasis on precise identification of disease processes, it's useful to remember that the word *diagnosis* derives from a Greek root meaning "to know thoroughly." In Ayurvedic medicine, this definition is understood to refer to the patient as well as to his or her pathology—and perhaps the physician's own level of self-knowledge would even be factored into a genuinely thorough diagnosis. These are elements that cannot be printed out by a computer, but they are vitally important to the healing process. With medicine's emphasis on the intricacies of disease and the associated technologies, we have devalued the nonquantifiable aspects of doctoring, and we are in danger of forgetting that health is more than the mere absence of a documentable illness.

It is important that the spiritual practice of medicine keep pace with the astonishing surgical and medical technologies of the late twentieth century. Radical and almost miraculous interventions are now available for conditions that once were hopeless, but the human spirit needs care to match that provided for the body.

In this connection, every doctor has seen cases of medical triumph but emotional failure. A few years ago, a retired engineer was diagnosed with advanced pancreatic cancer. Most often, such a diagnosis is more or less the end of the story. But this patient had been "a fighter" all his life. Rather than simply get his affairs in order, he sought other opinions. A famous surgeon told the dying man about a new procedure that had been known to save the lives of some patients with his condition. Of course, it was radical surgery, and would require a total change in the person's way of life, assuming he survived the operation. But the rage this old engineer had felt all his life, which may even have contributed to his illness, also got him through the surgery and a long stay in intensive care. But that rage did not permit him to make peace with his diminished pace of living, nor did he turn to the spiritual tradition in which he'd been raised, which might have aided him in his daily routine. He was alive, but he was a deeply unhappy man. The technology "saved" his body, but his spirit had not been healed.

On other occasions, a seriously ill patient may arrive at an outcome that is negative in narrow medical terms, but can be seen as successful in a broader sense. I recall a middle-aged man from Colombia who spent a week at our center after being diagnosed with advanced liver cancer. His personality was quite similar to that of the retired engineer described above. He was a combative person who had abused his body throughout his lifetime, while denying that someday there would be a price to pay. When his doctors told him that he was about to die, however, something changed in him. For the first time he began to concern himself with a spiritual element in his life, and it was this new viewpoint that brought him to us. While there was little we could do for the cancer that was taking over his body, we were able to introduce him to meditation and other integrated mind body techniques that made the end of his life not just more comfortable, but truly *healing* in terms of his relationship with the people closest to him, and even in the way he felt about himself. When we received a letter from his family informing us that he had died, we were of course disappointed that medical science had been unable to cure his illness, but it was extremely gratifying to learn that during his last months he had been, in the words of his wife, "the happiest I had ever seen him."

This man's physical body had succumbed to his illness, but his self was something more than his muscles, bones, and internal organs—and I believe that this larger self had been well served. Although in this instance the benefits of spiritual healing did not slow his already well-advanced disease, in many less dire cases the mind can do much toward healing the body.

Although the fathers of the great medical traditions around the world entreated us to remember that health was a dynamic interplay of spirit, mind, body, and environment, modern medicine's material view of human beings placed the highest priority on that which could be readily perceived and measured—the physical body with its tissues, cells, and biochemicals. Since we couldn't readily explain it, scientists stopped acknowledging the important role our minds have on physical health and disease. Yet, most of us know that our minds can influence our health, even if science has historically been unwilling or unable to validate this.

I can clearly remember my first glimpse of the mind's power to influence health:

I'm eleven years old and at a YMCA overnight summer camp that seems to me more like a Marine recruit-training depot. This is the first time I've been away from home for more than a couple of days and I am not a happy camper. I don't like getting up for the five o'clock morning run ending with a dive into freezing Lake Chippewa. I don't like sleeping on the bottom of a bunk bed with my upstairs neighbor needing to go to the latrine a dozen times each night. And I'm more than a little tired of singing, "Michael, row your boat ashore—hallelujah!"

By the third night, I'm committed to escaping this place at any cost and decide that the next morning I am going to feign the worst cold of my life so that my parents will have to rescue me. I fall asleep mentally rehearsing my agony. When I am awakened by the morning bugler I am surprised at how genuinely awful I feel. My throat is raw, my glands are swollen, and my body is on fire. I stumble into the infirmary, where the nurse diagnoses me with strep throat. A few hours later I'm in my parents' Chevy heading back to home sweet home. Although I'm feeling miserable, I'm amazed at my power to "really" make myself sick.

In the last decade a series of exciting discoveries has revolutionized our understanding of the mind body connection. These revelations have bridged the gap between natural healing technologies and modern biochemistry and physiology.

More than sixty different chemical messengers—known as neurotransmitters or neurochemicals—have been identified as "communicator molecules" because of their ability to conduct biological information throughout the physiology. Every thought, feeling, and experience that is generated in the mind correlates to a cascade of physiological and chemical changes in the body. These are awesome discoveries. For the first time it has been revealed that intangible, nonmaterial information can be transformed into a physical reality. Moreover, it has now been shown that a number of chemicals previously believed to originate only in the brain are actually produced by cells in other organs of the body. Since many of these substances are associated with cognitive and emotional processes, we recognize that intelligence is not localized in the central nervous system. We can now say with certainty that even such organs as the stomach and the liver are "thinking" entities. The entire body is a complex network of energy and information, which we in turn experience as consciousness.

A fascinating demonstration of this occurs when we go for a time without water. Every cell in our body becomes aware of our dehydrating state and responds to the best of its ability to conserve moisture. Our lungs release less water vapor in our breath. Our sweat glands reduce the amount of perspiration we produce. Our kidneys retain water so we produce more concentrated urine. Finally, when the congregated chorus of our bodily tissues' cry for water is loud enough for our conscious mind to pay attention, we have the thought, *Hmmm, I'm pretty thirsty. I think I'll get a glass of water.* (And with our first swallow, our cells must breathe a collective sigh of relief!)

Ayurveda teaches that consciousness is the basis for our experience of material reality, and twentieth-century physics is very much in agreement. Unfortunately, it's very easy to misunderstand and perhaps vulgarize the real meaning of this. The idea of a consciousness-based reality, for example, doesn't mean that "there's nothing out there unless I think there is"—nor does it mean "whatever I think about is going to be out there." Try as hard as you like to focus your consciousness and your intention on materializing a new Rolls-Royce in your driveway, but when you look out the front door you'll probably be disappointed. We are human beings, after all, and while our consciousness is indeed powerful, it is not *all-powerful.*

By way of contrast, the Bible tells us that God said, "Let there be light," and there was light—so for the Creator, mere intention instantly expresses itself as reality. Although no one that I know has yet reached that level, intention really does have organizing power. If you want to have a new car—even a Rolls!—and if the flow of that information through your consciousness is unobstructed, your desire will naturally express itself, for example, by your working in a job that creates sufficient income for you eventually to buy the automobile.

In a similar way, people can naturally maintain physical well being by living in a way that fosters good health. Nature provides certain internal signals, and when we heed them we are much more likely to have all our desires fulfilled. This does not mean that we never experience anger or destructive thoughts and feelings. But if we look deeply and honestly inside ourselves, there's usually a quiet voice directing us that allows us to structure the sequential steps to get our desires met. If we're also getting toxic external messages that distract us from our inner wisdom, genuine satisfaction will always remain elusive. We'll always be looking outside ourselves for the solutions to what are essentially internal needs.

In the great Vedic epic known as the Bhagavad-Gita, universal intelligence in the form of the god Krishna reveals to the warrior Arjuna a field of pure potentiality where the flow of Nature's intelligence organizes the universe. Here everything has a purpose, though from an individual perspective we may not be able to perceive it. And Arjuna quite naturally asks the question, "If Nature is organizing everything for a purpose, why do I have to do anything at all? Why not just let Nature take care of it?"

Krishna responds by saying that this is the ultimate paradox of life: that we are always subject to the direction of a cosmic intelligence, but at the same time we must make choices and assume control of our lives. As Krishna puts it, "Established in being, perform action."

To live with both universal and individual consciousness is one of life's great challenges. As individuals we eat breakfast, put gasoline in our cars, and do hundreds of other mundane tasks in the course of a day—but we can also be aware of being established in something that transcends the everyday world. There is a very practical benefit to this dual perspective: When you encounter obstacles in your daily life, then you can look beyond them and try to adopt the larger viewpoint.

As for doctors forced into aloofness or even isolation by the stress and structure of their role as physician, it's useful to remember the words of Galen, one of the earliest Western physicians, who observed that, "Where there is love of man, there is also love of the [physician's] art. For some patients, though conscious that their condition is perilous, recover their health simply through their contentment with the goodness of the physician." There is no larger picture without an intimate perspective. And just as life is more than a collection of vital signs, health is both a condition, a desire, and a cherished belief.

Similarly, society's evaluation of the medical profession derives not only from improved statistics on the survival rates of cancer patients or heart-attack victims, but from the feelings people have for their doctors as healers and as human beings. In their preoccupation with technological advances, many physicians have abandoned their traditional roles as bearers of compassion, wisdom, and even a unique kind of love. Although doctors are exasperated by the way the people seem to have devalued them despite medicine's improved statistics, it really is well within their grasp to regain public esteem *and* perform the clinical feats that technology has made possible.

ᔃ

During the late 1950s the polio epidemic is in full force. Parents are in a state of panic, fearing that the crippling virus lurks in every public place waiting to attack their vulnerable children. No one knows exactly how the disease is contracted, or what one must do to escape it, but many theories are circulating. The beach is deemed an especially dangerous place, especially if one comes into contact with another person's towel, and drinking water from public fountains is also considered hazardous. Although I remain healthy, my father develops a stiff neck and a fever. He is rushed to the hospital and, shockingly, I soon learn that my dad has polio.

As time passes my mother assures me again and again that Dad is doing well. Yet it's impossible to ignore the anxiety in her voice, and my father spends more than a month in the hospital. One day, at last, a car pulls up to our house and my father appears. He painfully makes his way toward the doorway, helped by two medical attendants and a cane. Later I'm captivated by his stories of the doctors and nurses who saved his life. As he describes enduring a series of spinal taps, I envision him pierced in the back by a yard-long needle.

Why did my father get sick while I remained unaffected? Why did he recover from polio, while others were severely disabled or even lost their lives? I asked myself these questions many times during the period of my father's illness and recuperation, and in my practice today I continue to ask them in a hundred different variations. I don't pretend to have found conclusive answers, but I'm convinced that the questions themselves can help reveal the supremely important connections between body, mind, and spirit. And I further believe that, by understanding these connections, we can begin to discover the most basic secrets of well being.

Modern medicine can recognize and describe illnesses with great precision. It can also recognize health, though this is considerably more difficult to define. But we really know very little about what lies between sickness and wellness. When, for example, does an illness really begin? Is there a moment when we're healthy and another when we're sick, or are we always somewhere in a gray area between health and disease? Do "germs" enter our bodies like an invading army breaching a wall, or are we always inhabited by organisms whose destructive potential is only activated when some other variable comes into play? Should we rely principally on objective tests—everything from thermometers to MRI machines—to tell us when we're sick, or can imbalances be perceived subjectively even in the absence of objective signs and symptoms? Patients have come to expect decisive answers from their doctors to important questions like these, but the truth remains much less clearly defined than we might wish.

The ambiguity that creeps into an honest consideration of sickness and health is also present in the distinctions between genuine prevention of disease and simply early detection of it. Western medicine has greatly improved its ability to discover the beginnings of illness—but what we consider "early signs" can be seen by other traditions as quite advanced stages of the disease process. I happened to be in India when President Ronald Reagan's colon cancer was discovered and treated by surgery. When the president's physicians expressed pride that the malignancy had been found at any early stage and had been prevented from spreading, an Ayurvedic doctor pointed out that, while he did not disagree with what was being said, the problem might have been avoided altogether if someone had spoken to Mr. Reagan about his diet forty years earlier.

My medical training taught me to approach new patients from a "worst-case" perspective. If I were examining a patient who complained of facial numbness, for example, my first priority would be to rule out the presence of a brain tumor or degenerative neurological disease. If someone reported rectal bleeding, I would investigate the possibility of colon cancer. While this is certainly a sensible and prudent approach, in actual practice it can foster an unfortunate psychology in the physician, especially one who is seeing scores of patients every day. Once we've checked for the most dire possibilities and eliminated them, we may find ourselves precipitously deciding that nothing at all is wrong. Quite often, in fact, doctors feel a certain disdain for patients who present suspicious symptoms without grave underlying medical problems. These patients can be seen as crying wolf—but just because there's no wolf at the door of someone's house doesn't mean that the roof isn't leaking, or that there aren't potentially serious cracks in the foundation. I once treated a young woman who arrived in the emergency room with an apparent epileptic seizure. Although it was soon evident to me that the problem was psychological rather than neurological, after talking with the patient it was also equally clear that the severe emotional difficulties in her life needed to be addressed. If they weren't, she would soon return to the emergency room with genuine physical problems that would be much more difficult to deal with—the effects of an attempted suicide were certainly one possibility. I know firsthand how overburdened doctors can resent patients who "waste our time" with pseudo illnesses. But the greater waste of time, to say nothing of the greater danger to the patient, really begins when we succumb to the all-or-nothing mind-set that can pervade contemporary health care. But that mind-set is inevitable in a system that attempts to understand people according to a purely mechanistic model of human health and the human body.

My intention here is not to minimize the successes of Western medicine, but to illuminate the sources of some great frustrations that patients and doctors feel, frustrations that I have experienced in my own practice. Again and again doctors meet patients who manifest, in body and in spirit, the effects of decades of self-destructive behavior. Yet many of these patients have seen no reason to consult a physician as long as they could at least still get out of bed each day. For millions of people, the time to see the doctor—or even to think about health issues at all—is when they're thoroughly, painfully, and perhaps desperately "sick." And for doctors, overworked and often under increasing financial pressure, it's difficult to spend time with people who are in the narrow sense symptom-free. Again, no one is to blame for this. It's simply the direction in which contemporary medicine has evolved, but I believe we can all benefit by changing that direction.

One of the most useful concepts in Vedic philosophy is *pragyaparadh,* which can be translated as "the mistake of the intellect." Pragyaparadh refers to the tendency of many people, and especially those who are very intelligent, to perceive or create divisions and distinctions where none ought to exist. Pragyaparadh can be found in the rigid dichotomy we've created between "being sick" and "being well," and it is also at the heart of other aspects of modern medicine. When, for example, we isolate and extract the "active ingredient" from an herb, when we refine it and concentrate it and market it as a drug, we are splitting off one element of a complex natural substance. What is the effect of doing this? What are the assumptions that underlie the process? How do these assumptions express themselves in other aspects of modern medicine? And most importantly: What can be gained by resisting our passion for making finer and finer distinctions, and by adopting a more holistic approach to illness, to therapies, to patients, to people, and to life?

I'm convinced it's important to ask questions like these, although as a doctor I've been trained to make pronouncements. Pronouncements are also what our patients have learned to expect from us, and they're what many patients frankly demand. In the warfare model of clinical medicine, patients are not only the "civilian population," but also the very battlefield itself. The struggle is being waged in their bones and tissues. Once this version of medicine has been accepted, the idea of the good doctor as a hard-hitting, decisive General George Patton follows quite naturally. Not someone who listens, but someone who gives orders.

The average time that a patient actually spends with a doctor during an office visit has been shrinking for many years. Doctors often cite financial pressure as a reason for seeing as many people as possible, but to a large extent this is a self-perpetuating problem. When I was doing my residency in neurology, I participated in a weekly clinic for seizure patients together with four other residents. Since more than fifty patients, most of them from low-income backgrounds, would typically appear at the three-hour clinic, a doctor was rarely able to spend more than five minutes with any individual. On one occasion, I examined a young epilepsy patient who was very uncomfortable taking his medications. Swallowing the pills made him feel different from other kids, stigmatized, and consequently he either pretended that he'd taken them or simply refused outright. Without the medications, of course, he experienced seizures and often required emergency hospital admittance. I spent approximately twenty minutes with this patient and his parents, listening to their concerns and explaining how the medications would actually reduce the level of difference the boy felt from other kids. By preventing the seizures and keeping him out of the hospital, the pills would free him to lead a normal life. After our talk, the young patient seemed much less anxious about his condition, and agreed to take the medications on schedule.

This seemed like a reasonable expenditure of my time, since a twenty-minute conversation with a resident was surely less costly to the hospital and the entire health-care system than repeated emergency-room admissions by an uninsured patient. Immediately after talking with this boy, however, I was chewed out by the furious chief resident for slowing down the assembly line of the seizure clinic. I felt like a foot soldier who had provided his general with an inadequate "body count."

When my father was being treated for polio, the doctors of whom he spoke so highly were hardly able to play the roles of generals. The support of the medical team was considered essential to my dad's recovery, yet its objective participation was limited to confirming the diagnosis of polio and prescribing physical therapy. Still, their explanations, counseling, and encouragement continue to be seen by my parents as critical to his recovery.

Even when specific medical interventions were not able to affect the course of an illness directly, the health-care team continued to provide comfort and support—and this was seen as an extremely important activity by both doctors and patients. Today, we have developed new diagnostic techniques that can make fine discriminations among pathologies, as well as drugs and procedures that can directly influence the course of an illness. But there has been a price. We have come to neglect the person who actually has the disease.

In searching for an alternative to the metaphor of doctor as battlefield commander, several options have presented themselves. For example, I once knew a very fine surgeon who, after grappling with the same problem, concluded that his job was not unlike that of an airplane pilot, and that if he could establish himself in that role with his patients, everyone's interests would be well served. Patients would instinctively trust him in a highly compliant way, and wouldn't bother him with questions—after all, no one boards a 747 with a dozen inquiries for the person flying the plane. The night before major operations, my friend would visit his patients in their hospital rooms. Everything about his manner and bearing conveyed absolute confidence and competence—and his parting words were always, "Just relax, and leave the flying to us."

Although the doctor-as-pilot model may well be appropriate for individuals facing surgery, it does relegate the patient to a thoroughly uninvolved, almost sheeplike role with respect to the authority figure who controls the powerful and incomprehensible machines. Is this really the feeling that we want to foster in people who are trying to get well? Very often a passive attitude about health has contributed to their becoming ill in the first place.

At one time I felt that a doctor should really be more like a gardener, and in some ways I still believe this is a useful metaphor. A gardener doesn't really grow his plants and flowers; rather, he builds a setting in which they can flourish. Although Nature is not really "rooting" for the roses any more than the crabgrass—nor, perhaps, for a patient any more than a malignancy—the caregiver does everything he can to create an environment that benefits one and restricts the other. But I became less fond of the gardener comparison because it too places the patient in a passive stance with respect to the physician. Plants do indeed grow—while airline passengers just sit there—but neither have any real give-and-take with the individual who is responsible for them.

Today I believe that a physician should really be a kind of teacher. A teacher imparts knowledge and perhaps even wisdom to students, but often gains as much as he gives. A teacher asks questions, but encourages pupils to ask challenging questions of their own. Moreover, a good teacher fosters love of learning by loving it himself. He is not only a giver of wisdom, he is an example of it.

I think this metaphor works quite well, although there is also a very personal reason for my attraction to it. It was a teacher who first led me to question some ideas that had always seemed very much like certainties.

I'm in the seventh grade, and we're talking about non-Western civilizations in social-studies class. Our teacher, Mr. Shakow, brings up the concept of meditation. He reminds us that in our society an active mind is most highly prized because we believe that having plenty of thoughts leads to creative innovations and technological advances. But he adds that, strange as it seems, there are people in India, Tibet, and Japan who believe that having a silent mind is the ultimate and most difficult of life's goals.

My energetic, all-knowing classmates and I snicker at the idea that it could possibly be difficult to stop thinking, but this attitude quickly fades when we are asked to close our eyes and see how long it takes before a

thought enters our minds. My cockiness evaporates as I realize that no mat-
ter how hard I try I can't shut off the constant stream of thoughts that is
always coursing through my head.

And then yet another thought appears: "Uh-oh, what if they're right!"

Our society prizes action, invention, accomplishment. The triumphs
of this value system are all around us, and it would be foolish to minimize the benefits of Western society's emphasis on practical results
and applied intelligence. The wellspring of these achievements is the
"active mind" that Mr. Shakow spoke of in his seventh-grade class-
room, but it's interesting to note that even within the Western tradition, the qualities of mind that are most admired have changed over
time. A prodigious memory, for example, was once thought to be the
true marker of high intelligence, and learned men and women of the
past took it for granted that they should know entire books by heart.
Today we attach similar importance to mathematical and scientific
ability: If you're good at math, if you can perform calculations
quickly and accurately, then you're really smart. When test scores of
American schools are measured against the educational systems of
other countries, it's now the "hard science" areas of the curriculum
that are emphasized and worried about.

In this environment, the notion of creating silence in the
mind—of slowing it down, or even bringing the onrushing train of
thought to a complete halt—may seem unnatural or perhaps self-
destructive. Nature gave us brains, after all. Since the purpose of a
brain is to think, the more we think and the faster we think the better
off we'll be. Like a child holding his breath, we may choose to amuse
ourselves by trying to "not think" for a few moments, but the idea that
there could be some profound benefit in this is quite outside our orientation. Beginning with that experiment in social-studies class, I
found myself trying to integrate my conventional academic aspira-
tions with a fascination and growing respect for the ideal of the quiet
mind—a mind in which every thought that arose expressed clarity,
perspective, and integrity, free of the anxious noise reflecting static,
fear, and confusion.

Perhaps because of my early impressions of the medical profession, I had always known I would be a doctor. However, I majored
in anthropology as an undergraduate, with a special interest in the

healing arts of non-Western cultures. I discovered that in societies throughout the world, the medicine man or shaman has traditionally been viewed as a figure capable of traversing the physical, emotional, and spiritual planes of existence in search of means to benefit suffering patients. For this purpose, practitioners could draw upon a vast array of therapeutic accoutrements, including chant, massage, visual symbols, foods, herbs, and scents. Cultural ideology, collective beliefs, and even highly dramatic performances contributed to the creation of a healing atmosphere.

For me, these were more than academic interests. I began a daily meditation practice during my sophomore year as an undergraduate, and in the three months between college and medical school I embarked on a program that included eight hours a day of meditation. By the end of that summer, I was convinced that I was ready to begin my formal medical training at the University of Chicago. After all, I had taken not only organic chemistry, but had written a thesis on shamanism as well, and had spent months deep in meditation. How much better prepared could I be?

But in medical school, of course, there would be no talk of anything "sacred" about doctoring or anything else. The word *healer* was never used, nor was *health, spirit, humanity, caring, compassion,* or *love.* During my months in dissection rooms, biochemistry laboratories, and genetics lectures it became clear that modern medicine was about fixing a physical machine known as the human body. The power of the mind was barely acknowledged as relevant to health, and any references to the "quiet mind" were best made very quietly indeed.

When I tried to introduce my spiritual interests into this environment, even these efforts seemed to increase the pressure. As a freshman medical student, I arranged for Dr. Hans Selye to appear at medical grand rounds. The great Canadian researcher was the preeminent authority on the harmful effects of stress, and faculty and students packed the auditorium for his noon lecture. Unfortunately, Dr. Selye was nowhere to be seen. Close to panic, I raced to a telephone and called his office in Montreal, where his assistant assured me that she had most certainly dropped him off at the airport the day before. But where could he be? Lost or kidnapped, perhaps. My long-standing interest in visualization now produced a clear image of myself apologizing to the entire school for this inexplicable confusion. When I returned to the auditorium, however, I was stunned to discover that Dr. Selye was there and had begun the lecture in my absence. Out of breath, my heart pounding, I got to my seat just as the world's leading expert on the stress response was describing its mental and physical components. He could have called me to the lectern as a case in point.

Over the next four years I was perceived as somewhat eccentric by my classmates, yet by the time we graduated I had instructed about a quarter of them in the techniques of meditation. The demands of medical school gave proof to the saying that "there are no atheists in foxholes." If they believed that some relief might come of it, my fellow students were quite willing to partake of methods that they might otherwise intellectually reject. In at least one case, even an eminent professor was open to explore this approach. Though born in India, Dr. Napoleon DasGupta had shunned meditation and the teachings of Ayurveda until he met me, a Jewish American third-year medical student. Like most cardiologists, Dr. DasGupta suffered from extreme stress. He asked me to teach him meditation as a relaxation technique, then took to it at once and practiced it regularly. I vividly recall a moment when I was waiting for an elevator in Billings Hospital. The elevator door opened and there was Dr. DasGupta, attended by his retinue of cardiology fellows, residents, interns, and medical students. The professor's face lit up when he saw me. He turned to his entourage and declared, "This is Dr. David Simon, my *guru*."

When first encountered in seventh-grade social studies, the concept of meditation had seemed like an intriguing but remote notion. It was a little mind game, like closing your eyes and trying not to think of a white elephant. Certainly, meditation had appeared to be far from the goals of an aspiring doctor in an achievement-oriented educational system. Now, at the other end of that system, the capricious notion of a mind at rest was demonstrating practical benefits of its own. Moreover, it soon became clear that these benefits could extend beyond the anxieties of medical students and their even more stressed-out professors:

During my first year of medical school, I search for a project that will draw upon my interest in the relationship between mind and body. I approach a cardiologist, Dr. Suzanne Oparil, who is studying stress and hypertension, and although she is skeptical as to the outcome, she agrees to sponsor me for a research project teaching meditation to inner-city African American women who have high blood pressure.

Soon I recruit a group of ten women and instruct them in a mantra meditation technique. They all agree to return a few days later for a follow-up session, but only half of the women actually do so. When I ask about the others, I hear stories of children injured in fights and of people evicted from their homes. And of the five women who have returned, only two have practiced their meditation. Clearly, with these subjects I am directly confronting the challenge of translating theory into reality.

Focusing on this core group of five women, I try to explain the benefits of taking time each day to quiet their minds and rest their bodies. After we participate in a group meditation, each woman promises to practice the technique for at least twenty minutes each day.

I continue to follow them for the next six months, and throughout this time they keep their commitment to daily meditation. Over the period of the study their blood pressure falls an average of fifteen points, reducing or eliminating their need for blood-pressure medication.[2]

Like a number of leading American universities, the University of Chicago was situated in the midst of an economically depressed urban environment. The area around the school was physically run-down, and so were the people who lived there. Without diminishing the importance of dealing with the material conditions in that part of the city or the tangible needs of the people who lived there, it seemed impossible to ignore the emotional and spiritual devastation that accompanied life in the area. The medications that were routinely supplied to hypertensive patients were no more effective in fundamentally bettering their lives than were the minimal resources of jobs, good housing, and healthy food that were available in the area around the university.

My experience with the five inner-city women provided an important insight. Just as a human being can be financially deprived or poorly fed, he or she can be emotionally and spiritually undernourished or malnourished as well—and the importance of this should not be underestimated. Mind body medicine is valuable not just as a gentler philosophy, but because it provides powerful and affordable alternatives to standard drug treatments. This can be especially valuable in areas where economic resources are scarce, and it's certainly a more humane approach than is typically found in overworked big-city hospitals, where the perception of the environment as a "battleground" carries over to the doctors who are treating the "casualties."

As is true with any war, the officers on the medical battlefield are continuously weighing the potential benefits versus the costs of utilizing the high tech armamentarium that is available. Victims of major traumatic injuries are brought into the emergency rooms of urban hospitals around the country every day of the year. When the chances for success are essentially nil, aggressive therapeutic efforts should be withheld. On the other hand, emergency rooms exist to provide heroic interventions that could be lifesaving. A memory from my early medical training highlights the challenges that are faced in deciding how medical care is administered and how our perceptions of suffering, life and death are formed.

I am a senior medical student doing my emergency-room rotation during the middle of a freezing Chicago winter. The paramedics radio in to prepare us for a homeless man they are transporting who is comatose and severely hypothermic with a core temperature of 92°! Minutes later the ambulance arrives at the emergency-room entrance, and the gurney carrying the raggedly clothed elderly gentleman is rushed into Trauma Room 1.

Almost immediately the cardiac monitor sounds its alarm as the man goes into full cardiac arrest. A breathing tube is placed, CPR is begun, and medications are administered through multiple intravenous lines. After five minutes of unsuccessful resuscitative efforts one of the emergency-room residents quotes a recent journal article that recommended pouring heated water into an open chest cavity to accelerate the warming of hypothermic patients. The chief resident grabs a chest-cracking instrument, the patient's chest is opened, and warm salt water is continuously poured over the heart as open-chest cardiac massage is performed. After a half hour of effort with no response, the proceedings are halted and the man is pronounced dead.

A few minutes later the emergency-room attending physician arrives and wishes to review the video recording of the resuscitation efforts. The next scene is indelibly etched in my memory: a dozen doctors, nurses, and students are watching a video while standing in several inches of bloody water in a room with a now-dead man whose chest is still spilling crimson water onto the table and floor, while the chief resident and attending physician dispassionately describe the sequence of events that has just transpired.

In many ways, the best and worst of modern medicine exist side by side in the ERs of our country, which can be seen as the microcosms of our health-care system. Our ability to treat acute life-threatening conditions successfully is unprecedented in the history of mankind. On the other hand, patients often feel that they are treated like broken machines on a conveyor belt. In emergency rooms this is in part due to the fact that there is usually no prior contact between the staff and the patient, the stress level is high, and the mission of an ER is to make rapid diagnoses and dispositions. There is, however, something more insidious taking place, which reflects our prevailing medical model. On the battlefield of acute-care medicine the civilian with the disease may be confused with the disease itself and be susceptible to "friendly fire." At university training programs, difficult or disruptive patients may receive the pejorative label of "gomer," which is an acronym for Get Out of My Emergency Room. The message to an admitting intern on a hospital service might be, "You need to admit this gomer with three alcohol-withdrawal seizures." The underlying communication accents the perceived imposition that the patient's self-destructive behavior places on the already overextended team. This subtle dehumanization pervades our health-care system and has become more evident as the pressures associated with managed care rise.

Suggesting that taking a consciousness-based or spiritual approach is a solution to this problem may seem naive or simplistic. An emergency-room physician may believe that attending to a gunshot victim's spiritual needs is irrelevant when the hemorrhaging has not yet been controlled. Yet, taking a spiritual approach does not necessarily imply discussing the meaning of life with each patient; rather, it means recognizing the underlying and unifying humanity of each person we encounter and remembering that healing is the result of a profound intelligence that goes far beyond the skills of a doctor.

Honoring our humanity and providing an opportunity to train young physicians requires striking a careful, thoughtful balance. Patients who suffer irreversible cardiac arrests in teaching hospitals may receive prolonged CPR efforts to allow students to hone their skills. Although these patients may be clinically dead, fourth-year medical students perform cardiac massage in order to gain experience. Here the turmoil of the inner city provides practice opportunities for future physicians. On one occasion, a fourth-year student became upset when it seemed to him that the true purpose of these cardiac massages was simply to coarsen the feelings of the students. Although I know this was not a conscious intention, in retrospect, I can see his point had some merit by the fact that he was labeled soft by the supervising medical housestaff.

Halfway through my third year of medical school, I decided that neurology would be my area of specialization. Here I could continue my exploration of the relationships between consciousness and physiology. Although I felt an affinity with the psychiatrists I met in medical school, they were viewed suspiciously and often seen as outsiders by the other specialties. Since I already felt somewhat alienated from my colleagues, I was in no hurry for an additional stigma. I felt like a "real doctor" and I wanted to be perceived that way by my peers.

I was very fortunate to receive my neurology training at the University of Colorado, where Dr. James Austin was chairman. Although he was internationally known as the discoverer of a genetic variant of a rare neurological disease known as metachromatic leukodystrophy, Dr. Austin was personally fascinated by the phenomenon of consciousness, and he often spent his vacations visiting with Zen masters. Once he began laughing in the middle of a discussion on the possibility of understanding higher states of consciousness by studying measurable neurophysiological responses. Dr. Austin, it seemed, had once had a similar conversation with a Zen Buddhist monk. The monk had told him that seeking to understand consciousness by studying the brain was like trying to understand a person's nature by looking under the hood of his car parked in a driveway!

My years as a neurologist in training allowed me to explore deeply what was known about the mind and its relationship to physical and mental illness. In contrast to my experience in medical school, many of my fellow residents had interests similar to my own. We discussed the foundations of awareness, language, emotion, and behavior, and felt scientifically safe in doing so as long as we reminded ourselves that we were "brain doctors" rather than philosophers or mystics.

There was another aspect of neurology that encouraged me to look beyond standard medical approaches. Unfortunately, since there were often no medications available to treat degenerative nervous-system illnesses, we were forced to seek other kinds of support for our patients.

During my neurology training, I spent a year as a Muscular Dystrophy Association fellow at the University of Colorado Medical Center. Dr. Steven Ringel, the medical director of the program, intuitively understands the importance of treating the patient as well as the disease. Since our ability to influence these genetic disorders remains limited, this is particularly critical for patients with inherited muscle diseases.

Shortly after beginning my work in the neuromuscular program, I take on a patient with a rare disease known as myasthenia gravis, or MG. In this condition, the body produces antibodies that work against normal functioning between nerves and muscles, and patients suffer from fluctuating weakness. This autoimmune disease can produce serious or life-threatening problems affecting swallowing and breathing. Mrs. Miller is a woman in her fifties who has suffered with MG for more than ten years, and she is on multiple medications. During her first two months as my patient, ever-worsening weakness causes her to be admitted to the intensive-care unit at least five different times. On each occasion, after fairly minimal adjustments in her medicines, her condition stabilizes and she is ready to go home in two or three days.

I notice that her health invariably deteriorates and she requires hospitalization on those weekends that I am not on call. Although I often hear from her during the weekends that I am available, I never need to admit her. Instead, I am able to reassure her or make minor changes in her medications over the phone. But whenever I'm not on call, I begin to anticipate that Mrs. Miller will be waiting for me in the hospital on Monday morning.

After this has happened three weeks in a row, I realize that I need to gain a deeper understanding of this woman and I commit to spending more time with her. One Monday I pull up a chair in the intensive-care unit and begin to get a sense of Mrs. Miller as a person. She reminds me that she had been widowed about five years earlier and had been living with her son until he recently moved in with his fiancée. She keeps herself busy by volunteering at a day-care center during the week but has minimal social contacts on the weekends.

She relates a remarkably consistent pattern of deterioration in her condition. On Friday evenings, her anxiety rises as she anticipates spending a weekend entirely alone. She notices some worsening in her swallowing and a rising sense of panic. She often calls to see which doctor is available, and if she doesn't recognize the name, she begins to medicate herself with extra doses of one of her prescriptions. Although the drug she usually chooses has short-term benefits, when taken in excess it also tends to cause sudden and rapid deterioration in her condition. Eventually this leads to a 911 call and an emergency admission to the hospital.

Armed with this information, I contact a social worker who helps me structure a viable program for Mrs Miller. We have a visiting nurse contact her twice each weekend, and I ask the resident on call to check in with her on Friday evening, assuring him that the few minutes spent on the phone can save hours of work in the middle of the night. With these simple human interactions, Mrs. Miller needs only two hospital admissions over the next six months, both for complications unrelated to her medications.

When contemplating patients such as Mrs. Miller, I sometimes feel that I'm completing a long, circular journey into the art of healing. It began with the house call of a suburban pediatrician. Because he was unable to intervene directly in the minor but frightening illness that had brought him to our home, he simply did what he could, which was to talk and to listen—and paradoxically, this seemed to bring about rapid improvement in the patient. In the years that followed, my introduction to the full arsenal of medical "weaponry" may have at times diminished the essential wisdom that was at work in that first encounter, while at other times my interest in traditional healing arts may have caused me to magnify the importance of the physician as a human or spiritual presence. I'm gratified that today I've arrived at what I hope and believe is a balanced view of the healer's many-faceted art. This is the view that I try to bring to my clinical work each day, and it's the perspective that I hope this book will convey.

A doctor's patients must sometimes endure a certain amount of pain. That's the way it is, and there is no benefit in being naive about it. When it's necessary to have blood drawn it stings when the needle hits your arm—and there are many other important and beneficial procedures that also involve some discomfort. But I've found that an awareness and even an honoring of patients' hopes and fears, as well as their physical pain, can have clear therapeutic benefits. Conversely, the denial of feeling that becomes established over the course of medical training can do a great deal of harm both to patients' health and to the effectiveness of the physicians themselves.

Pediatricians and pediatric nurses can clearly see when children are about to cry or hide behind the examining table. In these situations, it's obvious that a certain amount of emotional support will benefit the process. But for other specialists, the frightened child in every patient is much less obviously present. When a woman visits a gynecologist, for example, her first meeting with the doctor may come when she's flat on her back with her feet in metal stirrups. The nurturing that was clearly required for a pediatrician has turned into an order for the patient to put her body up on a table so it can be checked out. If I seem to be suggesting that physicians sometimes approach their patients the way a car mechanic looks at a vehicle in a service bay, this may be too generous an analogy. A more apt comparison might be to a policeman interviewing the victim of a violent crime. Often there's a sense that the victim must somehow be to blame: If you decided to walk your dog in the middle of the night and you got robbed, wouldn't you have been smarter to stay in bed? If you left your car unlocked, why are you surprised when it was stolen? If you're overweight and a chain-smoker and now you've got cardiovascular problems, wouldn't you have been better off eating fewer hamburgers? But now you expect your doctor to solve your problems for you.

Let me emphasize that I have no intention of gratuitously criticizing physicians, who are under constant pressure of all kinds. I'm well aware that what might be seen as callous attitudes are really defense mechanisms born of frustration and disillusionment. We are constantly called upon to put severely damaged people back together again, which only demonstrates that we've failed to create an approach to health care that prevents damage in the first place. Rather than confront this failure, with all the complexities that such a confrontation would entail, it's easier for many doctors to become fatalistic, or to conclude that sick people in some sense are getting what they deserve. And once that viewpoint becomes established, a doctor finds that taking care of patients' bodies is all he or she can handle. That a physician should also treat their *souls* seems almost ludicrous.

Yet we must of course become involved with our patients as spiritual beings, because in the end their emotional selves cannot be separated from their physical selves. Although this is being proven every day in studies that demonstrate the essential unity of mind and body, even doctors who acknowledge the so-called mind body connection find it difficult to translate this recognition into effective therapeutic technique. Is it enough to spend a few moments talking about a patient's personal history? Does nurturing a sick person's spirit mean holding his hand, or managing to smile when entering his hospital room, or taking notes on a yellow legal pad when he recites the names of his grandchildren?

The final stage—in a sense, the culmination—of my medical education was my introduction to Ayurveda. In Ayurveda, I discovered an approach to treating both the spirit and the body of every patient—or, rather, to treating the spirit and the body as one.

My experience both as a patient and as a doctor had taught me the importance of talking and listening to individual human beings. It had also taught me that simply talking and listening were obviously not enough when dealing with serious health issues. In Ayurveda, I found a view of human health that embraces the best aspects of contemporary medicine, that excludes nothing that can be of benefit to the patient, while at the same time emphasizing the need for understanding the unique nature of every person as well as the intricacies of diagnosis and disease.

2

Creating a Universe

"Each thing we see hides something else we want to see."

René Magritte

"The world is moving too fast," lamented the successful middle-aged stock broker. He had worked hard to achieve his senior status and his corner office, but now he complained, "I just don't feel I can keep up with all the changes that are happening." He was having trouble sleeping and getting migraine headaches almost daily. Although they were annoying during the week, they became almost explosive on Saturday mornings, requiring him to stay in bed a good part of each weekend. He gained partial relief by drinking coffee, consuming almost six cups each day. Although his house was paid for, his pension fully funded, and his children's college funds well stocked, he hadn't taken a real vacation in over four years.

From a Western perspective, this man was having caffeine-withdrawal headaches, exacerbated by his irregular sleep-wake pattern. From the Ayurvedic point of view this poor man's life was being ruled by movement without rhythm. The air element (Vayu) had become excessive and was carrying him away. He needed to come back down to earth (Prithivi), and recapture the steadiness, stability, and balance that had always been his character. He needed to remember what he was really made of and return to his true nature.

In every culture throughout history, human beings have speculated as to how the world began, and about the principles that continue to structure and govern it. Our fundamental human interest in the beginning is not just metaphysical. There has always been a sense that, by thinking about how things began, we can understand the powers that are still at work in our daily experience of the world. In ancient times these cosmic speculations were generally quite poetic and metaphorical. A Chinese creation myth, for instance, describes the universe as originating from a gigantic hen's egg, while a Norse myth refers to a primordial cow emerging from a block of ice. Both these stories imply that animals are vehicles through which supreme powers express themselves, and this veneration of animals manifested itself elsewhere in art, religion, and even in early medicine. The Judeo-Christian tradition describes the beginnings of the universe in more abstract terms, with the disembodied voice of God commanding, "Let there be light."

Anthropologists debate the extent to which the peoples of the past thought that their myths literally described the process of creation. In the case of the Scandinavian peoples and their story of the "ice cow," for example, it's clear that the myth was of primarily symbolic significance, and that its importance was in the psychological and perhaps subconscious connotations evoked by the narrative, not as a depiction of how the universe really began. But now, at the end of the twentieth century, there is no doubt that cosmologists believe the current scientific model of creation is intended to describe "what really happened." According to the so-called big bang theory, the universe began when an entity of incomprehensible density exploded, generating the matter that makes up the galaxies and propelling it outward at unimaginable speeds. Over time, primordial matter cooled and condensed, resulting in galaxies, stars, and planets. Most cosmologists believe that the universe will continue to expand, doubling its known size over the next ten billion years. Will gravitational forces eventually overcome the expansion of the universe, leading to a contraction back to the center? This concept of an oscillating universe that expands and contracts over eons of time evokes the Vedic image of a breathing cosmos—the exhaling and inhaling of Brahma, the primordial creator. Modern cosmologists continue to debate the ultimate fate of our universe.

⟆

Despite some dissenters, the big bang theory is the prevailing explanation of the origin of the cosmos. But although it seems to describe
fairly accurately the universe as we perceive it, the theory raises the
question of what preceded the cosmic explosion? Where did the original entity come from? How long did it exist before exploding? What
caused it suddenly to break apart?

Scientists respond to these inquiries in various ways. To the
physicist Stephen Hawking, such questions are very understandable
but scientifically naive. Asking what came before the big bang, he has
said, is like asking what's north of the North Pole.[1] And yet, great scientists, including Albert Einstein, have not so readily dismissed these
questions as they searched for a unified theory that would define the
essential "stuff" out of which the universe arose.

Ayurveda teaches that *consciousness* is, in effect, the unifying
principle that physicists are seeking. Consciousness is the organizing
essence of the universe that simultaneously transcends and creates
the world we perceive. The essential "stuff" of the universe is actually
"non-stuff." But this essential non-stuff is not the same as emptiness,
for within it is contained the potential for all that was, is, and will be.
The *seen* world has its roots in the *unseen* field of pure potentiality—
in consciousness. From this primal consciousness, the elements that
make up the universe come into being. Western science has not yet
named this unifying essence and might be reluctant to embrace the
terms *consciousness* or *pure potentiality.* Yet, when we look at the original Ayurvedic term for this primordial state from which the universe
arose, the Sanskrit word, *avyakta,* simply means "unmanifest." Contained within the unmanifest is the impulse to create, known in
Ayurveda as *prakruti,* or nature. In essence, Ayurveda simply describes
the universe as arising from a field of potentiality that has an intrinsic nature to create.

Modern physics also describes the universe—consisting of time,
space, and matter—as arising from a timeless, spaceless point. This is
the culmination of a long tradition in Western thought. Pre-Socratic
philosophers such as Heracleitus asserted the existence of a basic
substance from which all things came and to which all things
returned. Heracleitus called this primordial essence *logos,* which is
the root word of *logic* and *intelligence.* The logos of Heracleitus can be
understood as a cosmic governing and generating principle analo-

gous to the primordial consciousness of Ayurveda, and here the Western and Eastern traditions begin to sound very much alike.

The Ayurvedic concept of creation describes not only the beginning of the universe, but also a continuing creative process that is occurring at every moment. Ayurveda teaches that the entire universe unfolds through the interaction of three vital principles, which in Sanskrit are known as the *gunas*. They are *sattva,* the creative principle; *rajas,* the principle of maintenance; and *tamas,* the principle of destruction. Everything that we perceive through our senses, from elementary particles to galaxies, is born, has a life span, and eventually dies. In this dynamic cycle, the gunas are the principles that are continuously expressing themselves.

According to Vedic philosophy, the three gunas interact to create both subjective and objective realities. In the subjective realm, the five sense organs, five motor organs, and the conscious mind are brought into being. On the objective side, the gunas give rise to five great elements, or *mahabhutas,* and five subtle elements, or *tanmatras,* the quanta of perceptual experience that feed our five sense organs. The five great elements are the codes of nature that compose the world of perceived forms.

The Five Great Elements

The mahabhutas are not elements in the sense that Western science most often uses that word, meaning substances that cannot be chemically broken down into constituent parts. Water, for example, is a compound rather than an element. It combines atoms of the elements hydrogen and oxygen. The atomic nuclei of these most fundamental substances all contain the same number of protons. In the Western terminology, this atomic number is the identifying characteristic of an element, and science currently recognizes 109 of them. Textbooks often refer to them as the building blocks of the universe.

To suggest, as Ayurveda does, that the universe is composed of only five elements would seem to be an invitation to ridicule. But here the Ayurvedic viewpoint is actually much closer to the perspective of contemporary physics than to the conventional definition of elements presented in high-school science classes. Quantum physics teaches that the universe is governed by four basic forces: a strong

CREATING THE UNIVERSE
The Ayurvedic Model

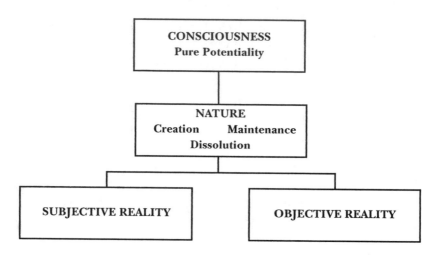

nuclear force, which binds together the particles of atomic nuclei; a weak nuclear force, which controls the process of radioactive decay in heavy atoms such as uranium; an electromagnetic force, which maintains subatomic particles in their orbits around the nucleus; and the force of gravity, which governs the attraction between large objects. Similarly, the Ayurvedic elements are the principles that underlie creation rather than the building blocks that make it up. Though Ayurveda does identify these principles with substances, it would be a mistake to understand this too literally. Charles Steinmetz, the great mathematician and electrical engineer who worked closely with Thomas Edison, believed that electricity was not really a substance like water or wind, but an abstraction, an animating principle behind the "way things happen." Though he probably never heard of Ayurveda, Steinmetz was really describing electricity as an element in Ayurvedic terms.

The five great elements are space, air, fire, water, and earth—and here again distinctions between Western and Eastern traditions of natural philosophy begin to blur. Aristotle, for example, taught that the universe was composed of these same five elements and he as well as other Greek philosophers may have been influenced by ideas from India that had reached Greece. A similar theory of the elements was the basis of the medieval science of alchemy, and a variation of this was employed by the brilliant sixteenth-century physician Paracelsus. According to Ayurvedic teaching, the five elements underlie our experience of the material environment. They are the principles structuring the world that is reported by our senses.

THE FIRST ELEMENT: SPACE (AKASHA)

Space in Ayurvedic terms is the emptiness in which unlimited potential resides. In this sense, space can be described as the outermost manifestation of the mind, which also encompasses infinite possibilities. Ayurveda teaches that space is the field of unlimited potential from which consciousness creates the material universe.

To understand this, it may be useful to refer to the French philosopher Henri Bergson's definition of consciousness as choice.[2] According to Bergson, people are more conscious than stones because human beings can experience various intentions, make selections among them, and act upon these choices. On the other hand, people are less conscious than God because our choices are not infinite. In Ayurvedic terms, space is the principle of unbounded choice-making potential—and it is literally everywhere, though our senses may deceive us on this point. For example, modern physics asserts that more than 99.99 percent of the material world is actually empty space, despite its apparent solidity. Even subatomic particles are only localized probabilities, and the vast emptiness between the electrons and nucleus of an atom is proportionately far greater than the distances between the planets of our solar system.

From a biological viewpoint, the element of space can be recognized in the membranes, pores, and receptor spaces of every cell in our bodies. If there is any obstruction to these areas, if passage through these spaces is somehow blocked, the cell will not survive. Even in the embryology of a human being, most major development consists of the creation of tubes to enclose and internalize space. As early as the third week of fetal life, cells on the surface of an embryo fold inward to create a groove that eventually forms the brain and nervous system.[3] Similarly, primitive cells create tubes that develop into the heart and blood vessels, the gastrointestinal tract, and the respiratory system. This enclosing, but not obstructing, of emptiness, of space, is a characteristic and essential feature of life.

THE SECOND ELEMENT: AIR (VAYU)

Air represents the principle of movement. Perhaps its presence is implicit in the element of space, for even as we envision a vast, empty expanse, we naturally imagine ourselves moving through it.

Movement is an essential feature of the universe, which is in a constant state of flux at every level. Vast galaxies are hurtling away from one another at unimaginable speeds, electrons are speeding around atomic nuclei, and, somewhere in between, people are driving along freeways in their automobiles. Even when material objects appear to be stationary, there is always activity at a subtler level. A piece of wood may appear to be stable, but the atoms that compose it are in continuous motion.

The human body perceives the element of movement through the sense of touch, through which tactile receptors register subtle fluctuations against the skin. At the microscopic level, this element expresses itself in the exchange of gases that is critical to each cell's functioning; cellular respiration is a magnificently orchestrated chemical symphony in which oxygen is utilized to extract energy and carbon dioxide is eliminated as a waste product. Movement is also represented by the continuous motion of molecules within and between cells. At every instant, DNA is zipping and unzipping to reveal vital genetic codes, proteins are being transported from their manufacturing plants to important cellular construction sites, and chemical messengers are delivering constantly updated packets of information.

THE THIRD ELEMENT: FIRE (TEJAS)

As consciousness increases in density and complexity, the Ayurvedic principle of fire comes into being. Once again, the existence of this element is implied by the existence of the previous one. Thus, fire is inherent in movement, for wherever there is motion there is friction, and friction in turn gives rise to heat and light.

Above all, fire is the transformational principle that changes states of matter from one form to another, and the addition or subtraction of fire reconfigures the atoms that compose a given substance. When fire is applied to a solid such as ice, for example, the solid becomes a liquid—and if fire is then applied to the liquid, it becomes a gas.

In biological systems, the fire principle expresses itself in the conversion of glucose, fats, and protein into energy. This conversion process occurs primarily in the mitochondria, the "energy factories" of the cell. The transformation of the chemical energy of food into the cells and tissues of a living being requires the orderly flow of intelligence through the chaotic field of all possibilities. This controlled production of heat and energy is a critical feature of living systems, which could not survive if the fire element were absent.

THE FOURTH ELEMENT: WATER (JALA)

Water represents the principle of cohesion and attraction throughout creation. Just as adding water to a bowl of dry flour causes the particles to stick together to form dough, water holds the individual impulses of matter together. Water keeps planets circling around the sun and keeps electrons within the influence of an atomic nucleus. It is also the elemental expression of emotional bonding between people, and as such it underlies the experience of love. Everywhere in nature there is a never-ending contest between the attractive influence of the water element and the freedom-loving impulse toward movement, which is represented by wind. When the cohesive forces dominate, there is an illusion of solidity; when movement dominates, there is an illusion of change.

Life itself originated in the primordial soup of the ocean, and an important aspect of life's evolution has been the development of efficient ways to internalize the sea. It should be no surprise, then, that human beings are primarily composed of water, which accounts for about 60 percent of our total body weight. In all living things, water is the essential cohesive liquid of the cell, and vital life-supporting functions occur within the cells' cytoplasm fluid. Quite literally, water is the medium that holds life together.

THE FIFTH ELEMENT: EARTH (PRITHIVI)

The earth element represents the material form of creation. As the water element releases energy, atoms approach one another to form objects of mass composed of the earth element. Earth represents all aspects of the material world that are localized in time and space, and it is the most consolidated form of consciousness. As such, it creates the greatest illusion of boundaries. But even the most dense substances—lead, for example—are comprised of atoms, most of which are vast expanses of empty space.

In the human body, the element of earth is represented by the various specific cell components and organelles that maintain independent structure. This includes cell parts such as the nucleus, Golgi apparatus, ribosomes, mitochondria, liposomes, and endoplasmic reticulum. Given the same genetic code and the same blueprint of intelligence, it is a remarkable feature of life that each cell can express its unique talent. Each of these discrete structures has its own reality in time and space, and this reality is an expression of the mass and the structure of the earth element.

The Five Subtle Elements and Our Remarkable Sensory Equipment

Ayurveda presents a fascinating way of describing our perception of the world. Just as we can organize the material universe into the five great elements, we can organize our internalization of the universe through the five subtle elements—*sound, touch, sight, taste,* and *smell.* These five subtle elements, or tanmatras, can be thought of as the impulses of experience that matter offers to the sense organs. The Vedic concept is that all matter, which in its essence is condensed consciousness, expresses itself through the subtle elements, which our five senses receive and convert into a mental representation.

The subtlest element is *sound,* known in Sanskrit as *shabda.* Sound is the first vibration that stirs from the field of silence. It is perceived to a greater or lesser degree by our organs of hearing, but we know that each living being can only perceive a limited slice of the entire vibratory symphony. The human ear can detect frequencies between fifteen hertz and twenty kilohertz. Dogs can detect vibrations up to fifty kilohertz and certain bats respond to frequencies well above one hundred kilohertz.[4] Regardless of the acuity of our hearing organs, sound carries information over distances, small or vast.

The subtle element of *touch* is known in Sanskrit as *sparsha.* Our ability to perceive and recognize cutaneous sensations is a feature of the receptors embedded in our skin. We have many types of receptors that respond to a variety of stimuli, including pressure, movement, and temperature. Perception of touch is a function of both the receiving apparatus and our attention. At every moment we filter out billions of bits of information before they enter conscious awareness. For example, you may not be consciously aware of the socks on your feet until reading this sentence, but through the simple act of placing your attention on any part of your body you can activate the sensory impulse that carries tactile information from that region.

The next subtle element is *sight*, or *rupa* in Sanskrit. Our ability to perceive electromagnetic radiation with our eyes is a remarkable and complex process. Fundamentally, the human visual system evolved in order to receive the energy of the sun. Although our visual capabilities are truly amazing, allowing us to see a light approximately 1/100,000,000th as strong as bright sunlight, we are still only able to register a small fraction of the visual information that is actually available. We receive visual energy in a relatively narrow band of the entire spectrum ranging from two hundred to seven hundred nanometers, or billionths of a meter.[5]

Human beings create the rainbow of the world from three basic colors perceived by our retina. Dogs and cats perceive a less brilliantly pigmented environment because they construct hues from only two colors. Some birds use up to five basic colors and may see a world much more brilliant than we could imagine. Insects and some birds and mammals seem capable of seeing ultraviolet light. And, the Australian silvereye bird appears to be capable of detecting magnetic fields through its visual system.[6] Although we'd like to think that "seeing is believing," we only see the narrow vibrations of light that our eyes can capture.

The subtle element of *taste* is known as *rasa* in Sanskrit. Taste operates through end organs on the surface of the tongue known as chemoreceptors, because they respond to subtle changes in the chemical environment. This is a critically important capability, because nature has coded information regarding nourishment or toxicity in the form of taste. Western science recognizes four fundamental tastes—sweet, sour, bitter, and salty—but Ayurveda adds two more, pungent and astringent. These last two create changes in the texture of the mucous membranes that provide the mind body physiology with important information on the nature of the substance being tasted.

The last subtle element is that of *smell*, or *gandha*. Smell is a primitive sense that allows us to sample the environment at a distance. In order for us to perceive a smell, an object has to release small particles of itself into the wind; moreover, the particles must be soluble in water or fat so they can dissolve in and penetrate the mucous lining of our olfactory receptors. Human beings are capable of perceiving thousands of distinctive odors and fragrances.[7] Because of the close relationship between smells and memory, familiar odors often trigger highly emotional associations. The aroma of freshly baked bread, the fragrance of lilacs at dusk, or the scent of rose cologne on the skin of a high-school heartthrob register impressions deep in our memory banks and may trigger cascades of memory when we encounter the smell years after the initial olfactory sensation.

The Vedic sages derived their insights into the nature of reality without benefit of sophisticated scientific instruments. They simply looked inside themselves, and discovered the secrets of the universe within their own physical beings and their consciousness. Their understanding of the world in terms of five great elements is at once simple and profound. Though this perspective is of ancient origin, the concepts are relevant to our current understanding of reality, and can even illuminate our understanding of Western scientific principles. We can, for example, describe chemical reactions as the application of the fire principle, or energy, to systems composed of the earth element, or atoms. This increases the movement principle (the air element) of the atoms, causing a reorganization of bonds (the water element), which results in a new substance.

Similarly, in nuclear reactions a powerful acceleration of the movement principle (the air element) within a system overcomes strong intranuclear bonding (the water element), liberating tremendous amounts of energy (fire) as subatomic particles are released from their bondage.

The theory of the five elements can be applied to human social systems as well. The fast-paced lives we live in the West, which are expressions of the air principle, are disruptive to the social cohesion (water) that bonds members of families, communities, or other organizations that are expressions of the earth principle. The absence of a unifying social fabric results in chaotic releases of emotional energy (fire) that are the bases of the unprecedented levels of violence in our society today.

By beginning to think of the world in terms of space, air, fire, water, and earth, we can gain insight into how the field of pure unmanifest consciousness interacts with itself to create manifest reality. This process is nothing other than the miracle of creation.

Vedic science teaches that we create our own reality. Consciousness, the field of all possibilities, systematically consolidates itself into the material world. The same field of intelligence that structures the galaxies, planets, mountains, and atoms creates living beings. The same intelligence that organizes the solar system, the seasons, and even the migration of birds is the origin of the creative thoughts that arise in our minds. This understanding is eloquently expressed in a Vedic poem:

> *As is the individual, so is the universe.*
> *As is the human body, so is the cosmic body.*
> *As is the human mind, so is the cosmic mind.*
> *As is the microcosm, so is the macrocosm.*

3

Personalizing the Universe

"Nature is made to conspire with spirit to emancipate us."

Ralph Waldo Emerson

Three people are listening to a political candidate describe his agenda for the future. The first listener is a musician. He is very sensitive to any evidence of aesthetic appreciation on the part of the candidate. The second listener, an attorney, is principally concerned with the logical foundation of the speaker's economic policy. The third voter is a retired grandmother who wants to know whether the candidate is a man of compassion who understands the concerns of the elderly.

Each listener hears the same words, yet each hears a different message. And each forms a markedly different opinion and interpretation. In a very real sense, each of the listeners experiences a different reality.

We rely on our senses and our emotions to tell us about the world. Everything we experience during the course of a day comes laden with physical attributes such as color, sound, or texture, and with emotional associations that evoke feelings such as happiness, sadness, or perhaps even both at the same time. But the sound of a car backfiring that one person finds disturbingly loud may be entirely unnoticed by another individual, while yet a third person may dive under the nearest table because of wartime associations conjured up by the noise. The facts of the backfire could be described numerically in terms of decibels and fractions of a second, but this objective rendering would in many ways be far less real than our personal interpretations of the event. A philosopher might even argue that the sound could not even exist in the absence of someone's response to it, just as a tree falling in the forest makes no sound unless someone hears the crash.

Reality is ultimately an act of selection and interpretation. The relatively small amount of information that enters our nervous system reinforces our learned notions of what we think is "out there," and whatever does not reinforce those notions is immediately edited out. In a somewhat similar way, primitive tribesmen who are unfamiliar with photography are not able to recognize even very familiar objects in a photograph; to them, everything in the picture is just a murky collage. Without our individually and culturally acquired interpretations, what we call reality "is a radically ambiguous and ceaselessly flowing quantum soup."[1]

Our interpretations shape our reality and if our interpretations change, our reality will change as well. Each ethnic group has its unique reality filters through which the world is viewed. There is some fascinating data about Chinese Americans facing life-threatening illnesses.[2] According to Chinese astrology, different signs predict good or bad outcomes for different diseases. First-generation Chinese Americans, who strongly adhere to their traditional beliefs, will die sooner if they have been born under a "bad" sign, and will live longer than anticipated if born under a "good" sign. Children and grandchildren in these families, who have less investment in the old beliefs, do not show this pattern. Similar patterns are found among Orthodox Jews, whose mortality rates drop 50 percent just before the Jewish high holidays but remain unchanged before Christmas.[3] Similarly, deaths among Chinese dip by 35 percent in the week before the Harvest Moon Festival and peak by the same amount in the week after the festival concludes.[4] Our reality maps are passed on from generation to generation, and are so deeply engraved into our collective psyche that we can barely consider the possibility that they may be incomplete.

Cultural and psychological learning limits the repertoire of what we acknowledge as reality, and we are further limited by our perceptual apparatus. Each of our senses has very significant limitations, and different people have different levels of capability. This is certainly true among different animals as well, where perceptions develop along lines of evolution. A bee does not have the receptors to experience the wavelengths of light that are visible to people—but because it can sense ultraviolet light, a bee can detect honey from a considerable distance. A snake can sense infrared radiation. A female mosquito can home in on heat radiating from our bodies from hundreds of yards away to feast on our blood. A bat receives information as the echo of ultrasound, which allows it to safely navigate very crowded airspace. A chameleon's eyeballs swivel on two different axes, so that we cannot even imagine what his lizard world is like!

What, then, is the "true" nature of reality? The answer depends on who is looking and what kind of instruments they are using. As human beings, our observations and interpretations are made by the set of instruments that we've come to call the nervous system. The forms and phenomena that we label as reality depend on the senses we use to detect them and the thoughts we use to interpret them. Perception depends upon what kinds of questions we are asking ourselves when we make the observation, most of which are outside our conscious awareness.

John Eccles, a brilliant neuroscientist and Nobel prize winner, recognized almost thirty years ago that our perception of reality is only a "symbolic picture" or "map." Eccles wrote, "Colors, sounds, smells, heat and cold . . . belong only to the perceptual world."[5] The external world has no real status independent of the observer. Out there beyond the limits of our perceptual apparatus is that radically ambiguous and ceaselessly flowing quantum soup. Like magicians, we transform the quantum soup into material reality through observation and interpretation. Throughout this book we hope to convince you that the waking state is only one mode of consciousness. Even our state of consciousness determines our perception of reality; only when we awaken do we realize that our exotic journeys were only a dream. Although we put such stock in the waking state, we can never know the true nature of reality, because even as we make the observation we are altering it.

How do these abstract ideas apply to healing? As a Western doctor I was trained to be an objective medical scientist focused on making an accurate diagnosis and developing a logical treatment plan. I learned to read a patient's chart and to "know" someone through the numbers generated through his or her various tests and diagnostic procedures. But this approach increasingly seemed incomplete to me. People are more than computer printouts or X-ray images. They could not be fully captured in objective terms, nor could my personal responses be fully suppressed as I interacted with them. Although it seems so intuitively obvious, my traditional medical training devalued the essential human component of a patient-physician encounter.

A fundamental premise of Ayurveda is that we are more than living machines that have somehow learned to generate thoughts. When I first began to study the ancient healing traditions, one of the things that interested me most was their use of a terminology that expressed the multidimensional nature of being human. According to Vedic teaching, we exist simultaneously on a number of levels, which are called *koshas* in Sanskrit. Layers of physical matter (anatomy), energy (physiology), emotions, beliefs, and our core desires and memories combine to form our being.

These layers are always in flux, constantly transforming themselves at various rates, but underlying all change is a foundation of non-change. This is the field of pure potentiality, which in Sanskrit is called *sat chit ananda,* or truth, existence, and bliss. It is also known as *Brahman,* or the universal field of consciousness, which exists as a silent witness to all the events of our lives. By learning to shift our awareness to this transcendent level, we can begin to experience change within the much larger context of timelessness, unity, and spirit.

How We Differ . . . and What We Share

Wrapped in the many layers of our being and cloaked in the various disguises that are superimposed upon our underlying unity consciousness, each of us experiences the world in a unique way. But for the most part, Western medicine has not placed much emphasis on individual differences. As a result, therapeutic interventions are typically based upon the particular characteristics of various diseases, not of the people who have them. Yet every doctor has seen patients who don't respond appropriately to treatment. This may take the form of

LAYERS OF LIFE

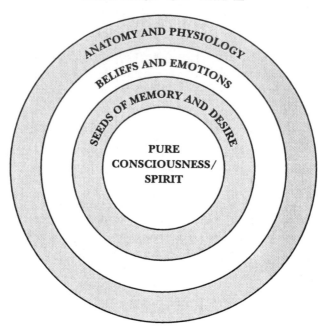

a "bad" reaction to a "good" drug, or even a response opposite to what was hoped for and predicted. Ayurveda seeks to avoid these complications by looking very closely at every person's unique mind body constitution as a first step toward diagnosis. As he meets with a new patient, the Ayurvedic physician's first task is to determine how this individual differs from all others. This is critically important, because the meaning and significance of any symptom can only be understood in the context of the patient's entire makeup.

In a case with which I'm familiar, an eighty-year-old woman visited her physician with complaints of insomnia and occasional gastrointestinal problems. She lived alone, had been widowed for many years, and her only child was now married and living in a distant city. In examining her, the physician noted that she had gained some weight since her last visit, that her blood pressure was mildly elevated, and that she was continuing to smoke between five and ten cigarettes a day despite repeated urgings that she quit.

The doctor now emphasized the importance of giving up cigarettes to this elderly lady, and this time she took his words to heart. Although she had enjoyed smoking several cigarettes in the evening while reading mystery novels, she resolved to forgo this pleasure for the good of her overall health. Unfortunately, she immediately began to consume more sweets, as well as salty snacks such as nuts and crackers. Her weight rose as the salt caused her system to retain fluids and she became more susceptible to the depression that had been stalking her. Except for the snacks, she even lost interest in food in an effort to avoid the temptation of smoking a cigarette after a meal. Within a few months she was hospitalized for congestive heart failure.

I see this as an example of imposing a categorical rule upon a patient without due consideration of her specific constitution and her way of conducting her life. Although cigarette smoking is clearly "bad" medically, and although this patient's years of tobacco use had undoubtedly contributed to her dangerous cardiovascular problems, there were other factors that deserved consideration. Cigarettes were a strongly entrenched habit for this lady—an addiction, in fact. Simply withdrawing them without addressing the needs underlying the addiction destabilized her mind body system, leading to the search for alternative sources of gratification. During sixty years of smoking, this patient's physiology had become accustomed to her habit and she had formed a strong emotional attachment to her cigarettes. Perhaps if alternative healthy choices had been suggested to substitute for giving up an indulgence, the transition away from smoking would have been smoother. But it takes time and attention to deal with all the emotional and physiological complexities that occur when people change their lives, so most physicians feel safer with a routine declaration of "Stop smoking."

Ayurveda emphasizes each person's uniqueness, and interventions that acknowledge one's special needs. In Western medicine different people with the same disease tend to be treated similarly, whereas in Ayurveda there may be substantial differences in therapeutic recommendations, based upon how the illness expresses itself in the individual. But, side by side with its acknowledgment of the many ways that each person is different from all others, Ayurveda focuses on characteristics that are shared. We have seen that Vedic science understands the universe as formed by the five great elements of space, air, fire, water, and earth. Just as the five elements structure the world around us, they are the building blocks of our bodies as well. In human beings, and indeed in all livings things, the five elements organize themselves into the three essential principles of *movement, metabolism,* and *structure.* These principles, called *doshas* in Sanskrit, underlie every aspect of Ayurvedic theory and practice, including all approaches to health and healing.

Vata Dosha—Movement and Change

Vata dosha is composed of the elements of space and air. Like the wind, Vata is characteristically light, quick, dry, moving, changeable, and irregular. It is responsible for movement in the body, whether in the form of circulation, respiration, or neuromuscular activity.

Vata creates movement and change in the physiology but may not be consistent in direction or intensity. When functioning in a balanced manner, Vata fosters energy and progress, but when out of balance it can cause the disruption of a gale-force storm.

Vata is responsible for mental activity and the movement of thought. Balanced Vata fosters creativity, energy, and fulfillment in the thinking process. When Vata is out of balance, mental activity may be disorganized, anxious, and erratic. The translation of thought into action is also a function of Vata, and all neuromuscular activity, including facial expression, hand gestures, and style of walking, is governed by this dosha.

The passage of air in and out of the lungs as well as cellular respiration are also under the jurisdiction of Vata. Inspiration, expiration, coughing, sneezing, and hiccuping all reflect various aspects of Vata in motion. Because the movement of breath mirrors the movement of our mind, imbalances in Vata will usually be reflected in agitation in both our breathing patterns and mental activity.

Movement in the gastrointestinal tract is a further expression of Vata. This includes the churning movement of the stomach, the transit of food through the small and large intestines, and the elimination of waste. It also involves the movement of gas out of the body. When Vata is balanced, the movement of the digestive tract is smooth and efficient. When there is imbalance in Vata, normal transit is disturbed with either too slow or too rapid motility.

Finally, the circulation of blood is also under the control of Vata dosha. This includes the pumping of blood through the chambers of the heart, its circulation to the body's periphery, and the eventual return of blood to the heart. Whenever there is the aspect of movement in the mind body physiology, Vata is behind the scene.

Pitta Dosha—Transformation and Metabolism

Pitta dosha is composed of the fire element and, to a lesser degree, of water. Pitta governs metabolism, digestion, and transformation. Through its general heating influence, Pitta is responsible for changing states of matter in a biological system. Applying the heat of Pitta to a solid substance can transform it to a liquid, while adding it to a liquid can change the substance to a gas.

Pitta governs all metabolic and transformational aspects of the mind and body. It is intimately concerned with digestion of food, ideas, and emotions. The light from Pitta's fire enables us to make careful decisions. It also governs the entire process of visual perception.

Chemical processes associated with digestion are an important aspect of Pitta. These include the secretion of stomach acid, pancreatic enzymes, and bile salts. The breakdown of food by the chemical fire of Pitta allows us to assimilate nourishing food substrates. Similarly, the process of breaking down new ideas so that we can "digest" them is a reflection of Pitta's functioning in the mind. Among its other functions, Pitta is responsible for bringing color to the skin and ensuring that body temperature is properly maintained. Pitta is like the fire in our furnace, keeping us warm in an environment that is usually cooler than our 98.6°F body temperature.

Kapha—Structure and Fluidity

Kapha dosha is composed of the elements of water and earth. This dosha is cold, heavy, stable, viscous, dense, smooth, and slow. It governs all processes related to structure and lubrication in the physiology.

In the nervous system, Kapha regulates the cerebrospinal fluid that nourishes and supports the neurons. In the digestive tract, Kapha is responsible for lubricating the mouth to facilitate the sense of taste, and for protecting the lining of the stomach and alimentary canal from the effects of digestive acids and enzymes. Kapha also governs fluid and salt balance throughout the body and plays an important role in the lubrication of the joints by governing the production of synovial fluid. Finally, in the respiratory tract, Kapha creates the mucus that cleanses and lubricates the airways, moistens the air, and assists in the removal of airborne particles. When Kapha is doing its job there is a smooth and continuous cleansing of the respiratory tract.

The Mind Body Questionnaire: A Snapshot of Your Current Condition

Ayurveda teaches that each of us inherits a unique proportion of the three doshas at the time of our conception. In Sanskrit, this personal balance point is known as *prakruti,* and it remains an important influence on your emotional and physical tendencies throughout your life. In accordance with the prakruti that was established at your birth, you may be "airy" by nature, and have Vata as your dominant dosha; or you may be more "fiery," with Pitta predominating; or you might be primarily "earthy," with a larger proportion of Kapha in your makeup.

All three doshas are necessary to maintain life, and Vata, Pitta, and Kapha are all present in every human being. Most people, however, express a single dosha more strongly, with the other two exerting a less obvious influence. When your prakruti—the natural proportion of the doshas in your system—is well maintained, you are mentally and physically in balance. Throughout life, however, as our choices and experiences interact with our basic nature, one or more of the doshas may become unbalanced. As a result, physical and emotional problems can appear. The Sanskrit word for these imbalances is *vikruti,* or "deviations from one's true nature." Unfortunately, almost everyone is experiencing vikruti to some degree.

Just as snow falling on a statue can change its appearance until the sun melts the snow away, a doshic imbalance can obscure the true nature of any person. For as long as the imbalance persists, the unbalanced dosha in effect becomes the dominant dosha in the physiology. An Ayurvedic physician's tasks, then, include identifying a patient's current imbalance, treating it, and restoring the prakruti that is the patient's true nature. All of this, of course, can very often be accomplished by the patient himself. Indeed, one of the central purposes of Ayurveda is educating and empowering individuals to take control, not only of their own health, but of every aspect of their lives.

The self-assessment questionnaire below can quickly provide insight into both prakruti and vikruti—that is, both the natural balance point of the doshas that was set at your birth, and any deviation from it that may be currently present. When you've completed the questionnaire and obtained the results, you can use the information that follows—on qualities of the dosha types—to enhance your understanding of where you began from an Ayurvedic perspective, where you are now, and where you want to go.

Remember, we *all* have *all* three doshas in our mind body systems but one tends to stand out more than the others. It is also common to find that features of two doshas are more or less equally represented in your physiology. If this is the case, you would be considered *bidoshic*. Less commonly, all three dosha qualities are present in fairly equal concentrations. Here the term *tridoshic* is applied.

MIND BODY QUESTIONNAIRE

The following questions are about you and your mind body nature. Using the following scale, indicate how characteristic each statement is of you. There are no right or wrong answers, so please answer each one as honestly as possible.

Section One

	CHARACTERISTIC OF ME . . .				
	NOT AT ALL	SLIGHTLY	SOME-WHAT	MODER-ATELY	VERY
• My mind is very active.	1	2	3	4	5
• I like trying out new ideas and having new experiences.	1	2	3	4	5
• I get restless if I'm not constantly on the move.	1	2	3	4	5

	CHARACTERISTIC OF ME . . .				
	NOT AT ALL	SLIGHTLY	SOME-WHAT	MODER-ATELY	VERY
• I speak quickly and am a lively conversationalist.	1	2	3	4	5
• Under stress, I worry or become anxious.	1	2	3	4	5
• I am a light sleeper.	1	2	3	4	5
• I am thin or underweight for my height.	1	2	3	4	5
• My appetite is variable; sometimes I am hungry and other times I have to force myself to eat.	1	2	3	4	5
• Under stress or when traveling, I am likely to have constipation.	1	2	3	4	5
• My digestion is frequently irregular with gas or bloating.	1	2	3	4	5
• My feet and hands are often cold.	1	2	3	4	5
• My skin is often dry or flaky.	1	2	3	4	5

Total for Section One   V =

Section Two

	CHARACTERISTIC OF ME . . .				
	NOT AT ALL	SLIGHTLY	SOME-WHAT	MODER-ATELY	VERY
• I have a very discriminating mind.	1	2	3	4	5
• I tend to be compulsive and have difficulty stopping once I've started a project.	1	2	3	4	5
• I am a perfectionist and am intolerant of errors.	1	2	3	4	5
• I often feel time pressure or become impatient easily.	1	2	3	4	5
• When stressed, I become irritable or lose my temper.	1	2	3	4	5
• I have a strong appetite and can eat large quantities of food if I choose.	1	2	3	4	5
• I often have indigestion or heartburn.	1	2	3	4	5

	CHARACTERISTIC OF ME . . .				
	NOT AT ALL	SLIGHTLY	SOME-WHAT	MODER-ATELY	VERY
• Under stress, I am more likely to get diarrhea than constipation.	1	2	3	4	5
• I feel rested with less than eight hours of sleep.	1	2	3	4	5
• My hair shows early thinning or graying, or a tendency toward a reddish color.	1	2	3	4	5
• I am most comfortable in cooler environments.	1	2	3	4	5
• My skin is sensitive, sunburns or breaks out easily.	1	2	3	4	5

Total for Section Two   P =

Section Three

	CHARACTERISTIC OF ME . . .				
	NOT AT ALL	SLIGHTLY	SOME-WHAT	MODER-ATELY	VERY
• I am sweet-natured and forgiving.	1	2	3	4	5
• I accumulate things; I don't like to let go of things even if I don't expect to use them again.	1	2	3	4	5
• I have difficulty leaving a relationship, even after it is no longer nourishing.	1	2	3	4	5
• I am a good listener. I tend to speak only when I feel I have something important to say.	1	2	3	4	5
• I am calm by nature and seldom lose my temper.	1	2	3	4	5
• I deal with conflict by withdrawing.	1	2	3	4	5
• Once I've learned something, I usually have good retention.	1	2	3	4	5
• I sleep deeply for eight or more hours each night.	1	2	3	4	5
• I commonly experience sinus congestion or excessive phlegm, or suffer with asthma.	1	2	3	4	5

	CHARACTERISTIC OF ME . . .				
	NOT AT ALL	SLIGHTLY	SOME-WHAT	MODER-ATELY	VERY
• My skin is usually soft and smooth.	1	2	3	4	5
• I gain weight easily and have difficulty losing extra pounds.	1	2	3	4	5

Total for Section Three   K =

V_____   P_____   K_____

How to Use Your Results on This Test

The total score for each section provides you with a snapshot of your current state of dosha balance/imbalance. If, for example, your results are:

V = 52   **P = 50**   **K = 30**

you would be considered a **Vata-Pitta,** with Kapha less prominent. Your overall focus, then, should be on balancing Vata and Pitta.

If one dosha is 5 or more points higher than the next, that dosha can be considered the most dominant. If this is the case, you could consider yourself primarily a single dosha type. For example, if your results are:

V = 52   **P = 44**   **K = 32**

you would be considered a **Vata** constitution, with Pitta and Kapha less represented.

If all three scores are within five points of each other as in the following example:

V = 48   **V = 45**   **V = 47**

you would be considered tri-doshic. If this is your situation, look at any symptoms you are experiencing in terms of a dosha that is out of balance. Also, pay attention to the season of the year, each of which can aggravate a particular dosha.

Vata Constitution—Movement Personified

Vicki was always on the move as a child and her anxious mom was perpetually concerned that she was too skinny. Her vivacious nature led her to go into advertising, where her work was at times inspired but somewhat inconsistent. Her many women friends appreciated her lively conversation skills but her love life was a steady succession of infatuations and disappointments. She came seeking help for her chronic insomnia and irregular digestion.

People who have Vata constitutions have the qualities of air and space most active in their natures. Their minds are characterized by restlessness, creativity, and enthusiasm. There is variability in everything they do and—again like the wind—their nature is to start and stop. Vatas rarely hold to a regular routine: They don't often eat at the same time every day, for example. If you're a Vata type, you may have deliberately skipped breakfast yesterday, but today you found yourself unable to function without a big breakfast immediately after awakening. Almost every other area of your life can be similarly variable, especially when your principal dosha is unbalanced. If someone with a preponderance of Vata is asked, "What time do you do this?" or "How often do you do that?" the answer will often be, "Well, it depends."

Although they may be either quite short or quite tall, they usually have a light, thin frame. Vata physiologies tend toward dryness, as it is the nature of the wind to dry things out; hair, skin, and even the digestive tract may be noticeably lacking in moisture. In addition to this dryness, there is often irregularity and constipation in digestive-tract functioning, particularly when under stress.

When functioning in a balanced manner, Vata natures are creative and enthusiastic. Indeed, Vata is the force that generates thought. But when Vata is aggravated or imbalanced there tends to be restlessness and loss of focus. Anxiety or insomnia is a frequent complaint.

Vata is the only dosha that is capable of movement. It is primarily responsible for creating change in the physiology. When Vata is in balance, change is creative and evolutionary. Out of balance, Vata may merely stir things up without any direction or fulfillment.

Temperament: Vata-predominant individuals are lively and energetic. They are expressive and engaging, although they tend to change their focus frequently. They are often physically and emotionally sensitive, responding to stress with anxiety and insomnia.

Activity Style: The irregularity of Vata tends to interfere with the completion of tasks. Often a new project is started before a previous one is completed. Vata types can be easily distracted, and usually do not require an orderly work environment.

Learning Style: Vatas have quick minds and are able to assimilate new information quickly. They are often able to learn as easily from casual listening as from reading or studying. But because of the changeable nature of the dosha, Vata types tend to forget quickly as well.

Appetite, Digestion, and Elimination: Irregularity affects all aspects of the digestive process in Vata people. Appetite, digestion, and elimination tend to be inconsistent and delicate. On one day a Vata type may eat three meals, and then not eat at all for the next twenty-four hours. Often they must "force" themselves to eat, and for this reason Vatas tend to be thin and to lose weight easily. Vata types often report lactose intolerance and allergies to many foods. They easily develop bloating and gaseousness, and may defecate several times one day and none the next. In general, excessive air dries out the colon so that chronic Vata imbalance results in constipation.

Sleep: Vata types often sleep lightly and awaken frequently. Sleeping problems are potentiated by Vata's tendency to maintain irregular daily schedules, with variable times of awakening and going to bed.

Hair and Skin: Vata hair is dry and tends to be kinky. Their skin often appears dry and flaky.

Temperature Comfort: Because space and air are associated with low temperatures, even a mild breeze can create a chill for a Vata person. They often complain of cold hands and feet. They often do well in tropical climates, however, as their thin physiques readily dispose of body heat.

Health Problems: Because of the constantly changing nature of Vata, people in whom this dosha predominates tend to have frequent health-related concerns. Emotionally, unbalanced Vata leads to nervousness and depression. Physically, Vata underlies many chronic-pain syndromes, arthritis, cardiac arrhythmias, and functional bowel disorders. When they visit medical doctors, Vata types are often frustrated by the number of their symptoms that cannot be ascribed to a specific diagnosis.

Pitta Constitution—A Worldly Appetite

Donald is a man with a strong appetite for life. Whether it is gourmet food, a new computer program, or a lucrative business contract, Donald approaches each venture with intense resolve. When his life is in balance, he is warm and friendly, a good leader and an articulate teacher. But when the demands on his time exceed his capacity to maintain control, he becomes irritable, sarcastic, and critical. While seeking medical attention for his recurrent heartburn, his blood pressure was found to be moderately elevated.

The strong internal fire of people with Pitta constitutions allows them to digest the world. Pittas tend to have strong appetites—be it for food, power, knowledge, wealth, or sex. When balanced, Pitta people can be alchemists, creating transformation for themselves and others. When imbalanced, the fire can be too hot, causing unnecessary singeing of their inner or outer environments.

It's heat that allows us to cook whatever we are choosing to put into our mind body system. When the heat is at the appropriate level, Pitta types are warm, intelligent, intense, direct, and good leaders. Physiologically, they can eat anything, have good energy, and maintain body warmth even in cold climates. But when the fire is too hot, Pittas burn what they are cooking. They become irritable, critical, and easily angered and have trouble with inflammations in their body. Hyperacidity, heartburn, diarrhea, skin rashes, and liver problems, resulting from the excessive heat in their mind body system, are more common in Pitta types.

Pittas often display intensity in their facial expressions and in their eyes, and there is a directness in their manner. They even walk emphatically, as if they don't want anything to get in their way. People with strong Pitta resent obstacles and hate feeling that anyone is taking advantage of them. If a Pitta is cut off in traffic by another driver, he may speed up and aggressively pass or tailgate the offender. In contrast, a Vata type will feel anxious. "Oh my God, I almost got killed," would be a typical Vata reaction.

Pittas are often good speakers: Their mental fire enables them to illuminate ideas for others. But if someone tries to disagree with a Pitta, he will tend to argue his point forcefully, even to the point of intimidation.

In its essence, Pitta in the physiology represents the power of digestion and metabolism. Pittas feel best when in pursuit of a goal. Thus, Pittas can be good leaders and "trailblazers." When Pitta is excessive and imbalanced, however, the fire can exceed its restraints and do damage. If something or someone is perceived as interfering with the satisfaction of a Pitta desire, the fire can flare up and scorch the apparent obstacle.

Temperament: When balanced, Pitta types are warm and friendly. They like to explore new ideas and are open to a healthy debate. When a Pitta person is under stress, he or she becomes angry, intimidating, and controlling.

Activity Style: Pitta creates orderliness and precision. A Pitta's desk tends to be clean and well organized. But, when excessive, Pitta creates the need for perfectionism with absolute intolerance for errors. Pittas are good at staying with a task until it is completed but they may become compulsive about it. If you suggest that someone with strong Pitta take a break before he has finished a task, there may be an irritated response.

Learning Style: Pitta types learn moderately fast and have fairly good memories. As they do in other areas, Pittas like to persevere in intellectual tasks until they feel mastery has been achieved.

Appetite, Digestion, and Elimination: The fire of Pitta creates a need for fuel in all areas of life, and strong appetite is a common feature of this dosha. When Pitta types are hungry, food will be the exclusive focus until their hunger is satisfied. Pittas can usually consume large quantities of food in a single meal. Pure Pitta types can often eat without gaining weight, but the addition of a significant Kapha presence may bring a tendency to obesity, particularly later in life. Similarly, Pittas usually believe they can eat anything, but this overconfidence leads to indigestion and heartburn. Peptic ulcers and inflammatory bowel disorders represent more severe cases of Pitta imbalance. Diarrhea is common, particularly under stress, as before public speaking or examinations. According to Ayurveda, one of the ways the body tries to eliminate excess heat is by speeding up the passage of food through the small intestines and colon.

Sleep: People with Pitta sleep soundly, and generally don't need much rest. Someone with high Pitta will report, "I feel fine with six hours of sleep."

Hair and Skin: Pitta hair tends to be thin and of red coloration, with early graying and baldness. Pittas sunburn easily and get nonspecific rashes under stress. Freckles and moles are common when Pitta is high.

Temperature Comfort: Pitta creates heat, so people with high Pitta like cooler weather. They tend to be uncomfortable in warm temperatures or hot climates. They also tend to perspire heavily.

Health Problems: Excessive Pitta leads to disorders that reflect too much fire in the system. In the digestive tract, this can mean indigestion, ulcers, inflammatory bowel disease, or diarrhea. On the skin excessive Pitta causes inflammatory rashes. In the circulatory system, it creates high blood pressure and coronary heart disease. Emotionally, it causes irritability and a bad temper.

Kapha Constitution—Solid, Like the Earth

Marvin's nature is to consider others' needs before his own. He is methodical without being compulsive, and he is an attentive listener. Beloved by his family for his nonjudgmental acceptance of others, Marvin is tolerant and forgiving to a fault. Overweight since high school, chronically trou-

bled by sinus allergies, he is urged by his wife to seek medical help for his loud snoring.

Kapha types are connected to the earth, and there is a solidity and stability in their nature. Their builds tend to be more heavyset, they are methodical and thoughtful in nature, and in groups of people they are generally less vocal than Vatas or Pittas. But when Kaphas do voice opinions, they are often so well thought out that listeners are likely to pay close attention.

Kapha digestion and metabolism is slow and steady, and weight can be put on easily. Western medicine is just beginning to recognize the role of slow metabolism in weight gain, but Ayurveda has long acknowledged this as an important characteristic of Kapha body types. In Ayurvedic terms, Kaphas have a tendency to hold on to earth; therefore they gain weight more readily than other dosha types, despite the fact that they may eat smaller quantities of food. They are reluctant to seek medical attention for any health problem, and when they do it is often at the urging of a family member.

The earthiness of Kapha people creates a sleep that is very deep and often prolonged, almost as if they're hibernating every night. Even after eight or nine hours of sleep, Kapha types may feel sluggish in the morning.

In contrast to Vata types, who become anxious, and Pittas, who get angry, Kaphas are generally able to stay calm under stress. "Live and let live" is the natural attitude of the Kapha type. In relationships, a person with Kapha predominance usually provides a stabilizing influence.

The stability and nourishing nature of earth and water as expressed through Kapha has long been cherished and sought after. When Kapha is balanced it brings calm and reliability to all aspects of life. An excess of Kapha dosha, however, can manifest itself as inappropriate resistance to change and evolution. When unbalanced, the Kapha tendency toward evenness can create dullness.

Temperament: Kapha dosha fosters an even disposition, and people with predominant Kapha tend to be sweet natured and forgiving. They may eventually lose their tempers, but they will tolerate uncomfortable situations for long periods before becoming angry. Kapha types are good listeners, speaking only when they feel they have something important to say.

Activity Style: Kaphas work in an even, methodical, slow-paced manner. They get things done but at their own pace. They have good endurance and consistent energy.

Learning Style: Kapha predominance does not produce quick learning ability, but once a subject is mastered it will not be forgotten.

Appetite, Digestion, and Elimination: Kaphas have relatively mild but steady appetites. They have a tendency to eat when there is food available and may not be aware of their true hunger levels. Because of their tendency to store energy, they can go for long periods without eating, but they also tend to gain weight rapidly if their level of food intake rises.

Kapha types may complain of heaviness after a meal even if relatively little was eaten. Kaphas tend to eat slowly and are often the last to finish a meal. The bowel habits of people with Kapha predominance tend to be very regular. Kapha types seldom pay much attention to this function, but if asked they will often respond, "Regular as clockwork."

Sleep: Kapha types sleep long and deeply. Even with eight hours of sleep, Kaphas are often slow to get going in the morning. Here a cup of coffee or tea may be very beneficial, with none of the negative effects noticed by Vata or Pitta. In fact, Kapha types can consider coffee or tea to be herbal nutritional supplements.

Hair and Skin: Kapha hair tends to be thick, dark, and wavy, and Kaphas often keep a full head of hair until late in life. Ayurveda compares the skin of Kapha types to fine porcelain, with a texture that is soft and smooth owing to the presence of earth and water elements. The qualities of their skin, hair, and eyes often lead others to describe Kaphas as having beautiful faces, despite their tendency to be overweight.

Temperature Comfort: Kapha qualities of cold and wet are balanced by warm and dry environments. Kapha people do not enjoy climates that are cool, damp, and cloudy, and they are uncomfortable when the sky is cloudy and overcast. But Kaphas rarely complain about the weather because they rarely complain about anything.

Health Problems: Out-of-balance Kapha tends toward congestion, which reflects accumulation of excessive earth and water. One of Kapha's roles is to lubricate the respiratory system, so mucus is a natural Kaphic aspect. But when Kapha becomes unbalanced, mucus is overproduced and allergies or sinus congestion can result. Obesity is another common manifestation of Kapha imbalance, again reflecting excessive storage of the earth and water elements.

Variety Is the Spice

In our fast-paced society, Vata has a tendency to be easily aggravated and those people with Vata constitutions get off balance most readily. Therefore, Vata concerns tend to bring more people to their doctors than imbalances in the other doshas. Pitta imbalances are the next most common. In contrast, those with Kapha predominance tend to have stronger constitutions, which insulate against many of the minor illnesses that affect the other doshas.

Faced with identical situations, people with each of the three doshas most predominant typically express themselves very differently. If as a Vata type, you are about to board an airplane when told that the flight is delayed due to mechanical problems, you may immediately and even frantically try to book a different flight. As a Pitta type, you will likely become angry at the ticket agent and demand better service. If Kapha is predominant in your constitution, you may welcome the opportunity to head casually for the ice-cream concession, using the delay to get some sweet refreshment. In all areas of life, the same external event will be processed by different people in very different ways owing to differences in their constitutions.

Learning from History

Information in a number of specific areas of a person's history can help to reveal a basic constitutional nature. Regarding sex, for example, Vata types tend to have variable sexual appetites, sometimes quite strong and sometimes weak. Owing to an often tenuous connection with their bodies, sex is usually not as important to Vatas. In contrast, Pitta types tend to be sexually intense and passionate; however, as soon as sexual desire has been fulfilled, Pittas are immediately on to something else, whether finding something to eat or getting back to work. Kapha types tend to be good lovers—slow and steady. Their passion builds up gradually and is sustained longer. But when Kapha is excessive, an individual's level of self-fulfillment may be so complete that he or she lacks motivation to provide loving attention.

Your attitudes about money can also be revealing. If you unexpectedly received an inheritance of two or three thousand dollars, how would you spend the money? Vata types will typically want to buy many different items without any clear plan; they're impulse spenders. Pittas will purchase some luxury item, a new car or piece of jewelry, after carefully researching the best buys. And Kaphas, who like to save, gain greatest enjoyment from knowing the money is in the bank.

MIND BODY CHARACTERISTICS

	VATA	PITTA	KAPHA
ACTIVITY STYLE	Active, restless	Sharp, precise	Calm, slow
DAILY ROUTINE	Variable	Precise	Methodical
UNDER STRESS	Anxious	Irritable	Calm
MEMORY	Quick to learn/forget	Medium	Slow to learn/forget
WEATHER PREFERENCE	Warm	Cool	*Not* cold and wet
PERSPIRATION	Less	More	Average
SLEEP	Light, interrupted	Little but sound	Heavy and prolonged
APPETITE	Variable	Strong	Slow, steady
DIGESTION	Variable	Strong	Slow
ELIMINATION	Constipation, variable	Frequent, loose	Regular, formed
MENSTRUATION	Spotty, irregular	Intense, heavy	Regular, smooth
SEX DRIVE	Low, variable	Passionate	Steady
FINANCIAL	Spends easily on trifles	Spends on luxuries	Saves

You Look Like a . . .

To help confirm the dosha information obtained from questionnaires, look over the physical attributes described below. How closely do your characteristics conform to those associated with your dominant dosha?

CHARACTERISTIC	VATA	PITTA	KAPHA
Frame	Light	Medium	Broad
Weight	Thin	Average	Heavy
Skin	Dry	Warm, moist	Thick, soft
Hair	Dry, kinky	Thin, reddish, gray	Thick, wavy
Eyes	Small, dry	Intense, fiery	Large, gentle
Teeth	Irregular	Yellow	White, even
Temperature	Cold	Warm	Cool
Tendons, veins	Visible	Moderate	Hidden
Nails	Brittle	Pink, soft	Thick, hard
Joints	Stiff, cracking	Flexible	Strong, solid
Abdomen	Thin	Muscular	Thick, soft
Speech	Talkative	Forceful	Deep, resonant

Perfection in Various Forms

It's important to emphasize the fact that there are no "good" or "bad" constitutional types. Regardless of which dosha is dominant in your nature, living in accordance with your prakruti, your ideal balanced state, will bring unbounded happiness to yourself and others. A balanced Vata person is lively, charming, enthusiastic, energetic, creative, and fun. A balanced Pitta person is warm, friendly, intelligent, insightful, competent, and a great leader. A balanced Kapha person is sweet, stable, reliable, compassionate, and loving. No type is more or less desirable than another. The goal is simply to develop fully the best features of whatever nature you have.

Think, for example, of three different kinds of automobiles: a Ferrari, a Firebird, and an old Mercedes. The Ferrari is quick and agile and delicate. The Firebird is powerful, passionate, and aggressive. The Mercedes is reliable, comfortable, and steady. We wouldn't want our Ferrari to run like a Mercedes and we wouldn't expect our Mercedes to throttle like a Firebird. The goal is to make certain that whatever vehicle we have, it is performing in its ideal running condition.

Infinite Flexibility

We've seen how the word *diagnosis* has traditionally been understood in Western medicine to denote knowledge of the disease process. In Ayurveda, diagnosis means to know a person's prakruti, which is his or her true nature. Each of us has a prakruti, which expresses the constellation of forces that we use to create ourselves. This inner life structures our temperament, our likes and dislikes, our behaviors, and our physical form.

The miracle of life takes the same basic constituents—the five elements and the three doshas—and synthesizes them into an infinity of possible patterns. Recognizing that the "stuff" that makes up the world around us is the same "stuff" that comprises our physical bodies is the starting point for a journey into deeper levels of life. As we proceed on the journey, we begin to see ever more clearly that our bodies and the bodies of everything around us are really different expressions of the same fields of energy and matter. But the impression of unity becomes even greater when we realize that the world of matter and our bodies of matter are merely consciousness taking on disguises for the sake of interesting diversity.

To become aware of both the unity of nonmaterial consciousness and the diversity of the vast material world is, according to Ayurvedic teaching, nothing less than the ultimate goal of life.

4

The Origins of Health and Disease

"Whatever notion is firmly held concerning the body, that it becomes."

Yoga Vasistha, Vedic sage

I am called to the emergency room of my hospital to see Thomas Atkins, a fifty-eight-year-old attorney complaining of trouble speaking and weakness in his right arm and leg for the past day. A self-described meat-and-potatoes man, Mr. Atkins has smoked a package of cigarettes daily since college.

As a neurologist I see that Mr. Atkins has suffered a cerebrovascular "accident" (stroke) due to atherosclerotic blockage in his carotid artery. His high-cholesterol diet and smoking were contributing risk factors. From an Ayurvedic perspective, Mr. Atkins's Majja dhatu (nerve tissue) was not receiving sufficient ojas (essential nourishment) due to the accumulation of ama (toxic residue) in his pranavaha srota (circulatory channel).

Both interpretations are valid and both lead to therapeutic interventions that are internally consistent, and more often than not, complementary.

You have probably heard your parents or grandparents say, "Nothing is more important than your health," or "If you have your health, you have everything," or "Good health is the most valuable thing in the world!" We often hear these exclamations from elderly people who are, unfortunately, no longer able to take good health for granted. If it's a cliché to say that good health is life's greatest blessing, as with most clichés there's a certain truth here. Yet if we ask a number of people what good health really is, the answers will probably be less lyrical than we might expect from a description of the most wonderful thing in the world. "Good health means you feel good," could probably summarize a majority of the responses—but most people would probably also add some version of the following sentence: *"Good health means you're not sick."*

This definition of health as the absence of disease is in fact a basic concept of Western medicine. In an earlier chapter, we have discussed how even the most advanced medical facilities are unprepared to devote much time to apparently healthy individuals when there are so many obviously ill patients who need treatment. Yet if we devoted a bit more attention to people when they are symptom-free, they would be much more likely to stay that way. And this would make our entire system of health care more efficient, more affordable, less painful in every way.

In American medical schools, it's almost a tradition for first-year students to begin their studies by dissecting a cadaver. This practice perfectly expresses the disease-directed orientation of Western medicine. Scrutinizing a dead person, after all, is no way to begin the study of health; rather, it once and for all shifts the focus toward the pathologies and "failures" of the human body, of which death is the ultimate expression. Though this is always left unspoken, the cadaver is actually presented as a kind of murder victim, done in by some as-yet-unidentified viral or oncological or cardiovascular perpetrator—and as any police officer can attest, there's usually an accompanying sense on the part of investigators that the victim was at least in part to blame for what happened to him. Medical students are almost always irreverent with their cadavers at times, and obviously this is in large part a defensive response. Although every student wonders about the person who once lived in the body laid open in front of them, the purely physical orientation of the gross-anatomy process marginalizes these human concerns. Detachment, cynicism, and arrogance insidiously creep in, widening the gap between the all-knowing doctor and the poor, hapless patient. Perhaps such feelings are inevitable in a system that begins the study of life with a self-contradictory inspection of death. Though dissection of a human body does have clear value in the training of a doctor, it's interesting to note that the ancient Greek physicians forbade dissection on the grounds that the practice showed disrespect for the human body.

Since its origins, Ayurveda has defined health not as the mere absence of illness, but as the dynamic and balanced integration between body, mind, and spirit. The original intention of Ayurvedic medicine, of course, was to free people from the burdens of ill health in order that they might better fulfill their spiritual potential. Nor was Ayurveda the only ancient tradition that saw a spiritual intention in the practice of medicine and the creation of health. In the fifth century B.C., the Greek physician Herophilus wrote, "When health is absent, wisdom cannot reveal itself, art cannot become manifest, and intelligence cannot be made use of."

With its understanding of mind and body as a unified whole, Ayurveda teaches that good health is really a higher state of consciousness. Health, then, is much more than just "feeling well" or being free of symptoms. It is a dynamic interplay among the environment, the physical body, the mind, and the spirit—a state in which we open ourselves to entirely new categories of creativity and vitality, including the ability to influence life processes through the power of our own awareness.

The Pathogenesis of Illness

Despite all that Western medicine knows about being sick, there is little understanding of how people actually move from health to illness. To illuminate this gray area, Ayurveda begins with the premise that consciousness, rather than biochemistry, is the true source of disease. Specifically, there are two key aspects of awareness that are of supreme importance to health and illness: These are *self-referral* and *object referral.*

Object referral is a process of relinquishing the identity of one's self to some object of reference, which may be an event, a person, or a thing. Once this has taken place—once the self has been exchanged for an external image—we begin to forget the true wholeness of our nature. By identifying ourselves with localized values of awareness, we begin the process that eventually gives rise to disease.

Every day we receive millions of messages from our environ-

ment urging us to identify with objects. We are told to buy a more luxurious car, drink a new beverage, own a bigger house, and get a better job, all with the promise that these choices will bring us love,
success, and happiness. And we all know the temporary pleasure that
these things bring to our lives. Yet most of us also know how material
objects fail to provide any lasting sense of value or even importance.
In fact, identification with an object that we treasure can actually lead
to greater anxiety and discomfort. What if the new car gets dented in
a parking lot? What if the diamond ring gets thrown out with the
trash? What if my beautiful, sexy lover falls for someone else?

According to Ayurvedic teaching, identifying with anything in
the world of name and form is a mistake. It means committing
ourselves mentally and emotionally to something that has a beginning, middle, and end—and endings usually bring sorrow and suffering. As mind and body are two fully integrated features of life,
any disease in the mind eventually is reflected as disease in the
body. Object referral, therefore, is held to be the ultimate source of
all illness.

This is a very important point. When remembrance of wholeness is lost, disease begins. Healing is simply the restoration of the
memory of wholeness. While it is very useful to understand disease in
terms of molecules, bacteria, and viruses, the ultimate cure at all levels of the mind body system depends on restoring the memory of
wholeness. This restoration must take place physically, emotionally,
intellectually, and spiritually. A fragmented approach cannot be successful or complete. Successful treatment of an illness requires a
holistic understanding that includes all aspects of human nature.

Four Key Elements of Health and Illness

In this next section, four key concepts of Ayurveda are introduced:
agni, or digestive power; *ojas,* or subtle life nourishment; *ama,* or
toxic residue; and *srota,* or circulatory channel. Whenever I present
these concepts to Western audiences, I am asked whether they have
any substantive objective basis or are best understood as abstract principles. My experience is that they serve best as cornerstones of a theoretical framework to understand health and illness. They are
inferred rather than directly observed. I do not anticipate that we will

be able to request an "ojas blood level" or perform an "ama biopsy" anytime soon, but these principles are key to improving well being nevertheless.

AGNI

Ayurveda teaches that good health depends upon our body's ability to metabolize material received from the environment. This includes not only tangible substances, such as foods and beverages, but also emotions such as anger or fear.

The metabolic power that accomplishes all this is called agni in Sanskrit. Linguistically, agni is the root of the English word *ignite,* and agni can be thought of as a kind of digestive fire: When it's robust and powerful, it can take in and metabolize a wide range of materials and use them to advantage. But when agni is weak, even potentially nourishing substances can't be properly utilized, and toxic by-products may accumulate. Similarly, when flames are roaring in a fireplace, even a damp log will burn down to a fine ash after providing heat and light. But if the fire is weak, the light will be limited, with an abundance of smoke—and if a log is just a little wet, it may put the fire out altogether, leaving a pile of charred remains.

Strong metabolic power allows us to metabolize all our life experiences fully. We can take whatever is nourishing and eliminate whatever is not. The ancient Ayurvedic texts even assert that when digestive power is robust, we can convert poison into nectar—but if digestion is weak, an opposite process will take place. We all know people who seem powerfully capable of processing everything that happens in their lives. They can eat anything, drink anything, and survive all sorts of harrowing personal trials. Of course, other individuals have highly delicate systems and have difficulty metabolizing even simple physical or emotional experiences.

Agni is also responsible for the healthy formation of tissues in the body. If the conversion power of agni is strong, we create healthy blood cells, muscle tissue, bones, and nerves. If agni's transformative potency is impaired, we create tissues that are weak, fragile, and vulnerable to illness.

It's easy to understand digestive power in terms of food, but it is important to realize that our minds and hearts are also continuously metabolizing energy and information. If this is the first time you've encountered the concept of agni, for example, your mental "diges-tion" is working right now to break down this new idea into basic components that can be assimilated intellectually. We also have emo-tional agnis. When these powers are strong, we are able to metabolize emotional experiences efficiently, extracting what is nourishing and eliminating any toxic feelings.

A number of simple but effective steps can be taken to strengthen agni. For example, it is very important that meals are taken in an atmosphere free of distraction or hostility. You may be eating a delicious meal prepared by your beloved, but watching a vio-lent television show at the same time will very likely negate any bene-fits to his system regardless of the quality of the food. When our awareness is settled, our agnis can focus their energy to create healthy tissues and create ojas, which, according to Ayurvedic teach-ing, is the true essence of life.

From a Western perspective, agni may be considered in terms of the millions of enzymes responsible for transforming biochemicals into more complex substances. We know that if a specific enzyme is faulty or produced in inadequate amounts due to an inherited or acquired process, illness may result. Someone with alcoholic pancre-atitis will not be able to digest his food properly due to a lack of pan-creatic enzymes. A child with an inherited muscular dystrophy will not develop normal muscles because he lacks the ability to create an essential protein. Both of these examples can be understood in terms of low metabolic power or weak agni.

OJAS

This is such a subtle substance that it can actually be considered non-material. Just as light can be a wave or a particle, ojas can be viewed as consciousness or matter, depending upon one's perspective. It exists at the junction point between mind and body. Vedic tradition states that we are born with a few drops of ojas in our hearts, and that its quantity increases or decreases with each of our thoughts. If our thoughts are of love, compassion, and appreciation, we create more ojas, while resentment, anger, or fear depletes it. When our agnis are healthy, ojas is brought into being at each step of the tissue-forming process. When ojas is plentiful and circulating throughout our system, it provides and strengthens immunity, which in Ayurveda is known as

HEALTH AND DISEASE

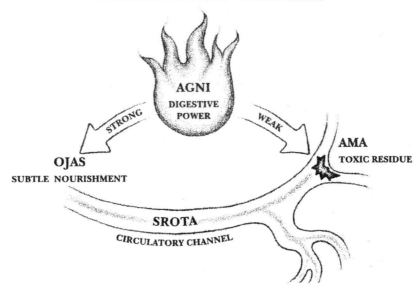

bala, or "strength." This empowers the mind body system to maintain equilibrium despite any challenges from the environment. So long as ojas permeates our physiology, we cannot be distracted from full awareness of life's unity. Ojas reminds each cell and tissue in the body that its essential purpose is to support the unity of the whole. When we exhaust all our ojas, our life force is exhausted and we die.

It is difficult to assign a physical basis to ojas as it vibrates in the boundary between mind and body. Some Vedic scholars have suggested that ojas perhaps represents the basic cholesterol molecule that is the chemical framework for many of our most important hormones, including cortisol, DHEA, estrogen, progesterone, and testosterone. Although we have tended to demonize cholesterol in our obsession with coronary heart disease, it is a biochemical that is essential to our survival—in the right amount. Others have suggested that ojas represents some fundamental neuropeptide, such as serotonin or an endorphin. Although I understand efforts to better define what ojas "really" is, I suspect that by its very nature, it cannot be localized to a single chemical.

AMA

When our agnis are weak and our metabolic processes are inefficient, Ayurveda teaches that a substance called ama, rather than ojas, is created as a by-product of metabolism. Ama is the Sanskrit term for toxic residue. It pollutes our system and blocks the free flow of information and intelligence. When ama accumulates in the physiology, a sense of dullness, lack of energy, and poor immunity are evident. Individuals with plentiful ama tend to be susceptible to every bacteria and virus. This can foster frequent colds and flu, but eventually more serious illnesses develop. And one also senses that there is not an abundance of happiness in people whose physiologies are dominated by ama. Ama is literally the foundation of disease.

Unfortunately, ama accumulation is almost universal in contemporary Western society, where few of us have consistent access to pure air, pure water, or, for that matter, to people who are pure of heart. This may affect an individual at the level of conscious awareness, but from an Ayurvedic perspective it is clear that negative influences are being introduced into awareness at a subtler level, which will ultimately foster the production of ama. There is a strong argument to be made, for example, that high levels of violence in the media do in fact contribute to the dangerous levels of real violence in our society. In every area of our lives, the more we favor choices that foster peace and purity in our awareness and in our bodies, the healthier we will be.

As our scientific understanding of degenerative illness grows, the concept of ama seems more and more relevant. We now know that illnesses ranging from arthritis to Alzheimer's disease are in large part the end result of cellular damage inflicted by free radicals. These highly reactive molecules, created through chemical reactions, damage normal cellular constituents. If our cells' free-radical scavengers are overloaded, we find ourselves with metabolic end products that cannot be eliminated from our tissues, resulting in dysfunction and, ultimately, cell death. In Alzheimer's disease, for example, a substance called amyloid is produced, which literally pollutes our brain cells, interfering with normal intellectual functions. Even the common "old-age spots" that many people develop on their hands are due to a chemical waste product, lipofuscin, which, once formed, cannot be eliminated. The recognition of the consequences of free-radical damage is very much in alignment with the Ayurvedic concept of ama.

SROTAS

Ayurveda understands the human body, and any other living organism, as fundamentally a network of channels through which biological intelligence flows. The srotas are an important Ayurvedic concept denoting channels of energy and information. When the channels are open and healthy, the life force is able to nourish the cells and tissues. But if the channels are blocked and the tissues are unable to receive nourishment, dysfunction and disease are the result.

There are thirteen major srotas through which the primary biological processes express themselves. Three of these roughly correspond to the respiratory tract, the digestive tract, and the circulatory system, which are responsible for bringing various forms of nourishment into the physiology. There are also seven channels dedicated to transporting the "essences" of the tissues; that is, the full range of energy and information that must come together in order to create a particular tissue category. For example, a "muscle-forming channel" accomplishes the delivery of amino acids to form the primary muscle proteins, together with iron to supply the myoglobin, a complex protein that binds oxygen. Clearly, a tissue-carrying srota can be a very abstract and technical concept. Rather than thinking of these tissue channels as anatomic structures, it may be useful to conceive of them simply as the orderly flow of biological intelligence.

The three remaining srotas carry sweat, feces, and urine out of the body, and any blockage in these channels will of course result in serious illness. Women have two additional srota channels for transporting menstrual flow and breast milk.

On a purely physiological level, Western medicine recognizes that blocks in circulation lead to illness. Urologists spend a good part of their working day relieving obstructions in the urinary tract, either due to swollen prostate glands or stones in the urethras. An ear, nose, and throat doctor understands the problems caused by swollen sinuses, which block the passages that drain mucus from the head and ears. Cardiologists are constantly seeking to identify and remove obstructions in heart vessels. The expansion of this idea to include all conduits for energy and information throughout the mind and body is a relatively small leap.

In considering these circulatory channels, the essential point is quite clear: Health requires the unobstructed flow of energy and intelligence. Any blockage of this flow results in disease.

The Six Stages of Disease

If a patient approaches a Western physician with a vague sense that something's wrong, the doctor may order blood tests, an EKG, or an X ray. All of these will probably be normal, and the patient will be told there's nothing wrong after all. But there is something wrong, of course, if the patient isn't feeling well.

Western medicine has difficulty addressing the initial stages of illness, before the appearance of manifest symptoms. In contrast, Ayurveda teaches that a disease is already in its *later* stages by the time it reveals itself at the level of the physical body. Illness first appears not as a sign or symptom, but as an *awareness*. Similarly, when disease begins to regress, the first changes occur in consciousness. The patient often knows he or she is getting better before the doctor can detect any changes in objective studies. When a patient with pneumococcal pneumonia receives antibiotics, he or she will improve days before there are any changes in the chest X ray, prompting the rule, "Treat the patient, not the X ray."

Ayurveda recognizes six stages of disease, each of which may continue for some time. The patient's intuitive awareness of each stage, however, always precedes any measurable or observable change. As you read through the descriptions below, notice how the first three stages of disease occur in the unmanifest field of the physiology, while only the final three stages occur at the material level.

- **First Stage—accumulation.** As a result of less-than-ideal choices, imbalance begins to accumulate somewhere in the body. The cause of the imbalance can be traced to some toxicity, which may be in the physical environment, in a food, or even in a relationship.

- **Second Stage—aggravation.** If the accumulation of toxicity progresses, the toxified dosha begins to distort normal functioning in a subtle manner.

- **Third Stage—dissemination.** At this stage, the imbalance is no longer contained. The patient experiences vague systemic symptoms, such as fatigue or generalized discomfort.

- **Fourth Stage—localization.** Eventually the toxic imbalance localizes in an area of the physiology where some weakness exists, perhaps due to an old trauma or some inherited tendency.

- **Fifth Stage—manifestation.** If the process is allowed to progress still further, an obvious dysfunction is revealed, perhaps as a flare-up of single-joint arthritis, an episode of angina, or the early stages of an infection.

- **Sixth Stage—disruption.** Finally, if efforts to reverse the disease process are not instituted, the stage of disruption is reached, with the arrival of a full-blown illness.

How can we use this portrayal of the progression of illness to understand and treat disease? A young man raised on cheeseburgers and ice cream ignores the occasional indigestion and bloating that he feels after a big meal. According to Ayurveda, he is *accumulating* toxicity due to poor food choices, which will lead to *aggravation*— more cholesterol than he can fully metabolize or eliminate. Over the next ten years, he moves to the next step, the *dissemination,* as landmarked by an elevated serum cholesterol.

Years later, he progresses into the *localization* phase, in which cholesterol is gradually deposited into his coronary arteries. By his mid-fifties, he shows *manifest* evidence of illness when he complains to his doctor of occasional chest pains when he mows the lawn. If the process continues, he is suddenly struck with the crushing chest pain of a life-threatening heart attack.

No one would argue that the seeds of illness were planted years before the full-blown expression of the disease. Ayurveda's major focus is on identifying the origins of illness in the choices we make and taking steps to prevent the inevitable progression that leads to sickness and suffering.

Etiology of Diseases

At a deeper level we could ask the question, why do we choose behaviors that are not good for us? Why do we eat foods that may not be good for us, ingest substances that are potentially harmful, or partake in behaviors that are risky? In an earlier chapter, we mentioned the concept of pragyaparadh—the "mistake of the intellect," the mind's temptation to create divisions where none exist. According to Ayurveda, forgetting the unified essence of life is a fundamental error from which all human suffering derives. Conversely, reestablishing connection with wholeness results in the melting away of all disease. *Object referral* is the single phrase with which Ayurveda accounts for the onset of the disease process—and the cure for all illness is expressed as *self-referral*. Object referral means that we seek fulfillment in things outside ourselves. Whether it is the promise of some intense sensory gratification, working late into the night to make more money, or using drugs to gain peer approval, the sacrifice of our self for our self-image is the seed of all suffering.

All Ayurvedic interventions are ultimately intended to transform object referral into self-referral, and to restore the memory of wholeness. We will always seek gratification in the world around us and we all deserve to have a good job, a safe home, and nourishing relationships. Ayurveda simply says that by themselves, our possessions and positions will not bring us true and lasting happiness. Therefore, for true health, we must seek to discover that aspect of ourselves that is universal. Then we remember that we are not physical beings having occasional spiritual experiences. Ultimately, we are spiritual beings having occasional physical experiences.

Ayurveda is also a very practical science, however, and it recognizes that potential causes of imbalance can exist at the physical level. Blatant abuse of the senses is one example: If you regularly attend heavy-metal concerts, for example, you will probably experience ringing in your ears or even permanent hearing loss. Seasonal changes are also a significant cause of illness, because each season has specific effects on the doshas that must be counterbalanced in order to maintain health. Many people, for example, suffer from frequent colds and congestion during rainy seasons. This is because Kapha has become dominant in the environment; even if a high proportion of Kapha is not usually present in your system, a very moist environment can foster Kapha accumulation, which underlies congestion and coughs. Similarly, sitting on the beach all day in the middle of the summer can create excessive Pitta in the system, which manifests itself as sunburn. Awareness of environmental influences on our mind body physiology is an important premise of Ayurveda, and minor modifications in our daily activity based upon the season are considered to be very important.

Ayurveda also recognizes that sometimes infectious organisms do invade our bodies. Though they were written thousands of years before the invention of the microscope, the ancient Ayurvedic texts describe entities that seem to resemble bacteria and viruses. There are also detailed descriptions of many parasites and the means for treating them. Parasites are usually discussed as the result of unwholesome contact with the senses, such as through improper food preparation. The Ayurvedic emphasis, however, always remains on the immune competence of the host rather than on the power of any invading germ. The soil, one might say, is always more important than the bug.

Mind, Body, Illness, and Health

Illness is the loss of the memory of wholeness, and health is the restoration of this memory. We lose the memory of wholeness when we identify with objects in our environment. When we become dependent upon people, circumstances, positions, or material possessions for our sense of security and well being, we run the substantial risk of losing the comfort when the external sources of satisfaction are unavailable. The only true and lasting source of peace is spirit. When we identify our essential nature with the field of pure potentiality, we are no longer vulnerable to suffering with every challenge we face in everyday life.

The goal of Ayurveda is always to raise the level of health throughout the course of life. Even if a person displays no specific illness, the state of well-being can still be enhanced. If a disease has manifested itself, the imbalance can be eliminated and wholeness restored. Of course, it is always easier and more effective to treat an illness at the earliest possible stage. If we can achieve balance before there is an abnormality on a laboratory test or X ray, we can avoid suffering and reduce the cost of health care as well. Thus, an Ayurvedic approach places premium value on identifying imbalances at early stages rather than waiting for more serious manifestations. We've seen how this concept has not been easily accepted by Western medical science. To suggest that chronic stress with its attendant imbalances in digestion, elimination, and sleep patterns can, over time, lead to serious and life-threatening illness is only now becoming part of the prevailing disease paradigm. A growing body of data, however, is concluding that most of the major causes of suffering and illness are the result of lifestyle choices and interpretations.

We in Western society are unique, in that so many of the illnesses plaguing us are the results of life-harming choices made by large segments of our culture. Technology has provided us with the luxury—or the liability—to ignore substantially nature's rhythms of sleeping, waking, and nourishing ourselves. As many of us have lost connection with the natural forces in our environment, we have simultaneously lost our connection to the natural healing forces within us. Mind body medicine describes how disease has resulted from this loss—and, perhaps more importantly, it also offers ways for us to reestablish our connection to nature in both our inner and outer environments.

PART TWO

BEYOND ILLNESS,
TOWARD WHOLENESS

Section 2 of The Wisdom of Healing *offers practical healing tech-niques in the context of a spiritual awareness that is fundamental to human health. These approaches are not intended as substitutes for conventional medical care but are explored as a means to expand the armamentarium of modern health care. Unfortunately, for much of the past half century, modern health care has been limited to the use of pharmacological drugs as the main treatment for illness. Consequently, we have tended to ignore other approaches to activate the intrinsic healing forces within people. In this section, I investigate complementary interventions that can reduce suffering and increase well-being without substantial risk or toxicity.*

Just as the line separating matter and perception has been blurred or even eliminated by quantum mechanics, the distinction between "method" and "mind" is out of place in a consciousness-based approach. In this sense, the material on herbs in Chapter 9 is no less consciousness oriented than the discussion of meditation in Chapter 5. The effectiveness of an intervention, be it the use of a nutritional herb or the practice of an advanced meditation technique, depends upon the ability of the body mind to translate the orga-

nizing power of a specific therapeutic approach into a healing influence in the mind and body. This is one of the key insights of mind body medicine: that ultimately all healing is the result of the return of the memory of wholeness. Without this understanding, we continue on our search for more drugs and new procedures. This approach will reap its rewards but ignore the potential to prevent illness and enhance health through the intrinsic and powerful self-balancing forces inherent in all of us.

5

Restful Alertness—
Eavesdropping on Silence

"Let us be silent, that we may hear the whispers of the gods."

Ralph Waldo Emerson

"Speech is of time, silence is of eternity."

Thomas Carlyle

I'm driving down the freeway, late for an appointment and traveling a bit over the limit. Suddenly I'm aroused from my preoccupations by the sound of a police siren. A glance into the rearview mirror causes a precipitous drop in my gut as I realize that a distinguished member of the California Highway Patrol is pulling me over for speeding.

Instantly, a torrent of physiological responses cascades through my mind and body. My pupils dilate, my heart beats faster and harder, my blood pressure rises, my breathing deepens, and my skin perspires as adrenaline and cortisol are pumped into my circulation. Every cell in my body is shouting, "Fight or flight! Fight or flight! Fight or flight!"

But despite all these urgent internal alarms, I carefully pull over to the shoulder of the highway, put on a deferential smile, and politely attempt to talk my way out of a ticket.

Our ability to react vigorously and decisively when we are at risk has been an essential evolutionary development, and we are hard-wired to initiate a "fight-or-flight" response when we feel threatened. Although it has worked for possums to "play dead" when in danger, the survival of our species has depended upon our skill in fighting when the odds are in our favor and running when they're not. This capability has been of tremendous importance to the human species at earlier stages of our evolution.

In his 1932 book entitled *The Wisdom of the Body*, the brilliant physiologist Walter B. Cannon described how the fight-or-flight response is programmed deeply into the oldest parts of our nervous system.[1] Ten thousand years ago, a human being confronted by a saber-toothed cat would quickly grab a big stick or run as fast as his legs would carry him. Today there are still situations in which wielding physical power or finding the nearest escape route is adaptive, but these days our primitive defense mechanisms often simply agitate us at times when the fight-or-flight option is inappropriate. At the checkout line of a supermarket, or when our phone call is interminably put on hold, stress responses flood our systems with hormones—yet there's not a saber-toothed cat anywhere in sight.

Perhaps because genuine physical threats have diminished, contemporary society seems addicted to simulations of danger and risk. Our children stand at video-arcade games for hours at a stretch fighting life-and-death battles, moving only their fingers. Millions of us attend movies featuring fierce violence and devastation. We sit quietly watching images on the screen, yet internally we may be close to panic, with stress hormones coursing through our veins. This frequent but suppressed activation of the fight-or-flight response contributes to a variety of illnesses. Hypertension, insomnia, anxiety, indigestion, irritable-bowel syndrome, and heart disease are just a few of the many health concerns that are linked to chronic stress.

The late Dr. Jonas Salk once wrote that the period of pure Darwinian "survival of the fittest" has largely passed, and that the ability to fight hard or run fast have to a great extent been rendered irrelevant by civilization's advances.[2] But, Salk suggested, if physical strength has become less significant, wisdom has become more important than ever before. We are now in the era of "survival of the wisest," and we would do well to cultivate our intellectual, emotional, and spiritual capabilities with the same diligence that our ancestors brought to hunting and gathering. This is a distinctly modern perspective, yet I believe the meditation techniques of Ayurveda and other ancient traditions provide some of the most powerful tools for satisfying the very real need that Salk addressed.

Silence and the Restful-Alertness Response

Along with the fight-or-flight response, human beings have a built-in ability to reestablish mental and physical equilibrium. This restful-alertness response is also programmed into our nature, and it too confers an evolutionary advantage. After conquering a wild boar in the jungle, our early ancestors were able to retire to a safe place, where they allowed their minds to become quiet and their bodies to relax. But while restoring their energy, they remained alert, ready to respond to the environment if necessary.

Meditation works in much the same way. As a child of the late sixties and early seventies, I was hungry for a natural means of expanding consciousness, and I began daily meditation during my senior year in college. I had visions of great spiritual masters who could travel celestial realms while their bodies remained in a timeless state of suspended animation, and I expected meditation to provide this sort of supernatural effect. But my experiences weren't at all "flashy." Instead, I found a sense of genuine calm, a feeling of truly coming home to myself. Though there was no chorus of angels, I quickly began to appreciate the value of centering and replenishing myself, and soon my daily meditations became indispensable.

The following summer, before entering medical school, I participated in a training course that included eight hours a day of silent meditation. The experience left me convinced that exploration of inner space through daily meditation is the most important thing anyone can do to enhance health and well-being.

I've found that almost everyone can readily experience restful alertness using basic meditation techniques. The process is simply intrinsic to our nature, and all effective meditation and relaxation techniques operate according to similar principles. As thoughts become disengaged from their associated emotions, the mind body physiology is gradually able to reestablish a profound state of inner balance.

Emotions tied to thoughts have a kind of activating charge, for each feeling is a physical sensation associated with an idea. As a result, emotions are experienced in both our minds and bodies, and every idea includes a taste of delight or disappointment, relief or anguish, hope or despair, love or fear. As you recall the birth of a child, for example, you'll remember not only the physical details, but also the powerful feelings evoked by the event. Or, if you think about the death of a friend or family member, you'll again see that both information and emotional energy are woven into the memory. This mixing of thoughts and emotions is also present in our desires for the future. If you imagine a vacation you are planning to Hawaii, you will also experience feelings about the journey to paradise. If you need to go to traffic court next week, there will be a quite different emotional flavor to the imagined event.

Each of our thoughts is an impulse of consciousness that expresses both meaning and sound. Someone estimated that human beings have about sixty thousand thoughts each day—but the sad news is that about fifty-nine thousand are the same ones as the day before. Beginning meditators often believe their minds should be absolutely quiet, and their many thoughts frustrate them. But thoughts are the natural expression of a conscious mind. We are all engaged in a continuous internal dialogue, in which the meaning and the associations of one thought trigger the next.

Our minds work something like this:

"I need to pay the phone **bill.**"

"Tomorrow is my brother **Bill's** birthday."

"What did he get me last year for my **birthday?**"

"**Last year,** I was in Hawaii at this time."

"I wonder what **time** it is."

During meditation, a new object of attention is introduced, which temporarily serves to disrupt the progression of one thought to the next. More specifically, this new object of attention is able to engage our attention, but lacks an emotional charge to trigger associations. The object may be a chant, a visual symbol, one's own breath, or a specific sound or mantra. By interrupting the usual meaningful progression of thoughts, it is possible to slip into the "gap" between our thoughts and experience the field of silence.

Verifications of the Meditative Experience

According to an integrated mind body model, mind and body are really two aspects of a unified underlying field of intelligence. The mind is a field of ideas and the body is a field of molecules—but both are manifestations of consciousness. If this intimate link between mind and body is really present, we should be able to measure changes in physiological functions during meditation that correspond to the ongoing mental experience. Indeed, over the past forty years many scientists have been intrigued by the remarkable changes that can be observed in experienced meditators.

During the 1950s, research on the Indian holy men known as yogis reported dramatic slowing of breathing rates and complete cessation of muscular activity for hours at a time.[3,4] When brain-wave-monitoring technology became widely available in the sixties, experienced meditators showed unique EEG patterns.[5,6] I was fascinated by the reports of mystics who could accomplish what seemed like miraculous feats of self-control. Some yogis could slow their breathing to two or three breaths per minute, while others appeared totally serene despite having their hands immersed in ice water.[7] I heard dramatic descriptions of yogis who meditated in airtight boxes and showed no signs of harm after hours of oxygen deprivation. Herbert Benson, M.D., a pioneer in meditation research, reported on Buddhist monks capable of raising their body temperatures in near-freezing weather to the point that they were able to heat up and completely dry icy sheets wrapped around them.[8]

These findings forced many Western scientists to reassess existing paradigms. Up until this time, it had generally been held that our nervous system has two distinct parts: a voluntary component through which we control movements of our muscles, and an involuntary, or autonomic, component to regulate blood pressure, heart rate, temperature, digestion, and other essential bodily processes that occur without conscious attention.

As information on advanced meditation practitioners came to light, neurophysiologists began to recognize that certain bodily functions that usually happen automatically can be brought under conscious control. Although it was initially believed that the ability to influence involuntary functions was exceptional and required years of austere practice, it quickly became apparent in the late sixties through studies on practitioners of transcendental meditation (TM) that any person with a mind has the ability to experience quieter levels of mental activity, accompanied by a state of deep physical relaxation.

Studies on newly initiated Westerners practicing a mantra meditation technique showed physiological changes surprisingly similar to those reported in experienced practitioners. Breathing patterns slowed, oxygen consumption fell, the heart pumped less blood, and brain-wave patterns became more coherent.[9,10,11] Of greater practical importance were studies showing that, rather than becoming recluses, people practicing meditation became less anxious, more sociable, and more successful in their worldly endeavors.[12,13] We have also learned that meditation can be helpful in the treatment of many common health disorders, including hypertension, anxiety, chronic pain, and infertility.[14-22] Meditation is now a component of mind body programs around the world.

Breathing-Awareness Meditation

The basic experience of meditation combines inner awareness with deep physical relaxation. This is very different from sleep, during which we have limited awareness, and from wakefulness, when we are physically active and our awareness is directed outward. In fact, studies have disclosed, there are sufficient distinctions between the physiological profile during meditation and all other known states of awareness that some researchers have suggested meditation represents a completely separate state of consciousness.

From the perspective of Ayurveda and mind body medicine, inner silence is fundamental to balancing, healing, and rejuvenating the physiology. From the silent field of pure potentiality, all energy and creativity springs forth, and the entire manifest creation flows from the silent unified field. Deep within each of us lies the ground state of consciousness, the realm of spirit that connects our individuality with universality. Through the process of meditation, this field of pure awareness can be found in the silent spaces between our thoughts. With the repeated experience of silence, the field of pure potentiality can become an internal reference point of inner stability and self-reference.

There are many different types of meditation for quieting the mind and expanding awareness.[23,24] Most techniques seek to focus attention gently on some physical or mental phenomenon, which may be an object, a sound, a thought, or a physiological process. Just by becoming aware of your breathing, for example, you can quiet your thoughts and create a deepening sense of relaxation.

As a first step in learning to meditate, try the simple breathing-awareness technique outlined below:

1. Close your eyes.

2. Gently focus awareness on your respiration. As you inhale and exhale, simply observe your breath.

3. Remain aware of your breathing, without trying to alter it in any way.

4. As you observe your breath, it may vary in speed, rhythm, or depth. It may even seem to stop for a time. Without resisting, calmly observe these changes.

5. At times your attention may drift to a thought passing through your mind, to a physical sensation in your body, or to some distraction in the environment.

6. Whenever you notice that you are not observing your breath, gently bring your attention back to it.

7. Relinquish any expectations you may have during the practice of this technique. If you find yourself being drawn to a particular feeling, mood, or expectation, treat this as you would any other thought. Gently return your awareness to your breath.

8. Continue for twenty minutes, then very slowly open your eyes, returning your attention to the sights and sounds around you.

Primordial Sound Meditation

Primordial sounds are the vibrations of nature that structure the universe. They are the root sounds of every language. We can hear these sounds in the songs of birds, the rushing of streams, the crashing of waves, and in the whispering breezes in the leaves of a tree. According to Ayurveda, listening to primordial sounds restores our sense of connection to the whole and enlivens our inner healing energy.

Primordial sound meditation (PSM) makes use of the seed sounds of the Sanskrit alphabet. These mantras, or vehicles of the mind, are mental vibrations that do not carry meaning. Because they are free of the associations that accompany the words we use in everyday speech, primordial sounds temporarily interrupt the otherwise continuous internal dialogue that progresses from one meaningful idea to another, and allows us to enter the silent space between thoughts.

Primordial sound meditation chooses an individual's mantra on the basis of Vedic mathematics. According to Ayurveda, each epoch of time has a particular vibratory frequency associated with it. A mantra that reflects the sound of the universe at the time of one's birth is identified and used in a silent, effortless meditation process. There are approximately one hundred classical mantras from which an individual's is chosen. The theory is that the sound of the cosmos at the time of one's birth reflects the vibration of moving from an unmanifest prenatal form to a living, breathing individual. By using this sound, it can serve as a vehicle to bring our awareness from individuality to universality. Simply stated, the mantra is used as a subtle vibration to create a quieting resonance in the mind. With practice, a true experience of silence is achieved.

What evidence is there that using a specifically chosen mantra is more effective than any randomly chosen one? From a scientific standpoint, the answer is—very little. In some studies on meditators, a control group of people who sat quietly with their eyes closed or read religious material generally did not show the same physiological changes as those practicing a specific meditation technique. In one of our recent studies, we taught our control members the Jacobsen progressive relaxation and fewer people stayed with it versus primordial sound meditation.[25] Dr. Herbert Benson has suggested that any pleasant, meaningless sound can be used to elicit a relaxation response, but we have decided to continue using an established means of choosing the subtle mental vehicles of the Vedic tradition. We know the traditional mantras work, and we find comfort and inspiration in the fact that they have been used in meditative practice for five thousand years.

What actually happens when one sits to meditate? Although each experience of meditation has its own flavor, mine tend to follow a general pattern. When I first close my eyes and introduce the mantra, a continuous stream of thoughts traffic is usually present, most often about a situation that is prominent in my life at that moment. Gradually my thoughts become fainter and blend together, as if I were watching a dream. Then, finally, thoughts seem to melt away entirely, yet awareness remains. While in this silent place, time and space are transcended, only to be reintroduced when I emerge from the internal silence. I may dip in and out of this state until it is time to resume the activities of my life. But I always feel a centering and a deep sense of rejuvenation as I reenter the world of activity.

Although taking time each day to access the inner field of silence and creativity is profoundly rewarding, the true value of meditation is not in the practice alone, but also in the benefits that it brings to everyday life. When we integrate meditation into our daily routine, the experience of silence begins to permeate our lives even outside of meditation. The expanded, nonlocal, blissful field we contact during the practice becomes established as an internal reference point. When you've begun meditating regularly, you're very likely to find that all your activities are performed with more awareness, balance, and joy. You'll be insulated from the hysteria of modern life, because on the level of your own experience you'll understand that your essential nature is silence.

Advanced Imagery

Once you've learned to enter the gap between your thoughts, you can begin using mental imagery to activate attention and intention at subtle levels, and to energize the deepest healing processes of your body. Some examples of mental imagery are provided below. Before making use of them, it's best to spend about ten minutes in breathing-awareness or a mantra meditation technique. Then the texts of these inner journeys should be read with a slow, soothing intonation. You can record your own voice, or ask a trusted friend to read to you.

Following each imaging experience, remain in a relaxed state for five minutes before opening your eyes.

Exercise 1—From Infinity to Infinity

This guided meditation provides the experience of going beyond our senses to embrace the timeless expansiveness of creation.

⌐⌐⌐

Imagine yourself lying atop a mountain on a clear, warm, moonless summer's night, gazing into the heavens. Your awareness begins expanding to fill the celestial sky. You begin traveling away from the earth as gravity releases its hold. You briefly glance back to see our beautiful blue planet diminishing to a tiny point of reflected light. As you expand outward across the solar system, you traverse the paths of the outer planets and soon the sun becomes just another star in the sky. You continue moving through the vast intergalactic space as you travel beyond the Milky Way galaxy with its millions of stars twinkling like fireflies on a summer night. Continuing to encompass more of the universe, you see other star clusters and nebulae as faint sparkles of light in the vast black sea of space. Eventually your awareness is filled with the cosmos and the cosmos is filled with your awareness.

Now, focus on the dimmest speck of light across the vast expanse of space and allow it to guide you across the universe as you retrace the path toward your home galaxy. As the light of the sun gradually glows brighter, you again see our azure planet floating in the blackness. Follow the path of a beam of light, back to your present space and time on earth. Now trace a light ray as it enters your eye and is absorbed by a vision cell in your retina. Follow a single photon as it moves through the cell membrane, through the watery bag of proteins, past the nucleus with its coiled genetic code, into a single molecule. Continue diving deeper into an atom as you cross a vibrating charged electron cloud. Penetrate the vast emptiness between the outer electrons and the minute, dense atomic nucleus made of protons and neutrons. You have now entered the shadowy zone between matter and energy. As you enter the subatomic realm, all illusion of solidity surrenders to evanescent bursts of energy. You find yourself once again in a boundless empty space glimpsing tiny flashes of light in a black sea of universal potential. Not only have matter and energy dissolved, but space and time as well.[26]

You now have direct experience of the Vedic verse:

> *"As is the individual, so is the universe.*
> *As is the human body, so is the cosmic body.*
> *As is the human mind, so is the cosmic mind.*
> *As is the microcosm, so is the macrocosm."*

What are the lessons of this exercise? If you allowed yourself to take this journey then it should be apparent that the reality you created was within your own awareness. Through memories and imaginations we create the substance of our lives, all the while believing that the quantum soup we interpret as "real" is immutable. The "solid" world of our senses, composed of molecules and atoms, is mostly emptiness. But paradoxically, this "emptiness" is actually full with the potential to create the infinite forms and phenomena of the universe.

When we enter the cosmic core, space and time lose their grip and we experience the beginning of the universe. The timeless womb of creation is present at every moment, engendering the world, but never surrendering its eternal, infinite potentiality. This field of pure intelligence is the source of the universe and the source of our individual minds.

Exercise 2—The Heart of Creation

In this visualization, you're encouraged to experience your connection to the universe with your heart, rather than with your intellect.

We will begin this journey to the heart of creation by traveling to a place that carries a special meaning for you. Envision a beautiful, natural environment that is safe and nurturing. It may be a lush beach on a tropical island, a natural hot springs deep in an old growth forest, or a pine-covered mountaintop with expansive views. Find your sacred place, spread a soft blanket on the ground, and make yourself comfortable, lying on your back, looking into the beautiful blue, sunny sky. As the sounds of birds warbling and the soft, warm breeze whispering through the trees fade into the background, close your eyes and allow the golden warmth of the sun to embrace and suffuse you. Feel the tension melting out of your body and allow the healing energy of nature to ease and comfort you. With each breath, release your fears and hurts, allowing them to evaporate in the purity of your nurturing, accepting surroundings.

Now envision the face of a loving celestial being coming before you, filled with tenderness, compassion, and forgiveness. Love and acceptance flow from the eyes of this being into your heart, bathing away your fears and pains. As you gaze into this angelic face you notice that it embodies other faces of people with whom you have shared true love. You may see a devoted parent, or a kind grandparent gazing into your eyes with unconditional acceptance. A childhood sweetheart smiles at you with the innocence of youthful love. A teacher or spiritual guide shares his compassion and deep knowingness with you. A spouse or lover honors your essence with his unwavering affection and appreciation. A child gazes into your eyes with trust and gratitude for your caring and commitment. Your dear friends express their unqualified appreciation of you.

Each of the faces offers love and forgiveness. As their healing energy permeates your heart, allow it to fill your being and radiate from you to all around you. The pain, grief, sadness, and fear that you have been carrying melts away and you feel increasingly light as your heart flows in love and gratitude. Surrounded by the caring people in your life, you realize that the love that unites your hearts is the same sacred essence expressing itself in various guises. The universe was created from love and the only real force on earth is the love we share with those around us. You have tasted the realm of spirit—this is wholeness—this is holy.

You probably found that this visualization had a different effect on you than the first exercise. This was a journey of the heart, which by its nature wants to overcome all boundaries and experience unity. Love is the sweetest essence of life. Although extremely delicate, love is invincible and imperishable for it is the vital force of the universe. In the Vedic tradition, spiritual seekers can be enlightened through knowledge or through devotion. This exercise provides a glimpse of the liberating and enlightening wisdom of the heart.

When you begin to own this knowledge, nothing in your environment can feel threatening to you. As a result, any fear of loss or separation will loosen its hold, and an unbroken flow of love and awareness will strengthen, inspire, and illuminate you.

Restful Alertness

As we've discussed earlier, Ayurveda teaches that the fundamental cause of all suffering and illness can be expressed in just two words:

object referral. If we choose to identify ourselves with objects—people, possessions, or emblems of status—we will eventually experience loss and pain as a consequence.

Self-referral, in contrast, is identification with the field of pure potentiality, the realm of silence and of spirit. Meditation allows us to experience directly the inner silence that is the ultimate source of all creativity and fulfillment. By devoting some time each day to meditation, we can reestablish contact with the underlying ground state of existence. This experience of inner silence connects each individual self with the infinite, immortal, cosmic intelligence. Directly experiencing the state of pure potentiality opens our individual awareness to universal awareness. By taking time to enter the gap between our thoughts—to settle into the silent ground state of existence—we can infuse all of our desires and intentions with the irresistible power of nature.

If you're accustomed to a fast-paced, tightly scheduled lifestyle, it may seem that meditating is simply "doing nothing" for an hour each day—and there is even some truth to this. While you're meditating, you're of no use to your friends or your family or your career. But when you arise from meditation refreshed, energized, centered, and creatively focused, you can become a powerful, beneficial force for yourself and everyone you encounter. Of all the mind body approaches discussed in this book, daily meditation is foremost.

6

Accessing the Inner Pharmacy
Through the Doors of Perception

"This life's five windows of the soul
Distort the heavens from pole to pole
And teach us to believe a lie
When we see with, not through, the eye."

William Blake

You're lying on a secluded beach in Acapulco. You hear the waves crashing onto the shore as the seagulls call to the wind. You feel the hot sand through your beach blanket while the warm tropical sun toasts your body. You see the sailboats leisurely carving through the surf as flocks of pelicans fly in formation overhead. As you savor the flavor of your sweet, delicious mango juice you catch a whiff of the coconut suntan lotion you applied earlier. The sensory world is a most captivating place.

We ingest the world around us through our five senses. The sounds, sensations, sights, tastes, and smells that enter our brain and register in our mind create the experiences by which we define ourselves and the universe we inhabit. Just as our bodily tissues are created from the food we eat, the substance of our mind is created from the sensory impressions we consume. The quality of these impressions determines the quality of our thoughts and feelings. If we wish to heal our minds and bodies, we need to substitute nourishing impressions for the toxic ones we've been ingesting.

Ultimately, our picture of the world is constructed in our consciousness. According to Ayurveda, there is a sequential unfoldment of the five sensory codes of nature. Undifferentiated consciousness interacting with itself creates sound, touch, sight, taste, and smell.

The Vedic seers exclaimed that the material world is simply condensed consciousness, foreshadowing by five thousand years Einstein's interconversion of energy and matter.

The German philosopher Martin Heidegger said, "Thinking is a subtle form of hearing." We *do* hear thoughts, and when they are powerful enough we feel them as well, and we call them emotions. This emotional category of thought is no longer just sound—it is also touch, as in the phrase, "I was so touched by your kindness." Here sound has become sensation, and thought has manifested itself as a molecule.

By understanding the transformation of sound into matter, we can gain insight into the basic mechanics of creation—because language does not just describe the world, language creates it. Think of the word *mother*. At first, you hear the thought as a sound, but almost immediately you literally feel the emotion that *mother* generates— sound has become joined with touch. Then, if you close your eyes, you will see *mother* as an image on the screen of your consciousness. According to Ayurveda, that image resides in your subtle body, in your mind's eye. The image is an expression of sight, a third code of intelligence that has been brought forth out of sound and touch.

These first three codes of intelligence—sound, touch, and sight—then give rise to *taste,* and these four codes in turn create a fifth, which is smell. All these codes of intelligence ultimately express themselves as the five Ayurvedic elements of creation: space, air, fire, water, and earth.

Space is just a name for matter in its quantum mechanical, unmanifest form. Air is a label for matter in the form of a gas; fire is matter in its metabolic form; water is matter in its liquid form; and earth is matter in its solid form. Everything in creation is a manifestation of these five great elements, the mahabhutas.

Healing Sounds

Sound has an important place in all the healing traditions of the world, including our Western tradition. In the New Testament, for example, the Roman centurion tells Christ, "Lord, I am not worthy that thou should come under my roof, but speak the word and my soul shall be healed." Anthropological studies reveal the significance of healing sounds in every indigenous society, from the Maoris in New Zealand to the Native Americans of the American Southwest.

Our experience of the world through sound begins very early in life. Our hearing is fairly well developed by the time we enter our second trimester in the womb. The drumming of Mother's heart and the gurgling of her bowels provide constant background music for our intrauterine life. The sounds outside Mother also filter into our watery incubator and provide us with an initial impression of the world awaiting us. If our earliest vibrations are soothing and comforting, we develop the sense that we will soon enter a nourishing environment. If the original sounds we encounter are hostile, violent, and associated with cascades of stress hormones released by Mother, our anticipation of the world takes on an entirely different tone.

Sound continues to be important once we enter the world. Newborns identify and prefer their mothers' voices within their first seventy-two hours of life, and mothers promptly and selectively respond to their babies' cries with increased blood circulation to their breasts, enhancing milk production.[1,2] Even unhatched baby chicks are capable of distinguishing their mother's chirps from those of other hens![3]

The concept that different sounds have different physiological effects is not foreign to us. If we are having difficulty sleeping at night, most of us would not choose to put on a John Philip Sousa military march or a heavy song, but would favor a Brahms lullaby or a gentle New Age musical journey. Just the thought of your schoolteacher screeching a piece of chalk across the blackboard could send shivers over your body, while recalling the pleasurable sounds of your lover can arouse a completely different physiological response.

Ayurveda teaches that every sound has a physiological effect, which may be either local or nonlocal. Vowels are nonlocal sounds. The sound *ahhhhhh*, for example, disperses from its source in all directions. But a nonlocal sound can be localized through attention. While making a vowel sound, attention can be directed to a particular area of the body and the healing influence of the sound will begin to take effect.

Nonlocal sounds are the basis of the overtone chants used by Tibetan lamas, Vedic priests, and Benedictine monks. In fact, the word *enchantment* refers to the magic of sound that leads to oneness;

enchantment literally means "one through chanting." Healing chants and music have measurable physiological effects. The chant is chemically metabolized into endogenous opiates that are chemically more powerful than any form of illegal narcotic, but they happen to be healing chemicals as well.

Unlike vowels, the consonant sounds of the alphabet tend to localize. They vibrate in certain parts of the body and spontaneously produce effects. Thus, the sound of the letter *n* produces a vibration that tends to go to the middle ear. The letter *m*, which vibrates in the sinuses and nasal cavities, can sometimes help to ease sinus congestion. *Ca, ga, gka* come from the vocal chords, localizing to the back of the throat; these sounds are used by professional singers who want to keep their voices young and vibrant. *Ya, yu, yea* mobilize the temporomandibular joint and can help to reduce tension in people who tend to clench their jaws.

Healing Music

The healing power of music has been recognized for thousands of years in Ayurveda. The Sanskrit word *rasa*, which is translated as "plasma" and "taste," also describes the moods that music can induce in us. Vedic musicians characterized the vibrational quality of times of the day and the seasons of the year and created musical pieces, or *ragas*, to reflect and harmonize with nature's cycles. A morning raga has an enlivening sound and rhythm while an evening raga may be settling and dreamlike. Modern musicians including Bruce and Brian BecVar have taken these ancient musical principles and applied them to contemporary melodies and instruments.

Music therapy is slowing gaining acceptance in modern health care.[4] People with movement difficulties due to Parkinson's disease or stroke have shown improvement in their walking when taught to entrain with music that has a great beat. Music is used to facilitate the various stages of labor and delivery and can reduce the need for pain medication after surgical and dental procedures. Children with cancer who participate in music-therapy classes show improvement in immune function, and heart surgeons perform tasks with greater accuracy when they listen to music they enjoy.[5] One of the most wonderful aspects of the human species is our ability to make and enjoy music. Vedic myths portray the universe as the dance of the gods. Our ability to resonate with nature's primordial sounds and rhythms is an innate gift that can provide us with joy and promote healing.

Primordial Sounds

In Vedic science, specific sounds called mantras are used to create vibratory frequencies in the nervous system. There are mantras for quieting the mind, expanding awareness, and for activating healing impulses. Mantras can be long or short and can be spoken aloud or used silently. Vedic literature describes hundreds of mantras, each with specific effects. This is an ancient form of healing that can have measurable physiological benefits.

The sounds of nature can also be used as healing instruments. Sounds such as waves breaking upon the shore or wind rustling through leaves are nature's authentic language. Human beings have heard these sounds through thousands of years of evolutionary time. Humanity has literally grown up with these vibrations, which are structured in our DNA. When we are completely cut off from the sounds of nature, as may be the case in urban environments, we are deprived of a form of nourishment that is essential to health.

The sounds of human language can be both healing and harming. I am frequently dismayed by stories I hear from my patients on how physicians have forgotten the powerful effect their words have on people. Recently, a young woman had an abnormality discovered on a mammogram, which was found to be cancerous when biopsied. She was referred to an oncologist who spent the rushed office visit bombarding her with statistics of her survival chances, based upon which treatment option she elected. Within moments after the lecture began, she found herself totally unable to absorb any information as her emotional defense mechanisms strove to protect her from the cold facts being presented. She was so terrified by the experience that she decided to avoid any medical care and began a quest for an alternative cure. When she came for an Ayurvedic program, it was clear to me that a combined Western/mind body approach would offer her the best chance for recovery. As I explained her options in words that she could hear, emphasizing the choices and opportunities that were available, she was very willing to accept the appropriate medical interventions. Using meditation, sensory modulation techniques, and massage, she tolerated her surgery and chemotherapy without serious side effects and is currently feeling well and empowered.

I recall a revealing story about the power of words.

A psychologist was attempting to sensitize the surgery department of a hospital to be careful about what was said in the operating room. Studies using hypnosis had revealed that even under anesthesia, people received powerful messages of hope or despair from their doctors and nurses. A heart surgeon became indignant that he was wasting his time listening to this "mumbo jumbo." He knew what was responsible for a patient's recovery—the technical skill of the surgeon, not insignificant words. The psychologist looked him directly in the eye and said, "I wouldn't expect anyone as arrogant and closed-minded as you to understand this concept." The indignant surgeon couldn't believe he was being addressed this way by a lowly psychologist. He promptly turned red in the face, began perspiring vigorously, and could only stammer a pitiful reply. The psychologist then calmly pointed out—with the surgeon as an example—how just a few spoken words could have a profound effect on another human being.

Pay attention to the sounds around you. Create a soothing auditory environment in your home, car, and workplace. Regularly take time away from urban noise and listen to nature's songs. Notice the effect that your words have on those around you and choose to communicate with sensitivity.

Healing Touch

The sense of touch can also evoke profound emotional and psychological healing responses. The skin, after all, is the largest organ in the body, and it is rich with nerve receptors, neurochemicals, and immune modulators. Possibly because it is derived from the same developmental layer as the nervous system, the skin contains almost every neurotransmitter that can be found in the brain. These include peptides closely related to antidepressants, which may explain why massage often induces an elevated mood. Natural pain relievers are also widely distributed in our skin, reinforcing my grandmother's prescription to "rub it" whenever I incurred a childhood soft-tissue injury.

Growth factors and growth hormones may be released with therapeutic touch so that premature babies who receive massage gain weight much faster than others.[6] Child psychologists have long recognized that loving physical contact between mothers and babies is essential for healthy growth and development and for maintaining good health. Baby rhesus monkeys who receive adequate food, water, and shelter but are denied the caresses of their mothers do not behave normally. Even after being reunited with their moms, they show signs of persistent fearful behavior and anxiety.[7]

Even humanely touched rodents have better health. At Ohio State University, rabbits who were petted and cuddled while being fed a very high-cholesterol diet had less than 15 percent as much hardening of the arteries as those animals fed the same diet without the compassionate treatment.[8]

Closer to home, therapeutic touch can lead to improved immune function, better sleep, and less arthritic pain. Touch can change us emotionally, physically, and biochemically.

We need loving touch throughout our lives as adults but we carry a lot of ambivalence and insecurity about it. Different cultures have different norms of tactile behavior. In many Latin American countries, it is natural for friends to hug and touch each other frequently without the fear that sexual boundaries are crossed. Friends and associates do not touch each other very often in the United States. We usually shake hands at the beginning and end of an encounter and occasionally give a hug, but if two men or two women are seen walking down the street arm in arm, a sexual relationship is usually assumed. In some societies, the boundaries of personal space are so tightly controlled that touching someone other than your spouse is a punishable offense. From an Ayurvedic perspective, healing touch is as important as nutritious food. We see the results of touch deprivation in neglected children and neglected seniors. We need to increasingly incorporate culturally acceptable ways to share this nourishing sense with each other.

In addition to the direct benefits of massage, the herbalized oils that are often used can provide benefits of their own. The skin absorbs these oils, which are free-radical scavengers and have antioxidant properties. According to Ayurveda, these oils help protect tissues from potentially harmful chemicals that can accumulate in the body following exposure to toxins.

Ayurvedic Oil Massage (Abhyanga)

An oil massage is one of the most enjoyable elements of the Ayurvedic daily routine. It benefits the nervous and endocrine systems, enhances circulation, improves muscle tone, and stimulates many other beneficial reactions throughout the mind body system.

Ayurvedic massage can be very gentle, or more vigorous in order to reach deep tissue. The kind of massage and the accompanying oils should be chosen based on an understanding of your dosha. For Vata types, massage should be relatively gentle, using heavy, warm oils such as sesame or almond. Pitta types benefit from deeper massages and cooling oils such as coconut, sunflower, or olive. Kaphas do best with a stimulating, vigorous massage that employs lighter oils such as safflower, sunflower, or warmer oils such as mustard or almond. A dry massage using herbal powders or a silk glove is also beneficial for Kapha types; this increases circulation and has an invigorating effect.

PREPARING FOR THE MASSAGE

Before it is used, oil should be cured once by slow and careful heating in a glass or metal pot. Place a few drops of water in the oil and remove the pot from the heat as soon as the water boils out of the oil. *The oil must be watched carefully while heating to prevent a fire.*

Just before beginning the massage, a small quantity of oil should be gently reheated by placing it in a plastic squeeze bottle, which is then warmed under hot tap water.

FULL-BODY MASSAGE (5–10 MINUTES)

Begin by pouring a tablespoon of warm oil onto the scalp. Using mainly the flat of the hand, massage the oil in vigorously. Cover the entire scalp with small circular strokes, as if shampooing.

Move to the face and ears, massaging more gently. Gentle massage of the temples and backs of the ears is especially good for settling Vata dosha.

Using both the flat of the hand and the fingers, massage a small amount of oil onto the neck, front and back, and then the shoulders.

Vigorously massage the arms. Use a circular motion at the shoulders and elbows, and long back-and-forth motions on the upper arms and forearms.

Avoid being excessively vigorous on the trunk. Using large, gentle, circular motions, massage the chest, stomach, and lower abdomen. Ayurveda traditionally advises moving in a clockwise direction. A straight up-and-down motion should be used over the breastbone.

After applying a bit of oil to both hands, gently reach around to massage the back and spine as best you can. Use an up-and-down motion.

As with the arms, vigorously massage the legs with a circular motion at the ankles and knees, straight back-and-forth on the long parts.

Use whatever oil remains to massage the feet vigorously. Pay extra attention to your toes.

Keeping a thin, almost imperceptible film of oil on the body is considered very beneficial for toning the skin, balancing Vata, and warming the muscles throughout the day. To conclude the massage, therefore, the oil should be rinsed off with mildly warm water and mild soap.

MINI-MASSAGE (1–2 MINUTES)

If there is no time for a full-body abhyanga, a short massage is still much better than none at all. The head and the feet are the most important parts of the body to cover, and this can be accomplished in a very short time. The mini-massage requires only about two tablespoons of oil.

Rub one tablespoon of warm oil into the scalp, using the small, circular motions described above. Using your palm, massage your forehead from side to side.

Gently massage the temples, using circular motions, then gently rub the outsides of the ears. Spend a few moments massaging the back and front of the neck.

With a second tablespoon of oil, massage both feet, using the flat of the hand. Work the oil around the toes with your fingertips. Then vigorously massage the soles of the feet with brisk back-and-forth motions of the palms.

Sit quietly for a few seconds to relax and soak in the oil, then bathe as usual.

Healing Vision

Our experiences are literally metabolized into our physical bodies. Fascinating studies on kittens in the late sixties clearly showed that their visual world directly determined how their brains developed. If they were only allowed to see horizontal stripes during the first months of their lives, the nerve cells in their brains that perceive vertical information failed to develop and for the rest of their lives they bumped into chair or table legs.[9] We become what we see.

We live in a very visual society. As we drive down any urban highway in the world, we are bombarded by images seducing our attention in hopes of selling us something new and indispensable. We sit transfixed watching moving images on a television screen for hours at a stretch, being visually transported to places and circumstances we might otherwise never encounter. We are such a visual species that our language reinforces our reliance on vision as the ultimate test of reality. We say, "Seeing is believing," despite the fact that our eyes tell us that parallel lines converge in the distance, the earth is flat, and the sun is revolving around our little planet.

Because of the constant bombardment of visual stimuli entering our eyes at any moment, our nervous systems have evolved sophisticated filters to distill information that is meaningful from that which is useless. Unfortunately, in our effort to dampen our exposure to the intense images surrounding us, we tend to overlook subtler nourishing visual treats. A wild flower blooming along a highway cannot compete with the sexy billboard for a new car. You may not notice a monarch butterfly fluttering past as you enter a dazzling modern steel-and-glass office building.

Healing implies returning to a simpler state of balance. Just as there are primordial sounds, there are primordial images that help us restore our memory of wholeness. People who have suffered heart attacks and are confined to coronary-care units recover more rapidly if their rooms look out onto a park as opposed to a parking lot. It is very healing to watch the clouds drift by, observe young children cavorting, or notice the chipmunks playing hide-and-seek. At least a few times each month, find a place where no matter in which direction you gaze, you can only see natural things. Take in these primordial images and allow them to nourish your body, mind, and soul.

Another technique for enlivening subtle vision is the science of *yantra,* which is the visual manifestation of mantra. As we've discussed, mantra is an instrument of the mind in the form of sound; yantra is a mental instrument in the form of a visual expression.

Every mantra has its own yantra. For example, *Aum* is the classic primordial mantra. *A* is a nonlocal sound, *m* is local, and *u* provides the unifying vibration between them. Aum spans the universe and collapses infinity into a single point, all at the same time. The yantra that corresponds to Aum is called the Shri Yantra, and it is the most important yantra in Ayurveda. Every mantra has its own visual form, because sound and form are intimately connected. Sound is information, and form is the matter that emerges from it. Try this simple visual meditation exercise using the Shri Yantra and notice how, with a little attention, we can expand the information and nourishment we receive through our sense of sight.

SHRI YANTRA

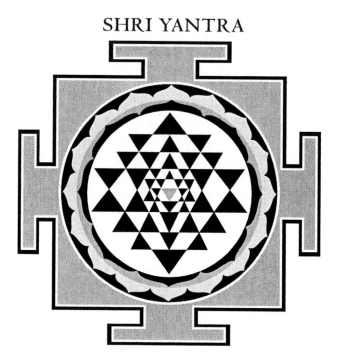

YANTRA MEDITATION

As you look at the yantra, allow your eyes to focus on the center of it. This dot in the center is called the Bindu. The Bindu represents the unity that underlies all the diversity of the physical world.

Now allow your eyes to see the triangle that encloses the Bindu. The downward-pointing triangle represents the feminine creative power, the upward-facing triangle represents male energy.

Allow your vision to expand to include the circles outside the triangles. They represent the cycles of cosmic rhythms. Within the image of the circle lies the notion that time has no beginning and no end. The farthest region of space and the innermost nucleus of an atom both pulsate with the same rhythmic energy of creation. It is all reflected right here. It is all reflected within you.

Notice the lotus petals outside the circle. Notice that they are pointing outward, as if opening. They illustrate the unfolding of our understanding. The lotus also represents the heart, the seat of the self. When the heart opens, understanding comes.

The square at the outside of the yantra represents the world of form, the material world that our senses show us, the illusion of separateness, of well-defined edges and boundaries.

And finally at the periphery of the figure are four T-shaped portals, or gateways. Notice that they point toward the interior of the yantra, the inner spaces of life. They represent our earthly passage from the external and material to the internal and sacred.

Now take a moment to gaze into the yantra, letting the different shapes and patterns emerge naturally.

Now allow your eyes to be soft, held loosely in focus. Your eyelids may droop a little. Perhaps your eyes will even seem to cross. Look at the center of the yantra. Now without moving your eyes, gradually begin to expand your field of vision. Begin to include the edges of the page, now objects in the room. Continue expanding your field of vision until you are taking in information from greater than 180°. Notice that all this information was there all along, you just became aware of it. Now slowly reverse the process by refocusing back to the center of the yantra.

Now gently close your eyes. Can you still see the yantra in your mind's eye? Is your vision limited to what you see through your eyes? Or is it greater than that?

Colors have noticeable effects on our well being. Warm, subtle tones can create a soothing, healing environment while harsh, glaring hues can be irritating. Colors influence and balance the doshas. Kapha types, who are hypometabolic, can be stimulated by colors that are warm and bright. Kaphas do well wearing and surrounding themselves with red, orange, and yellow. Pitta disorders can be cooled through greens and blues. Vata imbalances benefit from the calming influence of blue or from warming earth tones such as gold or brown. The colors of nature are balancing regardless of your mind body constitution. None of us is immune to the quieting and centering influence of autumn's crimson and gold colors or the rejuvenating effect of spring's verdant sproutings as teal blue hyacinths and lemon yellow daffodils burst from the earth.

Healing Taste

When we eat, we are processing the information of the universe into our bodies. Ayurveda recognizes six tastes—sweet, sour, salty, pungent, bitter, and astringent—each of which has a different effect on the three doshas. Chapter 8 presents a detailed analysis of how taste influences both the body and the mind.

Healing Aromas

Your sense of smell has a powerful influence throughout your body. The olfactory bulbs below the frontal lobes of your brain directly connect to the limbic part of the brain, which orchestrates behavior, emotion, and memory. By the fifth day of life, babies can recognize the smell of their mothers, and this important sense plays an essential role in bonding.[10] An aroma can trigger a cascade of memories, as when we walk into a bakery and remember our childhood, or smell a certain perfume and recall an old love affair.

The use of essential oils in aroma therapy is an ancient healing technology that is having a resurgence. Insomnia, anxiety, and depression have been treated with plant-derived fragrances, with some preliminary success. Studies from Japan have shown a positive effect on immune function in patients exposed to citrus fragrance.

The sense of smell has been used very effectively by Ayurveda to balance the doshas. Vata disorders are balanced by warm, sweet, and sour aromas, which are derived primarily from flowers or fruits. Pitta disorders benefit from sweet, cooling aromas such as sandalwood, mint, and jasmine. Kapha disorders are balanced by aromatic and spicy smells, including camphor, juniper, eucalyptus, and clove.

To relieve certain health problems, the sense of smell can be used in a process called neuroassociative conditioning. If you have a muscle spasm, for example, you can learn to place healing attention on the affected area during your daily meditation. If at the same time an aroma such as sandalwood is introduced over a number of sessions, a neuroassociative conditioning is created. Your brain will begin to associate the sandalwood aroma with relaxation of the spasm. Before long, when the pain of a spasm begins, it may be relieved by the aroma of sandalwood.

Making Sense of the World

The principles and techniques we've discussed in this chapter are well described in the Vedic tradition, but they are by no means unique to it. Leonardo da Vinci could have been referring to Ayurveda when he said, "I think with all my senses. When I have a vision of something, I can see it, I can touch it, I can taste it, I can smell it. I look for the hidden meaning behind everything, because I know that everything is connected with everything else."

We perceive and create the world through our five senses. They are the portals through which we ingest the raw material of the universe and create our picture of reality. Nourishing input through all the five senses is as important to our health as nourishing food. They are gifts of nature that allow us to open our minds and souls to the beauty in our environment. Take care to ensure that the food you take in through your senses will provide you with the joy that nourishes your body, mind, and soul.

7

Healing Breath and
Neuromuscular Integration
for Optimal Fitness

*"Health is the vital principle of bliss,
And exercise, of health."*

James Thomson

Ayurveda teaches that human life—*your* life—is a process of recycling earth, water, and air through the body's channels of circulation. The three basic elements are manifestations of the energy and information that make up the entire universe. As they pass through the channels of our mind body system, they literally put us in touch with the stars.

In Chapter 4, we introduced the concept of srotas, or channels of circulation. Although these streams of biological intelligence cross anatomic boundaries, they represent the network of information in the physical body. There is a corresponding system of circulation in our subtle body and these paths are referred to in Ayurveda as *nadis*. As compared to the thirteen channels of circulation in the physical body, there are reportedly seventy thousand channels in the subtle body! I find that the best way of conceiving of nadis is the recognition that almost every cell and every organ in the body has the capability of communicating with every other cell and organ. The body is a web of energy and information and each thread connecting one part with another can be thought of as a subtle channel. The subtle energy that flows through these subtle channels is our life force, which is called *prana*. Although it is sometimes defined as "breath," prana is actually the vital force that animates all living beings. Prana nourishes and supports every cell and tissue in the body, and underlies all the circulatory processes throughout our body. Prana is the primary energy impulse that moves us to take our first breath after leaving the womb, and leaves us at the moment of death.

Breathing with Awareness

Through the Vedic science of breath, or *Pranayama,* we can learn to activate, balance, and direct the life force consciously in order to expand awareness and increase our mind body integration.

According to Ayurveda, our mind and breath mirror each other. When our mind is agitated, our breathing becomes shallow and agitated, while when our mind is still, our breathing is quiet and even. By learning to regulate the breath, we can quickly and directly influence both our physical and emotional states.

Breathing is a beautifully complex process that connects our spirit, mind, body, and environment. It involves the full range of our body's capabilities, from the neuromuscular movements of the diaphragm and the rib cage to the subtlest cellular metabolic processes. With every breath, we inhale and exhale ten billion, trillion atoms of carbon, oxygen, and hydrogen. The atoms we take in are used to create our cells, tissues, and organs, while those that we release are the discarded building materials of our physiology. Breathing is the process of receiving nourishment and eliminating waste as we exchange our individual bodies with the body of the cosmos.

Most of the time our breathing occurs without our focused attention, but by using exercises to bring this function of the autonomic nervous system under conscious control, we can acquire a powerful tool for balancing the doshas and improving the energy patterns in both our mind and body.

Activating Breathing Exercises

Many different Pranayama breathing exercises are described in the yogic and Ayurvedic texts. Some of these are intended to calm the system, while others are more stimulating. Vigorous, forceful breathing exercises, for example, are useful for activating the physiology. These can be particularly valuable if you are a Kapha type, and feel a need for greater mental or physical energy.

The first of these activating exercises is called *Kapalabhati* in Sanskrit, which means "making the head shine." It consists of a very vigorous exhalation followed by an inhalation that is relatively slow and passive. Kapalabhati should be performed while sitting erect but comfortably, and all breathing should be through the nose.

The face and shoulders should be relaxed, and only the diaphragm should be used to expel the breath. Begin with a set of ten complete breaths, then rest for thirty seconds before repeating the cycle. After each set sit for about thirty seconds with your eyes closed, allowing yourself to feel the sensations that the exercise creates in your body.

A second activating and purifying exercise is called *Bhastrika,* or "bellows breath." It is performed by forcefully exhaling *and* inhaling each breath through the nose.

Bhastrika should initially be performed in sets of ten, with thirty-second rest periods between the sets. Once the exercise becomes comfortable it can be performed for longer periods, varying the depth and rate of the breathing pattern. It is important not to overextend. Return immediately to normal breathing if you feel faint or if any sort of discomfort appears.

Kapalabhati and Bhastrika are not recommended during pregnancy or if you are having your menstrual period. Since heightened levels of alertness may make sleep difficult, they should generally not be undertaken late in the evening. Also, you should not perform breathing exercises until your most recent meal has been digested, which is usually at least two hours after eating.

Calming Breathing Exercises

When your mind is agitated, perhaps as a result of a Vata imbalance, there are Pranayama exercises that can provide a calming influence. *Nadi Shodhana,* which means "cleansing the channels of circulation," is often known as alternate-nostril breathing. There are three basic ways to perform this technique, and in each of them the right hand is used to control the flow of breath through the nostrils. The thumb is positioned over the right nostril, while the third and fourth fingers are over the left.

In the first Nadi Shodhana technique, the closed-off nostril alternates at both the end of exhalation and the end of inhalation. In the second technique, the nostril is changed only at the end of inhalation. In the third technique, the same nostril is used for both inhalation and exhalation during three complete breaths, after which the other nostril is used. In all the techniques, breathing should be effortless, with the mind simply witnessing the process. Nadi Shodhana should be performed for five to ten minutes.

NADI SHODHANA

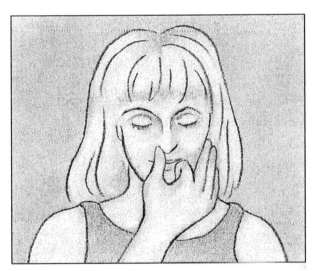

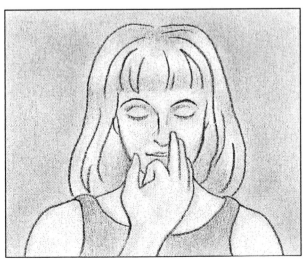

The second calming Pranayama exercise is called *Brihmari,* which means the sound of a bumble bee. It's a humming sound produced through the nose. Take a deep breath, then hum as you exhale. The vibration creates a very relaxing effect. It is particularly pleasant to perform Brihmari in a group. If everyone hums on key, a very expansive vibration fills the room, creating a tangible atmosphere of peace and harmony.

Breathing exercises can't change the circumstances that give rise to anxiety or agitation, but they can definitely change your reaction to those circumstances. Challenges can be met much more effectively when you're operating from a quiet, centered perspective.

Cooling Breath Exercises

When there is too much heat in your physiology, both mind and body are likely to become irritated. Pranayama breathing exercises that cool the system can calm these raging fires and prevent the scorching damage of aggravated Pitta.

The first exercise—called *Ujjayi* in Sanskrit—is performed by slightly contracting the back of the throat while inhaling and exhaling through the nose. This procedure creates a cooling sensation and a soft but audible sound that resembles light snoring. Ujjayi is best learned by first saying the sound *haaa* with the mouth open, and then continuing to move the breath while closing the mouth and partially closing the throat in the area of the soft palate. Ujjayi can be performed along with other activities, and we recommend using it while doing aerobic exercises. If your workout has become so vigorous that Ujjayi breathing can no longer be performed easily, you should probably reduce your level of exertion.

The second cooling exercise, called *Sitali,* is performed by breathing through the mouth with the tongue curled into a cylinder. If you can't comfortably do this, a similar effect can be gained by breathing in and out through rounded lips.

Sitali creates a cooling influence at the back of the throat—but part of the reason it quickly pacifies irritability may be the silly feeling that comes with making this face! You can use this cooling exercise whenever frustration or disappointment leads to anger. Your mind will become clear, and it will be easier to deal with whatever the real issues may be.

SITALI

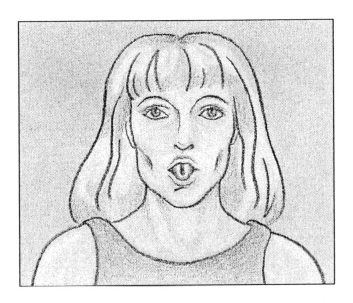

What does it feel like to perform these breathing practices? With the activating exercises (Kapalabhati and Bhastrika), there is usually a pronounced clearing of extraneous thoughts and a sense of witnessing. I suspect that physiologically, the deep ventilations reduce the level of carbon dioxide, which lowers blood flow to the thinking parts of the brain (cortex) without affecting the awareness centers. Therefore, most people have the experience of being very awake without a lot of mental noise. The calming exercises (Nadi Shodhana) create an influence similar to mindfulness meditation, with the rhythmic procedure serving as the object of attention to interfere with our usual thought associations.

Breathing Exercises as Preparation for Meditation

These breathing exercises have a profoundly balancing effect on the mind body physiology and can be valuable in preparing for silent meditation. They facilitate entrance into the "gap"—the silent space between thoughts, which is basic to the experience of restful alertness.

If there is time, perform one of the vigorous Pranayama techniques (Bhastrika or Kapalabhati) for five to ten minutes. Follow this with one of the calming techniques (Nadi Shodhana or Brihmari). Then meditation can begin.

Balanced Exercise

Physical exercise is good for you—but it does not necessarily follow that the more you do, the better it is. Two aspirin, after all, may relieve a headache, but five or six can cause an ulcer.

When you perform any exercise, you can ensure maximum benefit by paying careful attention to your body's responses. Use the following Ayurvedically based suggestions as a guide:

- During peak exercise, you should have a very thin film of perspiration, but you should not be sweating excessively.
- You should be able to hold a conversation while you are exercising. If you are unable to talk because you are short of breath, you should reduce the intensity of your workout.
- Above all, emphasize exercises that you truly enjoy.

It's even possible to elicit the restful-alertness response while exercising. One way to achieve this is through a traditional breathing mantra, *so hum*. Silently repeat *so* as you inhale and *hum* as you exhale. Other words or phrases repeated in a rhythmic manner can have a similar effect. Simply observing the breath can also establish inner silence in the midst of vigorous physical activity.

Body-Type-Specific Exercise

Choosing the appropriate exercise for your body type will ensure the most benefit and the greatest enjoyment. If you are performing some physical activity for the sake of your health but are finding it a strain, it will not provide the benefit you are seeking and you probably will not stay with it for very long.

Exercises beneficial for Vata types should focus on balance and stretching. They should generally be lighter than for the other doshas and may include easy walking, yoga, bicycling, and dance.

Their primary effects are to increase agility and coordination. Exercises for Pitta types should be of moderate intensity and noncompetitive. Brisk walking, jogging, skiing, mountain climbing, biking, and swimming are all beneficial to balance Pitta. They improve circulation and cardiovascular efficiency. Kapha-balancing exercises emphasize endurance and include vigorous running, bicycling, swimming, aerobics, and weight training. They are designed to increase strength and endurance.

The Sun Salute

From an Ayurvedic point of view, if you had to choose only one exercise program, it should be *Surya Namaskar,* or "Sun Salute." Though it takes only a few minutes, this set of twelve postures is rejuvenating, exhilarating, and is appropriate for all body types. Moreover, the Sun Salute encourages a sense of sanctity and reverence for the experience of being alive.

The twelve poses in the set should be performed twice a day, ideally at sunrise and sunset. They represent the full experience of human life, with all its highs and lows and ins and outs. The postures are also symbolic of the twelve months of the year, emphasizing the connection of man with nature.

Begin with your feet firmly planted on the ground in the (1) Salutation pose, inhaling and exhaling easily. Then, with the buttocks muscles tightened, begin stretching up toward the sky while inhaling into the (2) Sky Reach pose. Next, stretch gently forward, exhaling, placing your hands on the outsides of your feet, gently pressing your head toward your knees. You can bend your knees as much as you need to in this (3) Hand to Feet pose. Now stretch back your right leg while looking upward, breathing easily in the (4) Equestrian pose. Then, move into the (5) Mountain pose, with both legs straight and together, raising the buttocks into the air, stretching the arms. From this position, lower yourself gently to the ground touching your forehead, chest, and knees, while maintaining the bulk of your weight on your hands and toes. This is the (6) Eight Limbs pose. Move directly into the (7) Cobra pose, raising off the ground using only your back and chest muscles. Do not overextend by pushing off with your hands. Return again to the (8) Mountain pose and then again to the

SUN SALUTATION (*Surya Namaskar*)

1 RESTFUL BREATHING **SALUTATION POSE**	**2** INHALE **SKY-REACHING POSE**	**3** EXHALE **HAND-TO-FOOT POSE**
4 INHALE **EQUESTRIAN POSE**	**5** EXHALE **MOUNTAIN POSE**	**6** HOLD **EIGHT LIMBS POSE**
7 INHALE **COBRA POSE**	**8** EXHALE **MOUNTAIN POSE**	**9** INHALE **EQUESTRIAN POSE**
10 EXHALE **HAND-TO-FOOT POSE**	**11** INHALE **SKY-REACHING POSE**	**12** RESTFUL BREATHING **SALUTATION POSE**

(9) Equestrian pose with the right leg back. On the second round, the left leg is brought back during both Equestrian positions. The cycle is completed by returning to the (10) Hand to Feet, (11) Sky Reach, and back to the (12) Salutation poses.

The speed and vigor of the exercises should be adjusted to suit your body type. If you have a predominance of Vata, the postures should be performed in a very gentle, relaxed manner. If Pitta is dominant, be sure to focus attention on each individual posture, witnessing but not acting upon the impulse to race through to the next position or to approach the exercise competitively. Kapha types should make an effort to perform each pose vigorously.

It's best to start with a total of ten sets, five with each leg back during the Equestrian pose. As you become more comfortable, you can gradually increase the number to twenty. Breathe in harmony with the movements, so that you're inhaling each time the body is extended and exhaling each time you move into flexion. The postures are most beneficial when performed in a smooth, flowing, sequential manner. According to Ayurveda, if you do the Sun Salute every day of your life you will remain mentally young and vibrant and your body will be light and flexible.

Yoga

Yoga is much more than a set of physical exercises. The practice of yoga integrates body, mind, and spirit, and helps to activate the energy centers of the body by creating balance, flexibility, and relaxation. Yoga is definitely not a competitive sport. All the postures should be performed with a gentle, respectful attitude toward the body, and without any sense of strain. The goal is not a final perfect position, but awareness of the signals that the body is providing to activate energy and information.

While performing the postures, maintain awareness in the body, noticing any areas of tightness or blockage and allowing your attention to enter those places. Perform each position very slowly, as this encourages witnessing. Breathe easily during the postures, noticing how each position naturally encourages inhaling or exhaling.

During each set of postures, there should be a good balance of positions that encourage flexion and extension of the spine. The pace should be comfortable and unhurried, and always take a rest period after a yoga session before resuming normal activities.

Although there are hundreds of different positions, or *asanas,* in the yoga tradition, it's best to begin with a basic set that stretches and tones all parts of your body. With regular practice, the initial set will become easier, and more advanced positions can be added. Always remember that benefits are derived not from the final posture, but from the increased awareness that is gained by performing the poses with full attention and awareness.

If you have Vata predominant in your constitution, it's best to perform the postures slowly and with frequent rests. If Pitta is dominant, focus on each posture and gently resist the urge to race through the set and to push beyond your comfort zone. If Kapha is dominant, perform the positions with a flowing, active intention.

Several recommended yoga books and videos are listed in the references for this chapter. Most people find that taking a yoga class with an experienced instructor is the best way to taste the benefits of this ancient system of mind body integration.

If you have the time to perform yoga postures and breathing exercises before your meditation, we recommend that you start with the Sun Salutations, then perform a gentle set of yoga postures, then do five minutes of an active breathing exercise such as Bhastrika or Kapalabhati, and then five minutes of a calming breathing exercise like Nadi Shodhana. This will prepare the mind and body to quiet quickly, allowing you to experience the silent spaces between your thoughts when you begin your meditation.

Yoga in a Chair

The benefits of conscious movement and stretching are great and need not be missed just because of limited space availability. The following set of postures can be performed anywhere that you have access to a chair and can even be done while sitting on an airplane. The same principles apply to these postures as to all yoga poses—perform them consciously and without straining.

YOGA IN A CHAIR

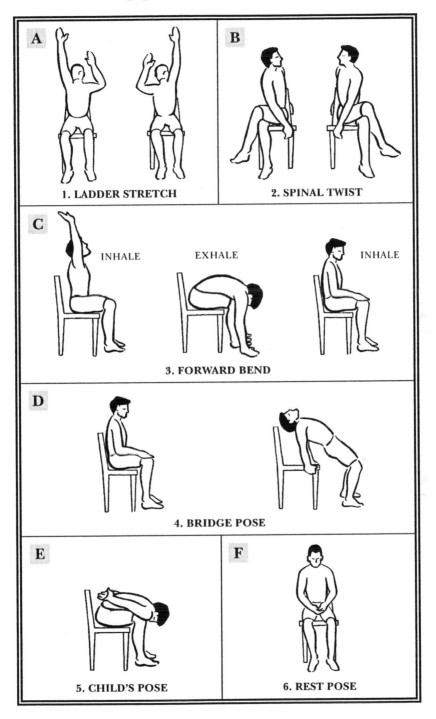

A 1. LADDER STRETCH

B 2. SPINAL TWIST

C INHALE   EXHALE   INHALE
3. FORWARD BEND

D 4. BRIDGE POSE

E 5. CHILD'S POSE

F 6. REST POSE

Mind, Body, and Movement

The nature of the body is to move. Our bodies rejoice when energy is flowing freely through our system. Motion is a feature of this universe, which is in a continuous cosmic dance. When we allow our bodies to dance with the universe through movement, we go beyond the limitations of individuality and become the dance.

To gain the most benefit from exercising our bodies, movement should be performed with grace, flexibility, and awareness. The adage "No pain, no gain," may be applicable to competitive athletes, but for most of us will not result in improved well being, vitality, or happiness. The mind body approach reminds us to listen to the wisdom of our bodies and heed its call to move with sensitivity and vitality.

The ancient mind body fitness program of yoga is more than a set of exercises to improve agility. At their essence, yoga poses are an opportunity to integrate body, mind, and spirit. When the movements and postures are performed with full awareness, we can transcend time and space and experience a state of "being" in motion. The true meaning of yoga is "union," which refers to the union of the individual with the universal. The key to experiencing the fullest value of physical movement is establishing our awareness in silence and then performing action.

8

Food as Medicine

"Let food be your medicine and medicine be your food."

Hippocrates

Sheila had a love/hate relationship with food. Her weight was always more than she felt comfortable with and if there was a new diet that promised an easy way to drop a few pounds, she was a willing subject. Unfortunately, as quickly as she lost, she regained.

When she came to me requesting an Ayurvedic diet, I asked her to forget about losing weight; rather, I asked her to focus on eating with full awareness. She learned to make her meals a meditation, listening attentively to her appetite and savoring every taste, smell, and sensation.

When I saw her again ten weeks later, she looked and felt terrific and hadn't stepped on a scale in over a month. Did she lose weight? Why do you ask?

As a physician, I frequently hear the accusation that medical doctors know nothing about nutrition. I used to be perplexed by this statement because I thought I knew a lot about nutrients. I studied biochemistry and could prescribe the precise intravenous requirements of calories, fluids, vitamins, and minerals for my hospitalized patients who were unable to eat. When I would see people in my office complaining of food allergies or vitamin deficiencies, I would check their immunoglobulin or vitamin levels and reassure them they were adequately nourished. Part of my resistance to dietary programs was that they were based on assumptions that were inconsistent with my understanding and experience. For example, I would see people who were told they had candidiasis and therefore needed to avoid any food that had yeast in it. I took care of people with systemic candida infections who were usually severely immune suppressed and invariably very sick. I could not fathom how sourdough bread would contribute to a significant health problem.

It wasn't until I began studying Ayurveda that I began to appreciate the subtle ways that food could be used to enhance health. Ayurveda provides a framework to understand the many concerns that patients voice about the influence of diet on their well being. It enabled me to grasp why different people had dramatically different experiences of how food impacted their lives. One person ate only pure organic grains and vegetables and was fragile and sickly while another ate burgers and fries and was vibrant. Ayurvedic nutrition made sense to me and did not require any major leaps of faith.

Ayurveda looks at life as the eternal recycling of earth, water, and air. Although our bodies may appear to be stable, we are continuously exchanging the raw material of our physical forms with the environment. We begin life as impulses of orderly intelligence on double-stranded DNA and wrap ourselves in molecules we derive from our surroundings in the form of food. This is how we create a body.

In order to maintain life, we must take something each day from outside ourselves and bring it inside, so that it can become part of us for a while. Since the ability to extract these codes of energy and information and convert them into biological intelligence is truly the foundation of good health, it's important to make use of the Ayurvedic principles that can help identify the best sources of nourishment and use them to our fullest advantage.

The Six Tastes

According to Ayurveda, there are six basic tastes into which all edible substances can be classified: sweet, sour, salty, pungent, bitter, and astringent. Long before the United States Department of Agriculture provided us with the recommended daily allowances for fats, carbohydrates, and proteins, we were sampling our environment with our taste buds. Nature packages its foods according to taste to tell us which ones are of benefit in high quantities, low quantities, or in very

minimal amounts. Generally, we consume high quantities of food
that are predominantly sweet in taste but small amounts that are bitter. The primary taste of a food, which in Sanskrit is called *rasa,*
begins to take effect on our mind body physiology as soon as it
touches our tongue. Although this may appear to defy physiological
principles, I'm sure that we have all had the experience of being
really hungry but instantly appeased by just a bite of a chocolate
brownie. According to Ayurveda, there are direct pathways that communicate the nutrient content of food to our nervous system via
taste, even before the biochemical substrates are released into the
bloodstream.

THE SIX TASTES

ENGLISH NAME	SANSKRIT NAME
Sweet	*Madhura*
Sour	*Amla*
Salty	*Lavana*
Pungent	*Katu*
Bitter	*Tikta*
Astringent	*Kashya*

Understanding the elemental composition of each taste allows
us to predict its influence on our physiology. Nature uses taste to
code the effects of food.

- The *sweet* taste (composed of the elements of earth and water)
  builds body mass and creates a lubricating effect.
- The *sour* taste (composed of earth and fire) contributes to mass
  and increases both chemical and physical heat in the body.
- *Salty* taste (composed of water and fire) is lubricating and
  increases heat in the system.
- The *pungent* taste (composed of fire and air) fosters heat and
  dryness.
- The *bitter* taste (composed of air and space) is the most drying
  and depleting to the system.
- The *astringent* taste (composed of air and earth) has a com-
  pacting, densifying effect.

THE ELEMENTAL COMPOSITION OF TASTE

Sweet	Earth and Water
Sour	Earth and Fire
Salty	Water and Fire
Pungent	Fire and Air
Bitter	Air and Space
Astringent	Air and Earth

Tastes and Doshas

Each taste influences the doshas in a particular way. Kapha dosha, composed of earth and water, is increased by tastes that have a predominance of those elements. Pitta dosha is increased by tastes that have the fire element. Vata dosha, which is made up of air and space, will be increased by tastes that have a predominance of air. For each dosha, there are three tastes that increase its power in the physiology and three that diminish it.

VATA

TASTES THAT INCREASE	TASTES THAT DECREASE
Pungent	Sweet
Bitter	Salty
Astringent	Sour

PITTA

TASTES THAT INCREASE	TASTES THAT DECREASE
Pungent	Sweet
Sour	Bitter
Salty	Astringent

KAPHA

TASTES THAT INCREASE	TASTES THAT DECREASE
Sweet	Pungent
Sour	Bitter
Salty	Astringent

The science of taste in Ayurveda may on first exposure seem complicated, but the principles that underlie it are actually very simple. They may be stated:

> Like qualities increase.
>
> Opposite qualities decrease.

Tastes with elements that make up a dosha will increase that dosha. Tastes with elements that do not comprise a dosha will reduce that dosha. For example, the taste of pungent chili peppers is composed primarily of the fire element. Therefore, peppers will increase Pitta dosha, which is made up primarily of fire. A sweet roll is composed of the earth and water elements; therefore, eating one will increase the Kapha dosha, which is composed of those two elements.

Tastes and Physiological Effects

In addition to its influence on the doshas, each taste has other effects on our mind body physiology. Although these physiological effects are mild, they can be used therapeutically. Some of the predominant influences for each taste are listed below:

SWEET	SOUR
Nutritive	Appetite enhancement
Soothing	Digestive aid
Softening	Carminative

SALTY	PUNGENT
Digestive aid	Digestive aid
Laxative	Diaphoretic
Mildly sedative	Expectorant

BITTER	ASTRINGENT
Depleting	Reduces sweating
Anti-inflammatory	Constipative
Detoxifying	Wound healing

Virya (Energy) and Vipaka (Postdigestive Effect)

Along with the effect of taste on the physiology, Ayurveda recognizes two other important influences that are present in nutritional substances: *energy* and *postdigestive effect*. In Sanskrit, these are known as *virya* and *vipaka*.

Virya refers to the intrinsic energy of a food, and can be characterized in several ways. The most common distinction is between the heating or cooling effects of a food. Substances that have a heating quality reduce Vata and Kapha, but increase Pitta, while those with a cooling quality have an opposite effect. Heating foods tend to contribute to the digestive process, whereas cooling foods require more energy for digestion. Most pungent, spicy foods such as pepper, chilies, and mustard are noted for their heating virya. Cooling foods include rice, wheat, and lentils.

The energy of a food can also be characterized according to whether it is heavy or light, and whether it is oily or dry.

Heavy foods increase Kapha but reduce Pitta and Vata. Examples include meat, cheese, honey, soy and garbanzo beans, beets, and carrots.

Light foods increase Vata and Pitta and reduce Kapha. Examples include nonfat milk, barley, millet, mung beans, leafy vegetables, and apples.

Oily foods increase Kapha and Pitta and reduce Vata. Examples include milk, butter, yogurt, meat, and eggs.

Dry foods increase Vata while reducing Kapha and Pitta. Examples include beans, cabbage, potatoes, and most grains.

Knowing the energy of a food can be useful in determining the most effective means to influence a dosha. For most purposes, knowing whether the virya is heating or cooling is of greatest usefulness. This understanding can usually explain why a food that you would think should have an effect on a dosha in one direction is classified in a different way. For example, you would probably assume that due to its sweet taste, honey pacifies Vata and Pitta and increases Kapha. Because honey has a heating virya, however, it actually slightly *increases* Pitta and *decreases* Kapha.

Postdigestive effect is the taste that emerges later in the digestive process. As a result of the metabolism of food, the influence of a food on the doshas will change as it moves down the gastrointestinal tract. Sweet and salty tastes usually result in a sweet postdigestive effect, with an overall nutritive effect on the physiology. Sour taste results in a sour postdigestive effect, which increases the fire in the system and often stimulates the desire for more nutrition. Pungent, bitter, and astringent tastes usually create a pungent postdigestive effect, which has a generally reducing effect on the physiology. Thus, the six rasas result in three vipakas. Even when a food has a number of tastes, there will usually be only one predominant postdigestive effect.

Knowledge of the vipaka can be very useful in determining a food's net influence on the doshas. For example, fresh ginger root has a pungent and sweet taste but a sweet vipaka. This sweet postdigestive effect allows ginger to be used in people with high Pitta who have weak agnis, as it can stimulate the digestive fire without aggravating the predominant dosha.

Another Sanskrit term, *prabhava,* refers to special effects of a food or herb that cannot be predicted on the basis of its rasa, virya, or vipaka. For example, the cardiotonic effect of foxglove (digitalis) is a special effect that can be used therapeutically, but would not be expected on the basis of its taste or potency. There are many examples of two substances that have the same rasa, virya, and vipaka but have different overall influences on the mind body physiology. Their special effects, or prabhava, result from subtler, intrinsic chemical properties.

Stages of Digestion

The six tastes can also be understood to reflect the various stages of digestion that food undergoes. For complete assimilation of nutrition, food must progress through all six phases in the gastrointestinal tract.

- Sweet taste is predominant in the mouth as salivary enzymes begin the digestion of carbohydrates.
- Sour taste is represented in the stomach with the secretion of gastric acid.
- Salty taste is expressed by the secretion of bile salts from the gallbladder into the duodenum.
- Pungent taste is reflected in the intense digestive enzymes of the small intestines.

- Bitter taste is expressed in the absorption of fluids, which results in the drying of stool in the large intestines.

- Finally, astringent taste is represented in the descending colon with the compaction of the fecal material in preparation for elimination.

Metabolism, and Eating with Awareness

According to Ayurveda, our ability to metabolize food is as important as what we choose to eat. Even normally healthy, nutritious food is of limited value when digestive power is weak. If food is not completely metabolized, healthy tissues cannot form; instead, there is an accumulation of toxicity. How we prepare and consume food is as essential to its nourishing influence as its carbohydrate, protein, vitamin, and mineral composition. Eating food with full awareness takes advantage of the enlivening power of attention.

There are some basic principles to follow in regard to the preparation and eating of a meal. We refer to these principles as *Body Intelligence Techniques* or *BITS*. If you pay attention to these simple principles, you can help your system extract the highest levels of nourishment from everything you eat.

BODY INTELLIGENCE TECHNIQUES (BITS)

1. **Eat in a settled environment.**
   If you are eating in chaotic surroundings, you are metabolizing the chaos along with your food. Try not to be watching a violent television show while eating dinner. Enjoy your meals in silence or with people that you love.

2. **Never eat when upset.**
   Although a pint of ice cream after a fight with your lover may seem like just the right thing to soothe your wounded heart, the powerful emotional chemicals that are released after an argument do not contribute to optimal digestion. Wait until you have settled down a bit, listen to your appetite, and then use food to fill your metabolic, not your emotional, needs.

3. **Always sit down to eat.**
   This doesn't mean eating a taco while driving on the highway. If you can't eat with your full attention on your food, wait until you can.

4. **Eat only when you feel hungry.**

Your appetite is your best friend when it comes to nutrition. If you think of your appetite as a fuel gauge with zero being empty and ten being full, wait until you are at a level two or three before eating and then stop when you are at a six or seven. This means eat when you are really hungry and stop when you are comfortably full. The only way to be clear about the level of your appetite is to check in regularly with your bodily sensations and eat with awareness. When we overeat, it is usually because we are doing something else while we are taking our meal and therefore, eat past our satiety point without noticing it until we are stuffed. If we eat consciously, we cannot miss the signals that a healthy physiology provides.

5. **Reduce ice-cold food and drink.**

For most of our evolutionary experience, we ate food at room temperature or hotter. All of our digestive enzymes work best at body temperature. It is only recently that we have consumed so many cold foods, particularly cold beverages. Ice tends to numb our taste buds, which may be why we are encouraged to drink alcoholic beverages and sodas ice cold—it may be the only way we would tolerate putting these nutritionally empty substances into our bodies. If we were forced to drink beer or colas at room temperature, our consumption would probably go way down. This doesn't mean we should never eat ice cream, but when we do consume cold food or beverages, it is best to do so when our digestive power is at its strongest—that is, during the noon meal.

6. **Eat at a moderate pace.**

This means neither too fast nor too slow. When you eat with awareness, the pace will be appropriate for maximal digestion because you will have savored each mouthful before you are ready for the next.

7. **Wait until one meal is digested before starting the next (two to six hours).**

This again requires us to be in touch with our bodies. It is useful to place your attention consciously on your stomach and even place your hand on your belly to focus your awareness. Eat only when your stomach is calling for more.

8. Sip warm water with your meals.

This helps the digestive process work efficiently. By avoiding ice-cold drinks your digestive enzymes can function optimally.

9. Eat freshly cooked meals.

The life force is greatest in meals prepared with fresh ingredients. The delicious smells and pleasing display of a freshly prepared meal stimulate the appetite and the secretion of digestive enzymes even before food is placed in the mouth.

10. Reduce raw foods.

Although there is no question that raw vegetables are richest in essential nutrients, if we cannot readily assimilate them, they are of little value. Appropriate cooking begins the digestive process, allowing us to extract maximal nourishment from our food.

11. Experience all six tastes at every meal.

If all six tastes are represented, you will be fully satisfied at the end of a meal. When you feel that you have eaten an adequate volume of food but still feel hungry, it usually implies that one of the tastes was missing. If you consciously identify and consume the missing taste, you will feel satiated.

12. Drink milk separately from meals, either alone or with other sweet foods.

Milk is a complete food in itself. Of course, if you are going to eat something with milk, the best choice would be cookies.

13. Leave one-third to one-fourth of your stomach empty to aid digestion.

Leaving some space allows the churning process to optimize digestion. This state of fullness can be recognized when you feel satisfied from a meal without being stuffed.

14. Sit quietly for a few minutes after your meal.

Eating is a sacred process. It is a magical transformation that allows for the energy of the universe to be transformed into the intelligence of our body. Savor the moments after a meal to appreciate the magic.

Herbal/Spice Blends

Spices add variety to life. Just as every food influences each mind body principle, so does every herb and spice. Blends of dosha-balancing seasonings are available or can be prepared to be used in cooking or sprinkled on food during a meal. These herb-and-spice blends ensure that each taste is represented in the right proportion. Vata, Pitta, and Kapha types eating the same pasta primavera can use the appropriate spice blends to personalize their meals.

In general, Vata-balancing spices are warm and sweet, Pitta-balancing spices are bitter and cool, and Kapha-balancing spices are light and hot. You can create your own dosha-specific spice-and-herb blends choosing from the ingredients listed below:

1. **Vata-Balancing Herbs and Spices**
   Basil, Bay, Black Pepper, Cardamom, Ginger, Marjoram, Nutmeg, Salt, Savory

2. **Pitta-Balancing Herbs and Spices**
   Cilantro, Coriander, Cumin, Dill, Fennel, Lemongrass, Licorice, Mint, Sugar

3. **Kapha-Balancing Herbs and Spices**
   Basil, Black Pepper, Caraway, Cardamom, Cayenne, Cinnamon, Dill, Fenugreek, Ginger, Mint, Mustard, Nutmeg, Parsley, Rosemary, Sage

Toxicity, and Dosha-Specific Diets

According to Ayurveda, a weak appetite is both a cause for and a result of an accumulation of toxicity in the system. The collective term for toxic residues, *ama,* is described by Ayurveda as cold, heavy, cloudy, malodorous, sticky, and impure. Certain foods are considered to be ama reducing and are recommended when your ability to assimilate nourishing foods seems weakened. A comprehensive ama-reducing program is presented in Chapter 11.

Once the signs of accumulated toxicity are reduced, Ayurveda recommends that you follow a dosha-specific diet—but only if you can do so with a sense of ease and joyfulness rather than strain or restriction. And always remember that the intention is to *favor* or *reduce* certain choices, rather than to completely eliminate variety from the diet. Your meals should be taken with a sense of appreciation, pleasure, and with awareness that the enjoyment of eating is as important to nutrition as the food that is eaten.

VATA-BALANCING DIET

Because Vata is drying, cooling, and light, you should favor foods that are oily, warming, and heavy. The best tastes for pacifying or balancing Vata are sweet, sour, and salty. Deemphasize foods that are pungent, bitter, and astringent.

RECOMMENDATIONS

1. To balance the lightness of Vata eat larger quantities, but do not overeat.

2. Dairy products pacify Vata. Heat milk before drinking it and take it warm. Do not drink milk at a full meal with mixed tastes.

3. All sweeteners pacify Vata and may be taken in moderation.

4. Fats and oils reduce Vata.

5. Rice and wheat are the best grains. Use less barley, corn, millet, buckwheat, rye, and oats.

6. Favor sweet, heavy fruits such as avocados, bananas, berries, cherries, grapes, mangoes, sweet oranges, papayas, peaches, pineapples, and plums. Reduce dry or light fruits such as apples, cranberries, pears, and pomegranates.

7. Cooked vegetables are best. Raw vegetables should be minimized. Favor asparagus, beets, and carrots. Other vegetables such as peas, broccoli, cauliflower, zucchini, and potatoes should be sautéed or steamed. Sprouts and cabbage tend to produce gas and should be minimized.

8. Spices known to pacify Vata are cardamom, cumin, ginger, cinnamon, salt, cloves, mustard seed, and black pepper. Vata spice blends are also useful.

9. All varieties of nuts are recommended.

10. Except for tofu and mung dahl, reduce the intake of beans.

11. For nonvegetarians, chicken, turkey, and seafood are best; beef should be minimized.

LIGHTER VATA-PACIFYING DIET

Although oily, heavier, sweeter, and richer foods are usually recommended to pacify Vata, there are circumstances in which lighter foods with Vata-pacifying qualities are desirable. People with Vata-aggravated minds who are overweight or those with high cholesterol levels who have been instructed to reduce their intake of fats and oils should favor a lighter Vata-pacifying diet.

RECOMMENDATIONS

1. Rice, wheat, and oats are the favored grains, prepared with reduced amounts of oil or sweeteners.

2. All sweeteners may be taken in reduced amounts.

3. Favor low-fat milk and lassi. Reduce your quantities of cheeses and cream.

4. All oils except for coconut can be used in small quantities. Small amounts of clarified butter (ghee) may be taken.

5. Green or yellow mung beans and red lentils are preferable. They are usually prepared by mixing one part dried beans with two parts water and boiling to the consistency of soup.

6. Vegetables should be well cooked and are best taken in soups, casseroles, and stews. Almost all vegetables are acceptable, with carrots, zucchini, asparagus, spinach, tomato, and artichoke most desirable.

7. Favor sweet, ripe fruits in season. Figs, pineapples, grapes, apricots, sweet oranges, papayas, and small amounts of raisins are acceptable.

8. The warmer and sweeter spices are useful, including ginger, cumin, cinnamon, cardamom, fennel, cloves, *hing* (asafetida), and anise. Salt, lemon juice, and tamarind are useful in small amounts.

PITTA-BALANCING DIET

Because Pitta dosha can overheat the mind and body, favor cool foods and liquids. Foods with sweet, bitter, and astringent tastes are best. Reduce foods that are pungent, salty, and sour.

RECOMMENDATIONS

1. To balance the heat of Pitta take milk, butter, and ghee. Use less yogurt, cheese, sour cream, and buttermilk as the sour taste aggravates Pitta.

2. All sweeteners may be taken in moderation except molasses and honey.

3. Olive, sunflower, and coconut oils are the best to pacify Pitta. Use less sesame, almond, and corn oil, which are more heating.

4. Wheat, rice, barley, and oats are the best grains to reduce Pitta. Use less corn, rye, millet, and brown rice.

5. The sweeter fruits such as grapes, melons, cherries, coconuts, avocados, mangoes, pomegranates, and fully ripe pineapples, oranges, and plums are recommended. Reduce sour fruits such as grapefruits, apricots, and berries.

6. The vegetables to favor are asparagus, cucumbers, potatoes, sweet potatoes, green leafy vegetables, pumpkins, broccoli, cauliflower, celery, okra, lettuce, green beans, and zucchini. Reduce tomatoes, hot peppers, carrots, beets, eggplant, onions, garlic, radishes, and spinach.

7. Pitta types need to use seasonings that are more soothing and cooling. These include cinnamon, coriander, cardamom, and fennel. Hotter spices such as ginger, cumin, black pepper, fenugreek, clove, salt, and mustard seed should be used sparingly. Very hot seasonings such as chili peppers and cayenne are best avoided.

8. For nonvegetarians, chicken, pheasant, and turkey are preferable; beef, seafood, and eggs increase Pitta and should be minimized.

KAPHA-BALANCING DIET

Kapha dosha is heavy, oily, and cold, so you should favor foods that are light, dry, and warm. Foods with pungent, bitter, and astringent tastes are most beneficial for pacifying Kapha. Sweet, sour, and salty tastes should be reduced.

RECOMMENDATIONS

1. Dairy products tend to increase Kapha, so low-fat milk is best. Boiling milk before drinking it makes it easier to digest. Adding turmeric or ginger to milk before boiling reduces its Kapha-increasing qualities.

2. Apples and pears, which are considered lighter fruits, are recommended. Reduce heavier fruits such as bananas, avocados, coconuts, melons, dates, figs, or sour oranges.

3. Honey is a sweetener that is said to pacify Kapha. Other sweeteners increase Kapha and should be reduced.

4. All beans are good for Kapha types except soybeans and tofu.

5. Favor the grains of barley, corn, millet, buckwheat, rye, and oats. Reduce the intake of rice and wheat.

6. Reduce all nuts.

7. All spices except salt are pacifying to Kapha.

8. All vegetables except tomatoes, cucumbers, sweet potatoes, and zucchini are suitable for Kapha types.

9. For nonvegetarians, white chicken meat, turkey, and seafood are acceptable. Reduce the intake of red meats.

A Word on Vegetarianism

We are biologically capable of eating just about anything—animal or vegetable. Although Ayurveda does not recommend a strict vegetarian diet, there are clear advantages to favoring a nutritional program that is high in whole grains, vegetables, and fruits and low in animal fats. There is now overwhelming scientific evidence that diet plays a significant role in heart disease and many forms of cancer. Vegetarians not only have lower incidences of these two major killers, but also show fewer occurrences of diabetes, gallstones, and osteoporosis.[1]

It is quite easy to obtain adequate protein and more than enough vitamins and minerals in a vegetarian diet. Primarily vegetarian diets are low in saturated fats and cholesterol and high in natural antioxidants. Pure vegetarians who consume no dairy will need to supplement with vitamin B_{12}, but Ayurveda supports the use of some dairy on a daily basis. A good time to drink milk is before bed when it can be heated with fresh ginger, nutmeg, and cardamom. The herbs along with the natural tryptophan in the milk promote a sound sleep. If you have an elevated cholesterol level, use low- or nonfat milk. If you have a definite lactase deficiency, you can add lactase enzyme or use a milk substitute made from rice, almond, or soy. There are increasing numbers of dairies that avoid pesticides and hormones and treat their cows humanely; they deserve our support even though the milk costs a little more.

From an ecological perspective, the consumption of meat is costly in terms of global food resources, as a pound of hamburger requires about sixteen pounds of grain. Ever since we moved from an agrarian to an urban-based society, most of us have lost touch with nature so that we seldom connect the steak on our plate with the beast that gave its life for our sustenance. Cultures that hunt or raise their own livestock invariably have genuine respect for their animals and acknowledge the sacrifice they are making. In most cultures where meat is an important nutritional component, it is one part of a diet that includes larger quantities of vegetables and grains. If you look at a plate in an American steak house, you may find a pound of sirloin surrounded by a couple of fried potatoes and a few string beans. In societies in the Middle East, Africa, and Asia, a smaller meat portion will usually be balanced with substantial helpings of grains and vegetables. As with every aspect of Ayurveda, the emphasis is on balance.

My main recommendation regarding vegetarianism is always to eat with awareness. Whatever you are bringing into your mind or body, do so consciously and with honor and respect, offering your appreciation to the source of your nourishment.

9

The Wisdom of Herbs

"Come forth into the light of things.
Let Nature be your teacher."

William Wordsworth

"You Herbs, born at the birth of time
More ancient than the gods themselves.
O Plants, with this hymn I sing to you
Our mothers and our gods."

The Rig Veda

The intimate relationship between the plants and animals of our earth began hundreds of millions of years ago, when early life-forms became organized into the predecessors of our vegetable and animal kingdoms. Without the magnificent botanical alchemy that captures the energy of the sun ninety-three million miles away and converts it into carbohydrates and oxygen, no animal could survive.

Mind body medicine recognizes and honors the interconnected relationships of all living beings on earth. No single individual or species is viewed in isolation from the larger ecology in which it exists. Within this context, plants are seen as sources of nourishment and healing. In every culture throughout history, human beings have honored plants and herbs for their medicinal value and have viewed them as gifts of nature. The plant kingdom has always been held in particularly high esteem by the Vedic tradition, and the Upanishads extol the role of plants in our universe:

The essence of all beings is earth.

The essence of earth is water.

The essence of water is plants.

The essence of plants is the human being.

It's only recently that the term *medicine* has been applied to synthesized drugs as well as to naturally derived substances. With the development of modern pharmacology and the appearance of "wonder drugs," botanical sources have been largely replaced as primary healing substances. But this abandonment of natural materials has extracted a toll in the form of drug-induced side effects on patients and increasingly drug-resistant forms of infection.

With our increased reliance on chemically synthesized drugs used in Western medicine, we tend to forget that over 125 medicines in current use are derived from over 40 species of plants.[1] Recent surveys have shown that almost 25 percent of all prescriptions dispensed in the United States contain products from botanical sources.[2] It is estimated that less than 10 percent of the world's estimated half a million plant species have been analyzed for medicinal activity, so that it is obvious that we have only scratched the surface of the potential healing power of our plant kingdom.[3]

I urge you to think of herbal substances as subtle forms of nutrition rather than as medicines. Herbs can be beneficial in early stages of physiological imbalance, and can complement other treatments when more advanced illness arises. I do not support herbal allopathy, in which a botanical formula is taken for every symptom without looking for the cause of the underlying imbalance; I do honor healing plants as a valuable part of a holistic mind body program.

Ayurvedic herbology includes almost twenty thousand plants, many of which have been categorized according to their benefit for more than four thousand years. This chapter provides an overview of some classical Ayurvedic formulas that we have been using, and that have been developed with the close assistance of leading Ayurvedic physicians. Once again, I believe these herbal nutritional formulas should be understood as providers of subtle nutrition to the cells and tissues, rather than as active pharmaceuticals. This is very much in keeping with the Ayurvedic approach that foods and herbs are part of the same continuum.

Twenty-five Important Ayurvedic Herbs

Throughout *The Wisdom of Healing*, I make reference to traditional nutritional herbs. The most commonly used Ayurvedic herbs are described in greater detail below. Each of the herbs is characterized according to its rasa, or taste; its virya, or potency for heating or cooling; its vipaka, or postdigestive effect; and its prabhava, or special action.

The Sanskrit name of each herb, its Latin name, and its English name (if available) are listed first. Each herb's energetics and influence on the three doshas is then presented, followed by the imbalances for which the herb is commonly prescribed.

Most of these herbs and spices are readily available in the West through local health-food stores, Indian and Middle Eastern food stores, and from nutritional herb and spice importers. Sources are listed in the reference section for this chapter. Again, we emphasize—these gifts of nature are not a substitute for medical care or appropriate medications. Before using these herbs and spices as part of a complete mind body program, please discuss them with your health-care provider.

1. *Ajwan* *Apium graveolens* **Wild celery seeds**
   rasa—**Pungent** *virya*—**Heating** *vipaka*—**Pungent**
   ↓ **K,V** ↑ **P**

Ajwan belongs to the Umbelliferae botanical family, which also includes anise, coriander, cumin, dill, and fennel. All these herbs are useful to enhance digestion and reduce bloating after a meal. A teaspoon of ajwan with a pinch of salt stimulates agni and reduces ama. In addition to helping with intestinal colic, it is commonly used to decrease respiratory congestion associated with colds, bronchitis, and asthma. An oil derived from the seeds has demonstrable tranquilizing effects.[4]

2. *Amalaki* *Emblica officinalis* *Emblic myrobalan*
   rasa—**All tastes** *virya*—**Cooling** *vipaka*—**Sweet**
   but salty
   ↓ **P,V** ↑ **K**

Amalaki is one of the most potent Ayurvedic rejuvenatives. It is the highest source of vitamin C known, with some laboratories reporting that it contains up to 720 milligrams of ascorbic acid per 100 grams of fresh pulp.[5] Its name in Sanskrit means "the sustainer," and it is traditionally used to provide nourishment to all the tissues. It has antibacterial and antiviral activity and is classically used in a wide range of debilitating conditions. It is commonly recommended to nourish the blood, skin, liver, and bone.

3. *Andraka* (fresh)   *Zingiber officinale*   **Ginger**
   Sunthi (dry)
   rasa—Pungent,   *virya*—Heating   *vipaka*—Sweet
   sweet
   ↓ V,K ↑ P

Ginger root is used in the culinary and healing arts around the world. Another name for ginger in Sanskrit means "the universal medicine." Fresh ginger strengthens the agnis without aggravating Pitta. It can be cooked in food or taken as a tea. When chewed with salt or lemon before a meal, it stimulates the appetite. Ginger reduces ama and helps with elimination. It is also an expectorant, is cleansing to the respiratory tract, and has been shown to reduce nausea associated with motion sickness.[6]

4. *Arjuna*   *Terminalia arjuna*   *Arjuna myrobalan*
   rasa—Astringent   *virya*—Cooling   *vipaka*—Pungent
   ↓ P ↑ K,V

Arjuna is the classical "heart tonic."[7] The traditional Ayurvedic literature does not discriminate among the many varieties of heart problems known to Western medicine. In fact, arjuna is used for both emotional and physical heart weaknesses. The Sanskrit word means "not twisted" or "open-hearted." Some studies have suggested that it has mild diuretic action and reduces blood lipids.

5. *Ashwagandha*   *Withania somnifera*   **Winter cherry**
   rasa—Bitter,   *virya*—Heating   *vipaka*—Sweet
   astringent, sweet
   ↓ V,K ↑ P

Ashwagandha has many uses in Ayurveda. Its leaves are said to be calming to the mind while the roots are used as a potent rejuvenative, particularly for men.[8] Its name in Sanskrit means "the smell of a horse," implying that its consumption imparts

the power of a stallion. It is used as a nutritive for the neuromuscular system and is traditionally used to relieve aches and
rheumatism.

6. *Bala*	*Sida cordifolia*	**Country mallow**
rasa—Sweet	*virya*—Cooling	*vipaka*—Sweet
V,P,K =		

Bala is related to the marshmallow plant. It is considered a rejuvenative for the heart and nervous system. Its Sanskrit name
means "provider of strength and immunity." It contains an alkaloid related to ephedrine, which may explain some of its ener-
gizing effects, but should also be used cautiously in anyone with
high blood pressure.[9] It has been classically used in people with
rheumatism and urinary-tract irritations.

7. *Bhringaraj*	*Eclipta alba*	
rasa—Pungent,	*virya*—Heating	*vipaka*—Sweet
bitter, sweet		
V,P,K =		

An herbalized oil of bhringaraj is widely used in Asia as a hair
tonic. It is also commonly applied to the scalp to relieve
headaches and calm an agitated mind. Internally, it is considered purifying to the blood and liver and has demonstrated
antiviral activity.[10] In Chinese medicine, it is recommended for
chronic pulmonary infections and hepatitis. It is found widely
throughout India and Pakistan.

8. *Brahmi*	*Centella asiatica*	**Indian pennywort**
rasa—Bitter	*virya*—Cooling	*vipaka*—Sweet
V,P,K =		

Brahmi is the classical Ayurvedic herb to nourish the nervous
system. Its name in Sanskrit means "that which expands awareness." It is used as a blood cleanser and in chronic skin conditions. It is cooling to the system and has a particular balancing
effect on Sadhaka Pitta, the discriminating aspect of the mind.
Studies have shown a calming effect on the central nervous
system.[11]

9. *Eranda*	*Ricinus communis*	**Castor oil**
rasa—**Pungent, bitter, sweet**	*virya*—**Heating**	*vipaka*—**Pungent**

↓ V ↑ P,K

Castor oil has multiple important uses in Ayurveda. Derived from the bean of the castor plant, the oil can be applied externally via massage for muscular aches and pains. Internally it is a strong purgative, acting on the small intestines by reducing absorption of salts and fluids and stimulating intestinal action. It is used in Ayurveda to treat gout and arthritis and in very small doses to treat food poisoning and intestinal colic. It should not be used on a long-term basis and is to be completely avoided in pregnancy as it can stimulate uterine contractions.

10. *Gokshura*	*Tribulis terrestris*	**Caltrops**
rasa—**Sweet, bitter**	*virya*—**Cooling**	*vipaka*—**Sweet**

V,P,K =

Gokshura is a plant that is commonly found wild in the United States. It is soothing to the mucous membranes and has been traditionally used as a rejuvenative for the urinary tract. It is lubricating to the throat and used in chronic coughs. Gokshura is also said to be calming to the nervous system. It has been found to contain essential oils and nitrates, which may account for its reputed diuretic action.[12]

11. *Guduchi*	*Tinospora cordifolia*	**Heart-leaf**
rasa—**Bitter, sweet**	*virya*—**Heating**	**moonseed**
		vipaka—**Sweet**

V,P,K =

Another Sanskrit name for guduchi is *amrit,* which means "immortality." It has a heating quality, which stimulates the agnis to digest ama, but it does not generally aggravate Pitta. It is sometimes known as "Indian quinine" for its effect on chronic fevers. It is traditionally used in people with skin disorders, rheumatism, and urinary problems.

12. *Guggulu*	*Commiphora mukul*	Indian gum myrrh
rasa—Bitter,	*virya*—Heating	*vipaka*—Pungent
pungent, astringent		
↓ K,V ↑ P		

Studies on this resin have demonstrated a measurable cholesterol-lowering effect.[13] In traditional healing systems it is used for a wide variety of complaints including arthritis, menstrual irregularities, and chronic infections of the lungs and skin. It can be used as a mouthwash and gargle for gingivitis and sore throats.

13. *Haridra*	*Curcuma longa*	Turmeric
rasa—Bitter,	*virya*—Heating	*vipaka*—Pungent
astringent		
↓ K ↑ P,V		

Turmeric has been used as a culinary spice, cosmetic agent, and medicinal herb. It holds an important place in Ayurveda as a natural anti-inflammatory, useful in rheumatic and skin conditions.[14] Its Sanskrit name means "carry away illness." It is a natural antibiotic and blood cleanser and is nourishing to all the tissues. It is traditionally used topically for skin eruptions.

14. *Haritaki*	*Terminalia chebulia*	Chebulic
rasa—All tastes	*virya*—Heating	myrobalan
but saline		*vipaka*—Sweet
V,P,K =		

Haritaki is held to be one of the most important Ayurvedic herbs. Like turmeric, its Sanskrit name also means "that which carries away disease." It is a powerful rejuvenative, particularly for Vata imbalances. It is a good astringent for external use. Haritaki is the basis of triphala, a widely used bowel tonic.

15. *Hing*	*Ferula asafoetida*	Asafetida
rasa—Pungent	*virya*—Heating	*vipaka*—Pungent
↓ V,K ↑ P		

Asafetida is a potent root resin that has been traditionally used as a digestive aid. It stimulates elimination while reducing and dispelling intestinal gas. When added to the cooking of beans, it reduces bloating and gaseousness. Among its many Vata-pacifying properties, hing is calming to the nervous system. It has anitmicrobial activity against diarrhea-producing bacteria.[15]

16. *Jatamamsi*   *Nardostachys jatamamsi*   **Muskroot**
    rasa—Bitter,   *virya*—Cooling   *vipaka*—Pungent
    astringent, sweet
    V,P,K =

Jatamamsi is another important nervine, or nervous-system bal-ancer. Its Sanskrit name means "clustered hair," which describes the roots of the plant. Although calming to the mind, it is said to promote awareness.[16] It has demonstrated antibacterial and antifungal activity. Jatamamsi has been shown to lower blood pressure in animal studies and traditionally has been used as a cardiovascular rejuvenative.

17. *Jatiphala*   *Myristica fragrans*   **Nutmeg**
    rasa—Pungent   *virya*—Heating   *vipaka*—Pungent
    ↓ V,K ↑ P

This tall tropical tree does not produce its fruit, of which nut-meg is the seed, until its ninth or tenth year. It has a calming effect on each physiological system it influences. When used for digestion, it relieves abdominal cramping and reduces diarrhea. Added to warm milk before bedtime, nutmeg has a soothing effect, inducing a sound sleep.

18. *Kapikacchu*   *Mucuna pruriens*   **Cow-itch plant**
    rasa—Sweet   *virya*—Heating   *vipaka*—Sweet
    ↓ V ↑ P,K

Kapikacchu is another useful nutritive herb that is classically used as a nervous-system and kidney tonic. It has been shown in some studies to have a mild positive effect in Parkinson's dis-ease.[17] It is often recommended by Ayurvedic doctors for weak-nesses in the reproductive system. Some reports have suggested that it can help to lower blood lipids.

19. *Katuka*   *Picrorhiza kurroa*

rasa—Bitter,   *virya*—Heating   *vipaka*—Pungent

pungent

↓ P,K ↑ V

Katuka, also known as kutki, is a powerful liver and gall-bladder detoxifier. It is a mild laxative in low doses and has a fever-lowering effect. It has been studied in people with infectious hepatitis and jaundice and found to accelerate their recovery.[18] It has also been beneficial in patients with asthma and can reduce serum cholesterol.

20. *Kumari*   *Aloe vera*   **Aloe**

rasa—Bitter,   *virya*—Cooling   *vipaka*—Sweet

astringent, sweet

VPK =

This popular succulent has been used externally in many cultures to hasten wound and burn healing. According to Ayurveda it is also useful taken internally as a juice and is considered to be an alterative, or "blood cleanser." Its Sanskrit name means "providing the energy of youth." Aloe is a tonic for all the agnis and is traditionally used as a rejuvenative for the liver and female reproductive tract. It has been shown to accelerate healing after burn and frostbite injuries.[19]

21. *Neem*   *Azadiracta indica*   **Persian lilac**

rasa—Bitter   *virya*—Cooling   *vipaka*—Pungent

↓ P,K ↑ V

Neem is highly prized for the bitter and aromatic flavor it imparts to food. It is considered one of the most effective food alteratives (blood purifiers) in Ayurveda. Extracts of neem have been shown to have potent antibiotic properties.[20] Neem has classically been used to reduce the heat of chronic fevers. It is one of the traditional herbs used in chronic skin disorders.

22. *Shankhapushpi*   *Canscora decussata*   **Dankuni plant**
    rasa—Astringent   *virya*—Heating   *vipaka*—Pungent
    ↓ V,P ↑ K

Shankhapushpi is one of the most effective Ayurvedic nervines. It has traditionally been used for neuralgias and in rheumatic conditions. It is nourishing to all the tissues and combines well with brahmi to quiet a restless mind.

23. *Shatavari*   *Asparagus racemosus*   **Indian asparagus**
    rasa—Sweet, bitter   *virya*—Cooling   *vipaka*—Sweet
    ↓ P,V ↑ K

Shatavari is the major Ayurvedic rejuvenative for women. Its name in Sanskrit means "able to have one hundred husbands," and it is said to be nourishing to the female reproductive system. Shatavari is soothing to mucous membranes and used to calm stomach upset. It is not recommended in fibrocystic breast condition or uterine fibroids. Extracts of Shatavari have been shown to slow the growth of certain cancer cells in tissue cultures.

24. *Tulsi*   *Ocinum sanctum*   **Holy basil**
    rasa—Pungent   *virya*—Heating   *vipaka*—Pungent
    ↓V,K ↑ P

Tulsi, which is a form of basil, has long been used for its purifying influence. In India, many families keep a plant in their homes, where it is held to create an atmosphere of peace and prosperity. As a tea, it has traditionally been used for children with stomach aches, and taken with honey, it quiets coughs and reduces congestion. A paste of the leaves applied externally is useful to reduce the irritation of insect bites. Essential oils derived from the leaves of tulsi have antibacterial and antifungal activity.[21]

25. *Yasti madhu*   *Glycyrrhiza glabra*   **Licorice**
    rasa—Sweet, bitter   *virya*—Cooling   *vipaka*—Sweet
    ↓ V,P ↑ K

Licorice is soothing to all the tissues, particularly the mucous membranes. It has been used in both Ayurveda and Western herbal systems to help liquefy and mobilize respiratory mucus.

Its name in Sanskrit means "honey stick." It provides relief for ulcer pain. Licorice has a deoxycorticosterone steroid effect, which may explain its traditional use in inflammatory conditions, but if it is overused it can cause fluid retention and electrolye imbalances.[22]

Simple Herbal Formulas

Below are several simple herbal formulas that can be helpful in a variety of minor health concerns. These nutritional aids have been readily available in India, and most are now more easily accessible in the West.

1. **Trikatu "The Three Pungents" Dry Ginger, Black Pepper, Long Pepper**
   Trikatu consists of the three hot spices. These are classically used to stimulate the appetite and increase the digestive fire in people with weak agnis. It burns away ama but must be used with caution as its strong heating quality may aggravate Pitta. If long pepper (*pippali, Piper longum*) is not available, cayenne pepper may be substituted.

2. **Triphala "The Three Fruits" Chebulic, Emblic, and Beleric Myrobalan**
   Triphala is the classical Ayurvedic bowel tonic. It can be taken on a daily basis before bedtime to ensure a regular morning evacuation. Triphala is an excellent and balanced rejuvenative and helps to remove stagnated ama.

3. **"The Three Cooling Spices" Fennel, Cumin, and Coriander**
   Roasting the seeds of these three herbs and taking a pinch before and after meals helps to stimulate the digestive fire without aggravating Pitta. If there is weak digestion but a sensitivity to hot spices, the three cooling spices can help improve the appetite and digestion without causing hyperacidity.

4. **"The Three Aromatics" Cinnamon, Cardamom, and Bay**
   These three spices help to improve digestion, absorption, and elimination. They are particularly helpful in reducing discomfort due to gaseous stagnation. A tea can be made to relieve abdominal bloating in individuals with delicate digestions.

Herbal-Combination Formulas

A fundamental principle in Western medicine is to use a single pharmaceutical agent whenever possible so the drug responsible for the
therapeutic effect can be identified. If the patient has an adverse
reaction, the physician can more readily identify the offending agent.
In herbal medicine, combinations are the rule rather than the exception. The combining of herbs into balanced recipes is consistent with
the view that herbs are subtle nutritional supplements. In the same
way that a nutritious meal has a blend of different tastes and textures,
an effective herbal formula is composed of a blend of balancing
botanical substances.

Ayurvedic formulas are traditionally used to nourish the mind
body physiology in a variety of situations. They should not be thought
of as pharmaceuticals and should not be taken as substitutes for any
medication prescribed by a physician. I look upon them as herbal
nutritional supplements for improving the quality of the tissues and
for balancing the doshas.

A general herbal tonic known as Chavan prash has been used for
thousands of years in the East. Named after the Ayurvedic physician
who developed it, this complex fruit-and-herb mixture has been
shown to have potent antioxidant properties. The principal ingredient is amalaki, which is the highest known natural source of vitamin
C. It is usually combined with sweetener, ghee, long pepper, and over
thirty other herbs. Widely available under a variety of labels, a teaspoon twice daily is recommended for general well being. It should
be avoided by diabetics due to its high sugar content.

Formulas combining herbs specifically for men or women are
commonly recommended. Ashwagandha, kapikacchu, and gokshura
are important constituents of a male tonic, which may be recommended to increase general vitality or sexual potency. Shatavari,
amalaki, rose, and aloe are often suggested for women with menstrual discomforts.

Digestive aids may include trikatu (ginger, black pepper, long
pepper) to increase digestive power, and shatavari, amalaki, and yasti
madhu to reduce excess stomach acid. A variety of herbal agents may
be taken in combination to enhance bowel regularity, including
haritaki, ajwan, hing, and psyllium.

Expectorant herbs combined with those that soothe mucous membranes can be helpful when a person is troubled by cough and congestion. The combination of basil, licorice, cloves, and ginger can provide relief for the symptoms of a viral upper-respiratory infection.

The above examples illustrate the possibilities of using the gifts of the plant kingdom to relieve human suffering. If you have the time and inclination, try creating and mixing your own formulas. Suggestions for other blends are described in the herbal reference books for this chapter.

Using the Right Tool

I have previously discussed the importance of using the best and most appropriate intervention for each problem, and this is particularly important when it comes to herbal supplements. In early stages of imbalance, herbs can be invaluable to provide the necessary nudge back toward homeostasis. Whether it is a mild agent to reestablish normal elimination or a calming herb to help with occasional insomnia, I deeply honor these gentle plants for the gifts they bring. It is equally important, however, not to expect more from these subtle agents of nature than they can provide. I fully support the usage of a medication when it is clearly indicated, be it an antibiotic for a bacterial infection or a chemotherapy drug for metastatic cancer. The science that led to the discovery of the important pharmaceuticals of our time is also a product of nature's intelligence and is worthy of respect. By expanding our repertoire of healing options, we can choose the approach that offers the greatest potential benefit for the least possible risk.

Understanding Biological Rhythms: The Keys to Balance

"To everything there is a season,
and a time to every purpose under heaven."

Ecclesiastes

"Of what is the body made?
It is made of emptiness and rhythm.
At the ultimate heart of the body, at the heart of the world,
there is no solidity . . . there is only the dance."

George Leonard

A friend of mine was in his forties when he become a dedicated runner. Though twenty pounds overweight when he took up the sport, he quickly achieved a high level of conditioning and really seemed to have an affinity for running. Before long he was able to run weekly mileage equal to his age, and there were days when he felt he could have gone twice that far. Usually he ran in the late afternoon or early evening, when the temperature began to fall. Running was a kind of meditation, a genuine form of rest-ful awareness. At the age of forty-five he signed up to run in his first marathon, and he trained diligently. Since the race would begin in the early morning, he rescheduled his final training runs for six A.M., rather than later in the day, as had been his custom. Running in the morning would be a new and enjoyable experience, with the sun coming up over the trees instead of setting behind them, and a morning run would be good preparation for the marathon itself.

By this time my friend was capable of running more than seventy miles in a week. But, almost incredibly, the first time he hit the trail at sun-rise he was barely able to run a mile before his legs cramped and his stom-ach ached.

Biological Rhythms

Life flows in patterns of rest and activity. According to the Bible, God's first creation after heaven and earth was light, which led to the twenty-four-hour cycle of day and night. According to Vedic knowledge, the entire universe is a symphony of rhythms. We are healthy when we are in synchrony with the dance of nature; we feel dis-eased when we have lost our rhythm. Almost everyone has had the experience of feeling out of sorts when making a cross-country journey. Our biological rhythms need to be in harmony with the environment, and until this occurs, we feel dissonant.

Most societies across time have recognized the need to be in tune with natural rhythms. Festivals celebrating the spring planting and the autumn harvesting are universal cultural events, because we have a fundamental human need to be part of the eternal cadence of the cosmos. The evolution of life on this planet is inextricably linked with natural cycles, so that inherent rhythms can be demonstrated in almost every plant and animal on earth, from one-celled organisms to human beings.

A branch of science, chronobiology, has evolved over the last several decades, dedicated to understanding biological rhythms. Cyclical patterns have been discovered in almost every aspect of life, from the division of cells to the secretion of hormones to the metabolism of drugs to the timing of asthma attacks. From day to day, and even minute to minute, our bodies are undergoing constant transformation. Most of us are aware of the most obvious changes—gaining or losing weight, for instance—and we may even recognize that changes in our diet or exercise underlie them. But there are other influences affecting the mind body system that most of us fail to recognize. In recent years, research on the causes of insomnia, jet lag, and depression have brought heightened awareness of biological rhythms in the West. Ayurveda can be of great value in this area, for it has always recognized that the "temporal setting"—the time in which an action is performed—is as important as the physical setting or any other element of the undertaking. Here too the Ayurvedic viewpoint is a genuinely holistic one, emphasizing that one aspect of an experience cannot be separated or isolated from others.

There are at least four oscillations that take place in accordance with distinct rhythms in the human body. The first of these is a twenty-four-hour cycle that Western medicine calls circadian rhythm, from the Latin words *circa,* meaning "nearly" or "approximately," and *dia,* meaning "day." Like the earth itself, each of us has a cycle of day and night, and this circadian rhythm can be identified at many levels. Many hormonal fluctuations follow twenty-four-hour rhythms, including the secretion of cortisol, growth hormone, insulin, and the sex hormones.[1] The enzymes in our liver wax and wane according to a twenty-four-hour cycle so that our ability to burn alcohol is greater at nine P.M. than it is at nine A.M.[2] Interestingly, however, our brain's response to alcohol also fluctuates throughout the day, so a glass of wine at eleven P.M. is much more likely to intoxicate than a glass at eleven A.M.[3] Our body temperature also goes through a daily cycle, peaking at about five P.M., while reaching its trough in the early morning.[4,5] Our moods, our mental agility, and our fine motor skills all cycle throughout the day with relatively predictable highs and lows. Our cells, even when removed from our body, have a twenty-four-hour rhythm with daily peaks and troughs of reproductive activity.[6]

The existence of circadian rhythms has important implications for the treatment of disease. Chemotherapy administered to animals may be lethal at certain times of the day, but at other times the same treatment can be administered with minimal toxic effects.[7] Awareness of this principle can help us minimize the side effects and maximize the benefits of potent anticancer drugs, for malignant cells usually lose their normal rhythms, multiplying at high rates throughout the day.

A second biological rhythm is based on the twenty-nine-day cycle of the lunar month. Pituitary hormones that regulate the menstrual cycle, LH (luteinizing hormone) and FSH (follicle-stimulating hormone), have monthly peaks that are also associated with subtle but reproducible changes in a woman's sexual desire.[8] Women's perception of pain also goes through a monthly rhythm, with peak sensitivity during the latter half of the menstrual cycle.[9] Surprisingly, our ability to perceive orange and red colors also oscillates on a monthly basis, being more acute at the time of the full moon.[10] There are also subtle changes in our body fluids and blood chemistry that seem to have a relationship to a monthly pattern.

Tidal rhythms are based upon the gravitational effects of the moon on the earth. These are the influences that govern the ocean tides, and in a sense each of us has an internal "ocean," which behaves similarly to the ocean outside. It's as if we, human beings, actually brought the ocean with us in our physiology when we emerged from the water millions of years ago. The tidal rhythms are most obvious in animals that live along the shoreline. Fiddler crabs, for example, hide in underground burrows during high tide but become very active during low tide, feeding, fighting, and mating. Amazing experiments have shown that you can remove these crabs from their natural environment and place them in containers with constant light and temperature, and they will still have bursts of activity during the times of the low tides even though they are far removed from the ocean's ebb and flow![11]

Annual cycles too affect us at all levels. People simply feel different during different seasons of the year, often falling in love in spring, getting depressed in winter, and tending toward laziness during the long, hot days of summer. In recent years a condition known as seasonal affective disorder, or SAD, has been recognized to cause depression during the short days of winter. Exposure to very bright lights can often benefit this problem.[12] Animals that hibernate will have annual bursts of feeding activity that cannot be easily altered, even if temperature and light intensity are controlled.

When each of these biological rhythms is in harmony, there is energy, joy, and immunity to illness. When they are disrupted for any reason, there may be fatigue, emotional instability, and even serious illness.

Entrainment

Entrainment takes place when the rhythms of our mind body system are in complete harmony with the rhythms of the environment— when the music inside our body is perfectly synchronized with the music of nature.

Studies over the last several years have suggested that there are centers in our brain that are responsible for keeping and calling out the beat to keep the cells in our body aligned with the cycles of the environment. A place at the base of the brain called the suprachiasmatic nucleus, or SCN, receives input directly from our eyes and responds to changes in the amount of daily sunlight.[13] Messages sent out from this biological conductor ensure that other parts of the brain are in tune with daily and seasonal cycles. For example, the chemical melatonin, which is receiving a lot of attention these days for its benefit in treating jet lag and insomnia, is regulated by the SCN.

Entrainment also takes place between people. Babies entrain to their mother's heartbeats while still in the womb, and the process of infant bonding can be understood as a continuation of this. Falling in love is another form of entrainment, with new lovers often experiencing similar sleep-wake cycles and emotional patterns. In environments such as prisons, dormitories, and convents, where groups of women live together for long periods of time, there is often a synchronization of their menstrual cycles.

We can entrain with the environment, we can entrain with each other, but Ayurveda suggests that the ultimate entrainment is between our individuality and our universality. Whether we call it God, spirit, or the field of pure potentiality, entrainment is an attempt to establish an intimate relationship with the source of our own being. At some level, all mind body techniques are designed to foster this experience. These techniques are intended to help our awareness to reach the silent field within. Meditation procedures in particular can allow us to directly contact the realm of pure awareness, from which all the laws of nature arise.

Daily Cycles and the Doshas

Ayurveda very specifically describes the effects of daily and seasonal influences on our doshas. Once these environmental effects are understood, it's easy to make life choices that enhance balance and promote good health.

DAILY CYCLES

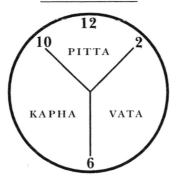

6 A.M. to 10 A.M. — KAPHA	6 P.M. to 10 P.M. — KAPHA
10 A.M. to 2 P.M. — PITTA	10 P.M. to 2 A.M. — PITTA
2 P.M. to 6 P.M. — VATA	2 A.M. to 6 A.M. — VATA

Kapha dosha predominates from six to ten in the morning, so between these hours your body is likely to feel slow, heavy, and relaxed. The period of peak metabolic activity and appetite occurs at noon, during the middle of the first *Pitta* period. Pitta, of course, is responsible for metabolizing food and distributing energy throughout the body. *Vata* dosha, which governs the nervous system, is predominant in the late afternoon, when mental activities and physical dexterity are most efficient.

The day's second cycle begins at 6 P.M., when the *Kapha* influence tends to create a slow, relaxed evening. During the nighttime *Pitta* period the physiology metabolizes the evening meal, but since the body is asleep during this 10 P.M. to 2 A.M. period, energy can be converted into warmth and the rebuilding of tissues. The early-morning *Vata* time activates the nervous system in the form REM sleep, during which a high level of dream activity occurs.

According to Ayurveda, you can encourage good health by synchronizing your daily routine with natural rhythms. Awakening before dawn during the end of the Vata period allows you to take advantage of the Vata qualities of alertness and energy. Eating your main meal during the noon hour when Pitta fire is strongest ensures strong digestion. Going to bed by 10 P.M. at the end of the Kapha period takes advantage of the slow Kapha qualities and fosters sound sleep.

Daily Routine

The schedule below is recommended for maintaining optimal physiological rhythms. Without becoming compulsive about it—which would create stress of its own—you should make an attempt to follow these suggestions.

ARISING: 6 TO 8 A.M.
- Wake without an alarm clock
- Brush your teeth and clean your tongue
- Drink a glass of warm water to encourage regular elimination
- Empty your bowels and bladder
- Massage your body with oil (abhyanga)
- Bathe
- Perform light exercise: Sun Salutes, yoga postures, breathing exercises
- Meditate
- Eat breakfast
- Take a midmorning walk

LUNCH: NOON TO 1 P.M.
- Eat lunch (the largest meal of the day)
- Sit quietly for five minutes after eating
- Walk to aid digestion (five to fifteen minutes)
- Meditate in the late afternoon

DINNER: 6 TO 7 P.M.
- Eat a light to moderate dinner
- Sit quietly for five minutes after eating
- Walk to aid digestion (five to fifteen minutes)

BEDTIME: 9:30 TO 10:30 P.M.
- Perform light activity in the evening
- Go to bed early, but at least three hours after dinner
- Do not read, eat, or watch TV in bed

Ayurveda stipulates that it's best to awaken without an alarm clock at about six A.M. However, there are people whose circadian rhythms have become so askew that they find it extremely difficult to get into this balance. If you have insomnia or if you have never paid much attention to any sort of lifestyle regularity, we recommend that you initially use an alarm clock and wake up very early (before five A.M.) every morning. If you follow this schedule for five days in a row and avoid napping during the day, you will definitely soon be drifting off to sleep by ten in the evening. This will reset your whole cycle.

Brush your teeth, gently cleaning the tongue if it is coated. The condition of the tongue in the morning is a gauge of how much ama, or accumulated toxicity, is present in the system. Ayurveda also recommends gargling with a small amount of sesame oil to lubricate the mucous membranes and protect your gums. Drink a glass of warm water after cleaning your mouth. This stimulates peristaltic motion so that you will be able to empty your bowels and bladder effortlessly.

You can perform a daily oil massage, or abhyanga, in just a few minutes before your bath or shower, and this has many benefits for your skin and general health (see pages 103–5). We also suggest a light set of yoga postures followed by Pranayama breathing exercises and a half hour of meditation. Then eat breakfast if you are hungry and take a little walk after your meal if you can.

Because digestive powers are strongest during the early afternoon, the noon meal should be the largest of the day. This was the natural practice in most cultures until the Industrial Revolution, when it became inconvenient for employees to take off two hours to eat a large midday lunch. A balanced, well-cooked meal at noon can have a very positive effect on your entire daily routine. Sit for a few minutes after lunch and take a short walk if possible.

Your second meditation period should take place in the late afternoon or in the early evening before dinner. This facilitates the release of accumulated stress and prepares you for your evening activities. Ayurveda recommends a light-to-moderate dinner around six P.M. Again, you should sit quietly for five minutes after eating and take a walk afterward to aid digestion.

Activity after dinner should be light. Bedtime should be no later than eleven P.M., and at least three hours after your last meal.

Seasonal Variations

Ayurveda recognizes that seasonal rhythms have important influences on our biological cycles. Each season expresses characteristics of a specific dosha. Autumn and early winter is Vata time with the cold, dry, and windy weather; the hot, moist summer expresses the qualities of Pitta; and the cold, wet weather of late winter and spring are expressions of Kapha in the environment.

Certain common conditions caused by a particular doshic imbalance tend to become aggravated during the season that expresses that dosha. Arthritis, for example, tends to worsen during the cold, dry Vata season. Tempers tend to flare and skin rashes become inflamed during the hot summer Pitta season. Colds and sinus congestion become common during the rainy Kapha periods. If you're a Vata type, you should be particularly careful about diet and daily routine in the autumn and early winter. This is the time to be certain to wear warm clothing, eat hot soups and casseroles, and try to get to bed at a regular hour. Pitta body types should be aware of the potential for Pitta aggravation during the summer. Here, the emphasis is on keeping cool. Regardless of your mind body type, you probably gravitate to the local Pitta-pacifying lake or ocean, eat cooling melons, and wear light clothing in the summer. For Kaphas, late winter and spring are times to take special care, making certain to stay warm and dry. This is a good time to increase your consumption of spicy foods.

Above all, we should never forget that the environment is our extended body and that nature has already provided everything we need in the appropriate place and at the appropriate time in order to sustain us. The more we are in tune with natural internal and external rhythms, the more we can accept and metabolize the nourishment that is so readily available.

The Cosmic Dance

Human beings evolved over millions of years in adaptation to a wide range of environments on this planet. Although our technology has been able to override many of the challenges of nature, our biology is still intimately connected with our pretechnological heritage.

According to Ayurveda, many illnesses reflect a lack of integration with our extended body. When we lose connection with nature, we lose connection with an essential aspect of ourselves.

Knowledge of how the rhythms of nature influence our mind body physiology can be used in very specific ways to enhance healing. Studies on people with allergies show that their sneezing, itchy eyes, and coughing have a circadian pattern, with most sufferers having their most troublesome symptoms in the morning (Kapha time). This suggests that interventions, either natural or pharmaceutical, should be instituted immediately upon awakening.

Many common medical problems, including asthma, high blood pressure, angina, and ulcer pain, all fluctuate according to fairly predictable daily or monthly patterns.[14] Knowing the specific cycle of an illness opens the possibility of new approaches to treatments that can take into account the rhythms of the person, the disease, and the therapeutic intervention.

This is particularly relevant to the treatment of cancer. Earlier in this chapter, I referred to studies on the application of chemotherapy at various times of the day. Unlike healthy cells, most cancer cells do not show a normal daily rhythm of rest and activity. They seem to be stuck in an "on" mode and consequently divide and reproduce in an uncontrolled manner. There are increasing efforts to time the administration of anticancer drugs or radiation therapy to take advantage of the resting phase of normal cells to minimize debilitating side effects.[15] Cells from different tissues seem to have different patterns, so a uniform time to administer treatment is not possible. Normal human bone-marrow cells, however, seem to have maximal activity in the hours around noon, with relative periods of rest around midnight.[16] Since chemotherapy attacks multiplying cells, providing treatment when normal cells are resting may minimize the toxicity. Although this effect is fairly well established in laboratory animals, it is just beginning to be explored clinically in people, so if you are facing cancer and possible chemotherapy, discuss the timing options with your physician.

Since it has apparently become so easy to ignore the natural rhythms around us, it may seem overly simplified to suggest that harmonizing with the rhythms of the earth, moon, and sun can improve our health. Yet, principles such as these can be found in every culture and every historical period. Benjamin Franklin's counsel of, "Early to bed and early to rise makes a man healthy, wealthy, and wise," may seem laughably naive today, but it expresses an important Ayurvedic principle. It's so easy to stay up late at night, sleep in during the day, and eat at all hours. We may not notice the incremental negative effects of these behaviors on our health—but loss of harmony with natural rhythms is often the start of a shift from balance to imbalance that can eventually affect every aspect of our lives. I encourage you to try some simple shift in your daily routine—get to bed a little earlier or try eating lighter at dinner—and see if you notice some benefit through harmonizing with your environment.

11

Detoxification, Purification, and Rejuvenation

"You can only cure retail, but you can prevent wholesale."

Brock Chisholm

When I was a medical student, I would sometimes hear people discussing the possible presence of toxins in their bodies. At that time there were a number of alternative health procedures that promised to eliminate putrefying matter from the system, and adventurous souls were beginning to try liver flushes, high-colonic enemas, and a variety of herbal cleanses. It was easy to visualize plaques of toxic matter lining the intestines like mud caked on the exhaust pipe of an off-road vehicle. By flushing out this fetid material, the various remedies offered more energy, greater happiness, and a new lease on life. I found it difficult to believe any of this, however. In my gastrointestinal service rotations I had peered into dozens of digestive tracts through fiberoptic scopes, and I had seen remarkably little evidence that our intestines were lined with pockets of compost heaps.

As a result of my clinical experience, I was initially skeptical about Ayurvedic descriptions of ama, and the attendant recommendations for eliminating these toxic residues. Since then, however, I've come to appreciate the subtlety of the concept of incompletely digested experiences, and I've also seen the benefits of taking steps to metabolize them more fully.

Ayurveda describes disease as the final expression of toxic accumulations in the mind body physiology. If we think of our bodies as systems that ingest, transform, and release energy, we can then envision situations in which the energy that enters the system overloads the capacity to either transform or release it. This indigestible energy destabilizes the system's balance, while procedures for releasing these accumulations can help us reestablish a healthy homeostatic state.

In order to clarify the cause and the treatment of these toxic accumulations from an Ayurvedic point of view, we should first briefly review the concepts of agni and ama. Agni, or "digestive fire," is the principle of conversion that metabolizes nourishment from the environment. When our agnis are strong, the packages of information and intelligence that we take from the environment are digested into their fundamental elements. These elements are absorbed into the mind body physiology, where they eventually become our cells and tissues. If we are healthy, any part of the digested material that is not useful is eliminated from the body.

The principle of agni is usually applied to the digestion of food, but it can apply to the metabolism of anything that enters into us from the environment. We can speak of intellectual agnis as the process of digesting new ideas, or emotional agnis whereby we metabolize feelings, or sensory agnis that process all sensory input. When we are exposed to a new theory or concept, for example, our mental agnis break it down into fundamental bits of information, process the conceptual elements, assimilate those that are nourishing to our "intellectual body," and eliminate those aspects that are not nourishing. All sensory input—sound, touch, sight, taste, or smell, as well as our emotional experiences—is processed in a similar way.

When agni is not functioning efficiently, toxins and impurities can accumulate. Ayurveda refers to these incompletely metabolized materials as ama, and their presence in the body's cells and channels of circulation disrupts the free flow of nourishment. Ama is described as heavy, thick, cold, and foul, while agni is light, clear, hot, and pure. Thus, there is a fundamental opposition between the two concepts, and the strengthening of agni will automatically diminish the presence of ama.

If ama has accumulated over a period of time our mental and physical functioning is diminished, because significant energy is required to overcome the obstructive effects of the toxicity. People with significant ama accumulation are often mentally fatigued, and they may experience generalized physical pain as well. Since the condition of the tongue reflects the presence of ama in the system, there is frequently an unpleasant white coating on the tongues of people with significant ama accumulations, which is particularly noticeable in the morning.

Since ama is usually associated with one of the three doshas, it's possible to have Vata, Pitta, or Kapha imbalances either with ama or without it. In any case, if there is significant toxicity in the system, it is difficult to restore balance to the doshas until the impurities have been eliminated. Ayurveda refers to this process of transformation as moving from a state of Sama (with ama) to one of Nirama (without ama.) Once the ama is reduced, more specific measures for balancing the doshas can be effective.

Keys to Ama Reduction

A healthy diet is one of the most important tools for reducing ama accumulation. If you feel that you have accumulated toxicity due to poor nutrition or the use of alcohol, cigarettes, or drugs, following an ama-reducing program for a few days or weeks can be a good start to a healthier lifestyle. Try following these recommendations, and notice any effects on your energy levels and general well being.

- Eat foods that are freshly prepared, nutritious, and appetizing; minimize canned foods and leftovers.
- Take foods that are lighter and easier to digest, such as rice, soups, and lentils.
- Favor freshly steamed or lightly sautéed vegetables.
- Avoid fried foods.
- Avoid cold foods and drinks.
- Temporarily reduce your intake of dairy products.
- Minimize fermented foods and drinks, including vinegar, pickled condiments, cheeses, and alcohol.
- Favor the lighter grains, such as barley or basmati rice.

- Reduce highly refined carbohydrates such as white flour and sugar.

- Reduce oily, heavy, or salty nuts; sunflower, pumpkin, or sesame seeds may be taken in small amounts.

- If animal products cannot be eliminated entirely, favor the white meat of turkey or chicken; minimize red meats.

Ayurvedic Detoxification: Panchakarma Therapy for Prevention and Treatment of Illness

The ancient procedures for eliminating accumulated impurities from the physiology are known in Ayurveda as *panchakarma*. *Pancha,* in Sanskrit, means "five," and *karma* means "action." Panchakarma, therefore, refers to the five actions that are considered the most powerful, purifying, and rejuvenative procedures in Ayurveda. In the ancient Vedic cultures, panchakarma was available only to the nobility. But now Ayurvedic centers are springing up around the world, providing unprecedented access to these powerful rejuvenative processes.

Traditionally, a few days of panchakarma are recommended at the change of seasons. Since the changing annual weather periods foster accumulation of a specific dosha, cleansing yourself at seasonal transitions can be very helpful for reducing or eliminating those accumulations. Thus, at the end of a cold, dry fall and early winter, Vata accumulates; at the end of a wet, cold spring, Kapha builds up; and by the end of a warm, humid summer, Pitta levels have significantly increased. These are the ideal times to undergo panchakarma to restore balance in the physiology.

Panchakarma is also a beneficial, powerful process for people who have manifest illness. At The Chopra Center for Well Being, many people facing serious diseases arrive filled with anxiety, fear, and pain; but after a week of these powerful cleansing and rejuvenative procedures their view of their problem is dramatically transformed. They begin to sleep better, their appetite improves, pain is reduced, and they are able to reach a higher level of well being. This shift, of course, occurs in both the mind and body of the individual.

Ayurveda emphasizes an active role for the patient in the care of his or her health. Panchakarma, however, is unique among Ayurvedic procedure in that the patient passively receives the therapeutic approaches of trained caregivers. The entire process is designed to facilitate the deep-rooted release of stress, and to encourage the patient to surrender to the healing process. There are three integrated components of the panchakarma process: the preparation phase, the principal procedures, and the post-procedure phase. In Sanskrit these are known as *Poorva karma, Pradhana karma,* and *Paschat karma.*

POORVA KARMA—PREPARATORY PROCEDURES

Poorva karma, which is designed to prepare the body for the elimination of imbalances, has two aspects: *Snehana,* or oleation, and *Swedena,* or heat treatment. Snehana includes both internal and external oiling of the system. According to Ayurveda, pure herbalized oils are able to permeate the cells and tissues, encouraging the release of stored toxicity. During the preparation phase, patients are instructed to take increasing quantities of herbalized oils by mouth, which are designed to lubricate the digestive system and mobilize toxicity so it can be eliminated. The clarified butter or ghee is herbalized with bitter Ayurvedic herbs; these enhance its ama-reducing qualities and also reportedly reduce its effect on cholesterol levels. If an individual has high cholesterol, however, ghee should be used very sparingly. As an alternative, chewing raw sesame seeds with raisins can provide useful internal Snehana and will not effect cholesterol.

Regardless of which oleating substance is used, the Ayurvedic therapeutic principle is always the same. The oils move from the gastrointestinal tract into the tissues. As they travel through the cells, they extract the accumulated ama, allowing it to be moved into the circulatory channels for elimination.

Oleation is also provided externally through massage. Ayurveda describes hundreds of massage therapies designed to loosen impurities from the tissues. The type of oil, the herbs used to prepare the oil, and the massage techniques all have specific effects. In panchakarma, massage serves principally as a technique for providing oil to the tissues, thus loosening impurities and allowing them to move into the gastrointestinal tract or the circulatory system for removal.

Swedena, or heat treatment, is the second component of the preparatory phase. It is also sometimes translated as fomentation therapy. The English word *sweat* is derived from the Sanskrit word *sweden,* and heat is an important preparatory aspect of panchakarma.

Many cultures have used heat therapeutically. Sweat lodges among Native American tribes provide a ritualized opportunity for physical and spiritual purification. Dry and wet saunas have been a standard feature of European health spas for centuries. Anyone who has experienced the relaxing pleasure of a steam room understands the benefit of therapeutic heat.

Ayurveda teaches that heating the system has two principle detoxifying effects: It facilitates the mobilization of ama, and it dilates the channels of circulation, thus speeding the elimination of impurities that have been loosened by oleation. Swedena techniques include hot baths, herbalized steam treatments, dry heat, hot-water bottles, very warm oils, exercise, exposure to the sun, pungent herbs taken internally, and the application of herbalized poultices. Particularly for people with Vata problems such as arthritis, chronic low back pain, or abdominal bloating, heat can provide prompt symptomatic relief.

To my knowledge, there is no scientific evidence that these elaborate oleation and heat treatments actually mobilize measurable toxic substances. It is, however, clearly obvious that these procedures create a profound state of relaxation in our patients. The rhythmic massages performed by paired Ayurvedic therapists provide synchronized nourishing stimulation to the nervous system, and the herbalized heat treatment provokes controlled sweating that is very purifying to the skin.

PRADHANA KARMA—PRINCIPAL PROCEDURES

Once the preparatory therapies have loosened and mobilized impurities, the principal procedures are begun in order to eliminate the toxins from the body. There are five classical elimination procedures, and these are known as panchakarma. At present, we are not using all five of these at The Chopra Center, but we will review them all here in the interest of providing a complete description.

Vamana is therapeutic emesis, or carefully controlled vomiting. It is traditionally used in severe Kapha conditions such as recurrent asthma, bronchitis, and sinus congestion. Because the stomach is one of the major sites of Kapha in the physiology, cleansing this region reduces the accumulation of ama associated with Kapha. The patient is prepared with oleation and heat, and is then given a large volume of herbalized tea to drink. Finally, a small quantity of a potent herbal emetic induces a smooth emesis, and the volume is recorded.

Although the induction of vomiting is not a major component of Western medicine, it is occasionally used when a noncaustic poison has been consumed. The most commonly used agent in the West is emetine, also known as Brazil root, an alkaloid derived from ipecac. Animals in the wild often eat plants and grasses to induce vomiting if something is upsetting their digestion, and this is occasionally seen in household cats and dogs as well.

Virechana means purgation. In the context of panchakarma it refers to the movement of gastrointestinal contents out through the colon. Most of the important Ayurvedic purgatives act principally upon the small intestine, which is a major site of Pitta. Virechana, therefore, is one of the most effective modalities for removing ama that is associated with a Pitta accumulation.

Before receiving an herbal laxative, the patient is prepared with oleation and heat. Increasing quantities of herbalized oil are provided for four to seven days, and a hot bath is recommended before the purgative is given. At The Chopra Center we tend to use either castor oil or senna, which stimulates several movements within four to eight hours after taking the dosage. The laxative is usually taken before going to bed so it will have an effect early the next morning.

We do not recommend taking laxatives on a regular basis as they can create laziness in elimination. We recommend that Virechana only be performed under the supervision of a trained health provider. It is traditionally used for relieving Pitta accumulations in people with certain skin rashes, inflammatory arthritis, migraines, or chronic irritability, and in women with severe premenstrual discomfort.

Nasya refers to the application of herbalized substances through the nasal passages. Many different herbs are used and for the most part are enjoyable to receive; they are very useful in cleansing the sinuses and in calming or clearing the mind. To begin, a vigorous head-and-neck massage with herbalized oil is provided. Then heat is applied in the form of herbalized steam and hot packs, which are placed over the sinus areas. Finally, drops of herbalized oil are gently introduced into each nostril, and the patient sniffs the oil back into the nasal pharynx.

Nasya can be very effective in the treatment of chronic sinus congestion and allergic rhinitis. Conditions such as anxiety, insomnia, and headaches can also be relieved with the appropriate application of Nasya, and the procedures can be easily performed at home to alleviate mild upper-respiratory symptoms. At the onset of a cold, inhaling the steam of boiling water to which a few drops of eucalyptus oil has been added can provide rapid temporary decongestion. If this is done several times a day, sedating over-the-counter remedies may be avoided.

Basti is the administration of herbalized enemas. According to Ayurveda, the colon is one of the major sites of Vata in the mind body physiology, and the application of herbs through the large intestines is the most effective way to balance Vata and remove impurities.

There are two types of Basti: *Anuvasana* and *Niruha*. Anuvasana Bastis are oil-based and are primarily pacifying to Vata. The oil-based preparations usually use sesame oil and are administered in quantities of approximately eighty cc's. They are lubricating to the rectal area and are very soothing for hemorrhoids and mild constipation. Niruha Bastis are water-based decoctions and are primarily eliminative. They are decoctions of five to fifteen herbs and are administered in volumes of about a cup. In addition to facilitating elimination, the water-based decoctions also have a nutritive effect.

Ayurvedic texts devote a great deal of attention to Bastis. In ancient times, administering medicinal herbs via the colon was a very effective means of making the healing herb available to the system, particularly if the patient was unable to take things by mouth. Preparing the herbs in water- and oil-based solutions significantly enhances their absorption. In modern practice, medications are sometimes applied rectally because they cannot be given intravenously. Valproic acid, for example, is an anti-epilepsy medicine that is sometimes administered via an enema in patients with uncontrolled seizures, and it has been shown to achieve therapeutic blood concentrations.

The fifth and final purifying procedure is *Rakta Mokshana,* or therapeutic blood cleansing. Although historically this has involved the removal of small quantities of blood, this has not been routinely practiced in India for centuries and is not an acceptable method in the West. We apply the principles of these purification procedures by using natural herbal formulas that are considered alteratives, or blood cleansers.

Interestingly, although bloodletting sounds very primitive, modern medicine does make use of the practice in a number of conditions. Hemodialysis for renal disease, and plasma exchange for a host of neurological conditions, can be considered forms of blood detoxification; in certain hematological conditions such as polycythemia, where there is excessive production of the red-cell line, regular removal of blood is performed. Regular removal of blood is therapeutic for hemochromatosis, a condition in which excessive iron accumulates and results in liver damage. There is even a revival of the use of leeches to remove toxic blood and enhance revascularization after limb-amputation surgeries.

Because Rakta Mokshana is so rarely used, even in India, some authorities consider the five karmas to be: Vamana, Virechana, Nasya, Anuvasana Basti, and Niruha Basti. With these five procedures, ama can be eliminated and all three doshas can be balanced using the appropriate combination of herbs and oils.

What do I, as a scientifically trained physician, make of these rather esoteric approaches? As medical director of our center, I have supervised almost a thousand people going through the panchakarma program, and I've been consistently impressed with the normalization of basic biological functions that I've observed. Patients' digestive and elimination problems improve, healthier sleep patterns are restored, and emotional well being is consistently enhanced. Is this due to a specific effect of the panchakarma treatments, or to the more general benefits of total immersion in a nurturing, loving, healing environment? I don't know for sure, but I suspect that both influences are at work.

Mrs. Sterling was going through a rough year. Ten months ago her husband of forty-five years passed away from cancer and last month her only daughter had a second miscarriage. She recently moved from her large house into a more manageable apartment but was missing her familiar neighborhood. Her rheumatoid arthritis, which had been under good control, flared up, requiring higher doses of anti-inflammatory medications. Her sensitive stomach acted up, requiring new medications to treat the side effects of the other drugs. Her appetite was affected and she was sleeping poorly.

During her week with us, she was taught meditation, participated in yoga classes, and underwent two-hour daily panchakarma treatments. The Ayurvedic name for arthritis is amavata, *which means "the deposition of ama into the joints responsible for movement." The massages, heat treatments, and herbalized therapies were designed to eliminate toxicity and reestablish balance in her mind and body. By the end of the week, she was sleeping better and her joints were less swollen. Within a month, her rheumatologist was able to reduce her medications and she felt she was establishing a new rhythm in her life.*

I have seen benefits from these intensive treatments in a variety of health conditions. For people with common digestive disorders, the procedures directed toward the gastrointestinal tract, combined with a simplified diet, seem to have a "resetting" effect, normalizing digestion and elimination. The Nasya treatments seem to help clear the nasal and sinus passages in people with allergic rhinitis and sinus congestion. People with a host of chronic-pain disorders benefit from the massage and heat treatments. There is no question that being touched and cared for in a sensitive, ritualized way simply feels great and almost certainly enhances production and release of our intrinsic healing chemicals such as endorphins.

Over the past few years, I've met growing numbers of health-care providers who consider themselves holistically oriented. These are people who accept the existence of a mind body connection that can be useful in the healing process, and certainly this shift in awareness is critically important. But I also believe it's essential that we have a systematic means for providing patients with the experience of substituting nourishing experiences for toxic ones, and for allowing them to see how this can benefit their mental and physical health. Panchakarma therapies meet this need. They offer a way to directly and powerfully influence a patient's sense of well-being.

PASCHAT KARMA—POST-THERAPY PROCEDURES

After the preparatory procedures and the principal elimination processes, Ayurveda recommends a systematic rekindling of the agnis to prevent unhealthy accumulation. This is accomplished through nutritional herbs such as fresh ginger or trikatu (three pungent spices) to stimulate digestion. The diet in general should be primarily ama reducing, with a minimum of fermented, raw, or heavy foods. Meditation, daily oil massage, Pranayama, and yoga can all help to keep the channels of the mind body constitution clear, and to prevent the reaccumulation of toxins.

PANCHAKARMA THERAPIES—INTENSIVE PREVENTION

Panchakarma treatments are powerful procedures for eliminating deeply stored toxins and impurities from the mind body physiology. Each of the three doshas can be influenced, depending upon the procedure and the nutritional herbs that are used: the Kapha zone, which is from the diaphragm upward, is best treated with Vamana and Nasya; the Pitta zone, between the diaphragm and the navel, is addressed with Virechana; and the Vata zone, below the navel, is best treated with Bastis. In all cases, the mind body system must be carefully prepared with oleation and heat to gain maximal benefit from the main procedures; then, after the elimination process has taken place, digestive power must be reconstituted. Lastly, but of great importance, the patient should be provided with information for making healthy life choices that will prevent the reaccumulation of impurities.

Ama-Reducing Herbs

Herbs are an important component of an Ayurvedic program to

reduce and digest ama. Bitter herbs help to separate ama from the tissues, as their dry, light nature helps to reduce the heaviness associated with toxicity. Examples of readily available Western bitter herbs include aloe vera, barberry, golden seal, and echinacea, while the classical Ayurvedic bitter herbs include *manjishta* and neem. Pungent herbs are also useful for digesting ama, but they must be used carefully so as not to aggravate Pitta. Agni-stimulating spices include ginger and cayenne; fresh ginger and long pepper are especially valuable as they stimulate agni but do not exacerbate Pitta.

Gentle liquid fasting can also be valuable in reducing accumulated toxicity. Kapha-type individuals can tolerate several days of liquefied diet each month, but Vata types should fast sparingly. Fresh fruit and vegetable juices encourage the cleansing process without creating any deficiency of essential nutrients. Apples, carrots, and grapefruit are very commonly used, but almost any fruit or vegetable is appropriate. You can also make very thin, blended vegetable soups, which are purifying and nutritious. A liquefied regimen usually begins after dinner, continues through the next day, and ends at breakfast the following morning.

Rasayanas

Rasayanas are nutritional herbs that have a rapid rejuvenative effect on tissues. The word *rasayana* in Sanskrit means "that which enters rapidly into the essence of the physiology." Rasayanas penetrate rapidly and nourish the subtlest aspect of our psychophysiological being. Their purpose is to enhance the functioning of cells, tissues, and whole systems in order to support the highest level of awareness.

Many formulas have been used for thousands of years in Ayurveda. In the chapter on herbs, I discussed Chyvan prash, derived from the amalaki (Emblic myrobalan) fruit. Considered among the most valuable rasayanas, one hundred grams of the fresh pulp has over seven hundred milligrams of vitamin C, which is more than fifteen times that found in an orange. Reputed in the ancient texts to enhance immunity, Chavan prash's strong antioxidant properties have been confirmed in modern studies. One to two spoonfuls of the Chavan prash jam twice per day is recommended. It can be mixed in hot milk or water.

Brahma rasayana is another classical herbal nutritional formula that nourishes the mind and nervous system and enhances mental clarity. The principle ingredient is brahmi (Centella asiatica). This is said to awaken the highest energy centers and is useful before meditation.

Although rasayanas can be viewed as tonics with general benefit, specific nutritive herbs are also used for individuals with a predominance of certain doshas. Some of these are listed below:

VATA: Ashwagandha (*Withania somnifera*), Guggulu (*Commiphora mukul*), Haritaki (*Chebulic myrobalan*)

PITTA: Amalaki (*Emblic myrobalan*), Brahmi (*Centella asiatica*), Shatavari (*Asparagus racemosus*), Kumari (*Aloe vera*)

KAPHA : Bibhitaki (*Beleric myrobalan*), Guggulu (*Commiphora mukul*), Pippali (*Piper longum*)

Rejuvenation

Once the toxic accumulation has been reduced, steps can be taken to help cells and tissues return to their optimal state. This rejuvenating process involves choosing nourishing behaviors as well as nourishing foods. Thus, the regular practice of meditation is an essential component of any rejuvenation program. Yogic breathing exercises and postures energize and balance the mind body physiology, and a daily oil massage assists in the elimination of toxins and stimulates the release of healing chemicals from the skin. It is also extremely important to recognize the extent to which nourishing and supportive relationships provide mirrors of our own nature, allowing us to recognize and take appropriate responsibility for the conditions that we have created for ourselves.

A subtle but very enjoyable way to derive nourishment from the environment is to consciously allow your attention to go to the five natural elements. These life-force-enhancing exercises are rejuvenating and fun to do on a regular basis.

- Walk barefoot on the earth for at least ten minutes every day.

Have your attention on your feet and the earth with the intention to absorb nourishment from Mother Earth.

- Walk along natural bodies of water. Allow the cooling, coherent influence of water to infuse your being.

- Allow the light and warmth of the sun to permeate you. Acknowledge the energy-giving force of the sun, the source of all life on earth.

- Take a walk where there is abundant vegetation and deeply inhale the breath of plants. The ideal time to receive the life force of plants is right before dawn and right after sunset.

- Gaze into the heavens at night. Let your awareness touch the stars and the furthest reaches of the cosmos.

- Eat locally grown, fresh, and lovingly prepared fruits, vegetables, and grains, which imbibe the life force of all five elements.

Ayurvedic techniques of purification and rejuvenation can be studied in great detail, but the most important principles can be expressed in just a few words: We can improve our health by changing the material that we bring into our bodies and our minds, and by strengthening our ability to digest that material. By being fully present in all aspects of our lives, we can metabolize the gifts of nature into a sublime essence, a nectar that will bring us well being and joy.

Responsibility, Compassion, and Freedom

"If anybody achieves at least endurance of misery, he has already accomplished an almost superhuman task."

Carl Jung

A very kind and spiritual man in his mid-forties developed a pain in his neck. He was a longtime vegetarian, practiced meditation regularly, and rode his bicycle at least fifty miles a week. At first he thought he had strained his neck riding, but when the pain persisted for two months he sought medical help. He underwent an MRI scan, which, to the dismay of all, showed a malignant tumor. A complicated course of surgery, radiation, and chemotherapy followed, but eventually his medical doctors admitted there was nothing more they could do for him. He sought a variety of natural healing therapies including herbal medicine, acupuncture, and energy work, each of which provided him with some temporary relief. Sadly, however, after an agonizing two-year illness, he died quietly at home surrounded by his family and friends.

If a person who abuses alcohol develops cirrhosis of the liver, or if someone who smokes two packs of cigarettes a day contracts lung cancer, our sense of cosmic order is not challenged. But when a serious illness emerges without any obvious justification in someone we know and love, we quite naturally feel threatened. In order to rationalize the inexplicable, we mobilize our psychological defense mechanisms. This is a natural human response—for if we accept that something bad can happen despite someone doing all the right things, we are forced to confront our own vulnerability. We would like to believe that eating healthy foods, avoiding toxic substances, dealing appropriately with stress, and exercising regularly protect us from sickness, but this simple prescription for good health only works *most* of the time. As a physician, I have had to accept the reality that sometimes there is just no clear explanation for why someone gets sick.

Ayurveda acknowledges this mysterious fact of life by ascribing certain illnesses to *karma*. The Sanskrit word *karma* means "action." Vedic knowledge teaches that every action sets into motion an infinity of probable effects, like a pebble dropped into a still pond creating circular radiating waves. The effects ripple across time and space, interacting with other waves in complex and convoluted ways.

With respect to illness, the law of karma teaches that people's afflictions derive from sequences of events, but that does not necessarily mean that we, as human beings, will be able to understand the reasons for the illness, or even to discern the sequence of events that led up to it. There is a Vedic expression that says, "Unfathomable is the field of karma." Every human event is another link in an endless chain of circumstances, but it is impossible for any human mind to comprehend fully the process of cause and effect.

Consider the sequence of events that may have led to your reading this sentence at this moment in time: You picked this book out of the tens of thousands in the shop you visited; you may have visited the bookstore because you were taking a plane trip; you may have been taking a trip to a health conference because fifteen years ago you decided to go to nursing school; you chose nursing because, when your mother needed surgery twenty years ago, a hospital nurse was kind to you; and so on, and on, and on. An infinity of prior happenings precedes every current situation and circumstance. And even when we think we understand why something has occurred, we are really seeing only a tiny piece of the puzzle.

I sometimes hear well-meaning people tell those who are suffering that they "created their own illness." The ensuing discussion often includes the idea that patients develop illnesses in order to have some need met. If they were just willing to take responsibility for their lives, the reasoning goes, they could eliminate the sickness just as they created it. I was recently visited by a young woman with swollen lymph nodes in her neck. Despite three different biopsies and opinions by a half dozen doctors, no one had been able to diagnose her illness. Early lymph-node cancer was a possibility, she had been told, but the pathology reports were not definitive.

As people often do when faced with this type of uncertainty, the young woman sought alternative medical opinions. Again and again, albeit with the best of intentions, she was told that she was choosing to have this condition. If she really wanted to be healed, she could do so simply by changing her attitude. When she came to see me, she was interested in a mind body approach but was also very sensitive about the idea that she had somehow decided to be sick. She was happily married, had two young children whom she adored, and she viewed her condition as a nuisance that she would be happy to see behind her. There was no part of her conscious mind that was making a choice to be sick.

Ayurveda would agree with her. Just as people can be injured in an automobile accident due to a drunk driver or killed in an airplane crash, we can become ill through no apparent fault of our own. Does it make sense to say that an infant born through a complicated pregnancy chose to have cerebral palsy? If we are making such a choice, it is certainly not with our conscious mind. Perhaps on the level of our soul we have selected experiences in order to learn certain lessons, but this is a level beyond most people's ability to access or understand.

When I encounter people with such illnesses, I feel it is important to acknowledge that we may never know why the problem arose. This does not imply that we cannot find meaning in every circumstance of our life, because, ultimately, it is our interpretation of the situation that creates our reality. As medical director of a stroke-rehabilitation program for many years, I saw the different ways people respond to the challenge of neurological illness. One individual with a very mild weakness might go into a deep depression, unable to accept the slightest decline in physical ability, while another patient with much more severe impairment would remain positive, continuing to look forward to a meaningful future.

If we shift the focus from *why* the disease arose to *how* we can better deal with it, there is much to be gained from a mind body perspective. As a physician, I know that telling someone to change his or her attitude will have very limited value. We cannot alter our experience of the world by simply assuming a different mood. If you wake up in the morning with the commitment not to lose your temper at work today, it will probably last just until you find that someone has parked in your parking space. We all have good intentions to be loving, accepting, and nonjudgmental, but our mind body physiology may not so easily support this balanced style of functioning.

This is why mind body medicine and Ayurveda emphasize more than just having a positive mental attitude. Improving health requires us to make certain commitments: to take the time to meditate, to eat with awareness, to go to sleep at a reasonable hour, and to seek out sources of nourishment in all aspects of life. More than just talking about living a balanced lifestyle, we must actually live the principles that create health—and when we don't, we may get a reminder. I recently came down with a cold about three days before I was scheduled to teach a week-long course on mind body medicine. I was embarrassed that as a supposed expert on health, I was not able to prevent myself from getting sick. I was forced to take stock of my lifestyle and realized that over the prior three weeks I had taken two red-eye flights to the East Coast, had been working until midnight to finish a newsletter article, had been skipping lunch, eating a big dinner, and waiting until bedtime to do my second meditation. My body decided it was going to remind me to "walk my talk," and I was literally forced to spend a day resting, eating simple meals, and getting to bed on time. By the start of the conference, I was just about myself again.

Patience

Compassion and patience are virtues that are essential to the healing process. Compassion expresses the wise understanding that ultimately our bodies exist in space and time, and like all space-time events they have a beginning, middle, and end. Patience reflects a similarly wise understanding that "this too will pass." We were all born with a remarkable power for metabolizing the ups and downs of life. Whenever we fully digest an experience, we are able to gain knowledge, understanding, and wisdom. In the midst of a challenging life episode we may be unable to imagine any possible value to it—but if we can remain open to the possibility that we may learn something that will help us grow, we will rarely be disappointed. Sometimes, what appears to be a tragedy turns out to be a blessing, and vice versa. This is illustrated in a classic Vedic story.

A wise man had two things in life that he treasured—his son and his pony. One day, his son had left the gate to the corral open and the pony escaped. His neighbors, hearing that he had lost his prized possession, came to offer their condolences, to which he responded, "We'll see."

The next day the pony returned, and following it right into his corral were three beautiful wild horses. When the neighbors heard of this fortuitous turn of events, they paid him another visit to congratulate him on his good fortune. Again, he responded, "We'll see."

The following day, his son decided to try and ride one of the new horses, but on his first attempt was thrown to the ground, breaking his leg. Again, rather than judging the event, the wise man considered the situation with patience and acceptance.

Sure enough, the next day the army came to town and rounded up every able-bodied young man to fight a battle. Because of his injury, the son was left behind.

Not many of us have this degree of equanimity in the face of adversity, but we have all had painful experiences that later reveal themselves as essential steps to greater joy, love, and well being. It may have been a relationship that we obsessively held on to, but once we let go we were able to meet someone capable of truly engaging in a loving, nourishing connection. It may have been a job that was bridling our creativity. Leaving the job meant a loss of security and income, but it also opened the way to work that allowed our true talents to flourish.

This same pattern can be present in dealing with an illness. Although none of us would choose to develop cancer, I often hear people retrospectively describe their cancer experience as a true life gift. For many survivors of a serious disease, the illness was a pivotal point in reordering their priorities and consciously choosing to make each day meaningful. Often they take on new roles as teachers or supporters of others who are going through a similar trial.

Metabolizing Time

Over the centuries there have been many attempts to explain illness
and aging. According to Ayurveda, the aging process is an expression
of how our physiology metabolizes time. When time is metabolized in
a conscious, accepting manner, life is experienced with *timeless awareness.* The opposite of this is *timebound awareness,* in which time is
poorly metabolized and its lingering effects accelerate the aging
process and susceptibility to sickness.

By fully and completely experiencing each moment of every
day, we can eliminate the residual influences of time that can diminish us later on. This is particularly true of emotional experiences,
because the presence of toxic emotions has a toxic effect on our physical body. Ayurveda has a very simple approach to preventing the
accumulation of emotional toxicity. In Vedic philosophy, life is
known and experienced through contrast: between light and dark,
between up and down, between cold and hot—but perhaps most
importantly between pain and pleasure. All human behavior is motivated by pursuit of one and avoidance of the other. This makes obvious good sense, but according to Ayurveda the natural impulse to
avoid pain can be taken too far.

If we can truly experience an emotion, even a painful one, we
can then release it and move on without a buildup of emotional toxicity in the body. But if there is pain that we fail to acknowledge—
pain that we do not become intimate with, pain that we do not
embrace—then that pain will become suffering.

There is an important distinction between pain and suffering. A
wise person may experience pain, because pain is a physiological fact
of life, but he or she will not suffer. A wise person confronts pain,
embraces it, becomes intimate with it, and is then able to release it
once and for all.

The anger and hostility that we carry with us are expressions of
pain that was not confronted, embraced, and released at the time
that it occurred. When we anticipate that we will face similar pain in
the future, we feel anxiety and fear. When we hold on to the pain,
unable to forgive ourselves for the role we played in the creation of it,
we direct it inward in the form of guilt. The energy that we expend
defending ourselves against the full impact of the pain depletes our

life force and results in depression. All these apparently different disorders—anxiety, fear, guilt and sorrow, anger, hostility, and depression—are actually brought on by avoiding pain in the moment when it occurs.

Seven Steps to Process and Release Emotional Toxins

Keeping our emotional body clear is essential to our good health. Undigested emotions, just like undigested food, result in the accumulation of toxicity in our physiology. Yet we may hold on to emotional hurts, betrayals, and disappointments—perhaps because many of us have not been taught effective ways of dealing with them.

Dealing effectively with emotions requires knowledge and practice. I recommend becoming intimate with the following program to prevent and release emotional toxicity.

1. *Identify* the emotion. All of us have experienced some emotional pain, disappointment, and betrayal during our lives, beginning in our childhood. As children, we have many desires, limited power, and undeveloped skills of discrimination and are dependent upon the grace of our caregivers for love and nourishment. We learn patterns of behavior from our family, and these may not always be healthy or useful in our other relationships. These less-than-ideal interpersonal skills may subject us to repeated hurts, disappointments, and betrayals.

   When we experience emotional wounds as adults, we often tend to deny and defend against the hurt. If we do not fully embrace the pain at the time we encounter it, however, we may store it in our emotional body where it continues to fester. This accumulated toxicity, which we may refer to as emotional ama, interferes with our ability to be fully present in the moment. We become trapped in a pattern of reactivity due to our past traumas.

   Whenever you find yourself in a state of emotional turmoil, find a quiet place and identify the emotion. Say to yourself, *"I feel _____."* It may be angry, sad, hurt, betrayed, rejected, etc. As clearly as possible, define and describe what you are feeling.

2. *Witness* the feeling in your body. Emotions are thoughts associated with physical sensations. A memory of another emotionally charged situation may be triggered by the current circumstance. These thoughts trigger bodily reactions that we call "feelings." We experience the memory in our mind and the sensation in our body. By calling up the memory and allowing our attention to go to our bodies, we are able to release the toxic effects of the memories themselves. Placing our awareness in the body and opening to the feelings and sensations that arise allows the pain to dissipate. Being fully present with the emotions that are experienced, without resistance, while witnessing the physical sensations in the body, enables both our minds and bodies to shed the burden of carrying the toxins born of past hurts.

    The chemistry associated with emotions has a life of its own that must be acknowledged before the emotion can be processed further. So just observe the feeling. Allow your attention to embrace the sensation. Breathe into the feeling. By simply allowing your awareness to experience the physical sensations, you'll find the charge of the emotion dissipates and you'll be able to distinguish the feeling from the one who is witnessing the feeling.

3. *Take responsibility* for what you are feeling. Taking responsibility means that we have the ability to respond in new and creative ways. One of the most important aspects of healing the emotional body is understanding that we have a choice in how we respond to and interpret our experiences. At every moment of our existence we choose either to extract nourishment or to store toxicity from our experiences with people or circumstances. Most often these choices are made below the level of conscious awareness; therefore, we are often not aware that we are even making a choice. Someone uses a word to describe us and we feel insulted; someone else uses another word to compliment us and we feel flattered. But, we are actually making a choice in these situations. Eleanor Roosevelt once said, "No one can make you feel bad without your *consent*." We may not be able to influence the people and circumstances we encounter in our lives, but we can directly influence the way

we respond to people and situations. We are each responsible for our own feelings.

To help yourself take responsibility for your own feelings, review the following affirmations:

- I do not blame anyone for my situation, for I understand that everyone is always doing his best from his level of consciousness.

- I do not blame myself for my situation, for I understand that I am always doing my best from my level of consciousness.

- I recognize that no one can make me feel a certain way.

- When I become upset or frustrated by a person or situation, I realize that I am not reacting to the person or situation but to my own feelings about the person or situation.

- I recognize that my feelings about any situation, circumstance, person, or thing are my responsibility and that I have the ability to respond creatively to any challenge.

4. *Express* the emotion, in private, to yourself. You can write about your feelings or speak them out loud. Keep a special journal just for this purpose. Use the language of your heart to express your feelings. Describe the situation or circumstance and the effect that it has had on your heart and soul. While you are writing, new details may emerge—describe them as well. Freely elaborate on your memories while you are writing, allowing whatever details and insights that arise to be expressed.

   Describe the feelings in your body as you are recounting the event. Where do you feel it? How does it feel? Where are you holding the pain? Use words to express the subtle sensations in your chest or gut or head. Allow the words to serve as a conduit to release the emotional toxicity.

5. *Release* the emotion through some ritual. Physical exercise is usually best for this. Exercise, dance, walk, pound a pillow, get a massage, do some breathing exercises—anything that will help you to discharge the emotion from your physiology. Allow your body to detoxify. Acknowledge the release of the emotion

as you are doing the activity. If you are uncomfortable with moving your body, put on some rhythmic music and simply allow yourself to flow gently with the beat. Begin by closing your eyes and simply move your hands to the music. Feel the energy moving and allow your arms to flow with the music. Soon your body will begin to move as the ego gets out of the way and the joy of release takes over.

6. *Share* the emotion with the person involved in the situation once you have calmed down. If you have gone through Steps 1 through 5, you should be able to share it without blame and without trying to manipulate the person for approval or pity.

   If you find that the person involved has no space for you to share your feelings, even though you have taken full responsibility for them, if he or she says things like, "That's your problem, you deal with it," then alarms should go off in your mind that this is a toxic relationship! We would encourage you to take a strong look at whether this relationship is adding to your quality of life or just providing a distraction.

7. *Rejuvenate!* Do something nice for yourself. Get a massage, listen to music, buy yourself a present, eat a delicious meal— nourish yourself. If you've gone through Steps 1 through 6, you deserve to be rewarded—so reward yourself for your good work. During the process of physical Panchakarma, after the deep rooted toxins are eliminated, rasayanas or rejuvenatives have their greatest benefit. This is also true for the subtle body.

Follow these steps when you find yourself reacting strongly to anyone in your life: your husband or wife, your child, your boss, your best friend, your car mechanic—even your doctor! It's not always easy to see the whole world as your mirror, but it is essential for your evolution. The people in your life that annoy you can be gifts. They may trigger strong feelings in you but they are not responsible for them being there in the first place. When you are truly able to accept responsibility for your emotions, you will experience a new level of freedom. Then, your state of happiness will not be dependent upon other people changing their behavior. Shifting your awareness from object referral to self-referral is the basis of liberation.

Individual and Universal

The great paradox of life is how we can be singular beings, with our own needs, memories, desires, fears, and hopes, while at the same time established in the universal field of intelligence that transcends our individuality. Each of us knows that we are mortal, yet none of us can remember or imagine a time when we didn't or will not exist. It has been said that "The past is history, the future is a mystery, and all we really have is the present." When we're able to embrace the present moment through conscious choice making, a strange thing occurs. The pains of the past that we're escaping and the fears of the future we're resisting all dissolve as one. And when we transcend time through present-moment awareness, the deepest level of healing is enlivened. In the process of giving up everything to the present, we gain everything we have longed for.

PART THREE

THE SCIENCE OF
MIND BODY INTERACTIONS
IN ILLNESS

Part 3 of The Wisdom of Healing *deals with specific health issues. Each chapter defines and describes a specific disease topic, reviews the current approaches of Western scientific medicine, and presents our understanding from the perspective of mind body medicine.*

My goal is to demonstrate that the theoretical framework that underlies mind body approaches is very consistent with modern scientific theories. The role of the mind on our physical health has been a tenet of Western medicine since the time of Hippocrates; however, with the rise of modern synthesized pharmacological agents, nondrug approaches have been relegated to a minor and often denigrated status. In this section, I reference scientific studies that support the emerging field of mind body medicine. To some extent this documentation gives Part 3 a more academic texture that is not present elsewhere in the book. Readers who do not feel their needs are served by this more rigorous presentation can feel free to pass over this section, or simply to consult it regarding questions on individual topics. I hope, though, that the great majority of readers will be interested to discover the scientific underpinnings of mind body medicine as it applies to a variety of health issues. For health-care professionals looking to reconcile mind body concepts with the information they received in their training, I hope that this knowledge will be informative and reassuring.

At the end of each chapter, I offer a simple mind body prescription for each condition. Some of the recommendations are generally applicable, because the focus of these complementary approaches is on treating the person, not the disease. Interventions such as practicing daily meditation, following the Body Intelligence Techniques, and maintaining an ideal daily routine are beneficial regardless of the malady one is facing. When utilizing the specific recommendations offered for each condition, I suggest that you try one or two interventions for a month at a time. If you notice some benefit, you can add additional approaches later. Please coordinate any new health-enhancing procedures you are considering with your health provider.

There is no contradiction between mind body medicine and the scientific principles and procedures of mainstream Western health care. I believe that Part 3 of The Wisdom of Healing demonstrates that a consciousness-based understanding of medical issues provides a complementary perspective that furthers the quality of health care in our society. I hope that the information in Part 3 will be of interest and value for all readers, and that health-care practitioners will gain confidence in the validity of mind body approaches for a wide range of maladies.

The Epilogue to the book deals with the experience of death, and with the fear that is so intensely linked with the awareness of our mortality. This is an especially important topic for those who have chosen to work in health care, but it will also, ultimately, be of great relevance to all of us. Unlike many of the medical issues we have considered, death cannot be avoided, but it can in a real sense be healed. To do so is the final challenge, and perhaps the greatest achievement, of mind body medicine and of The Wisdom of Healing.

13

Psychoneuroimmunology—
Mind, Body, and Immunity

*"I have the conviction that when physiology will be far
enough advanced the poet, the philosopher and the physiologist
will all understand each other."*

Claude Bernard

By now it must be obvious that I am a firm believer in the concept
that our mental state influences our physical well being. This is the
premise of mind body medicine and this is a fundamental tenet of
Ayurveda. Only recently, however, has this seemingly commonsense
and ancient understanding begun to receive serious scientific attention in the West. For many years, there had been an almost cynical
rejection by medical science of the popular notion that good
thoughts can influence disease and healing. A 1985 editorial in the
New England Journal of Medicine, the Bible of Western medicine, characterized the *presumed* relationship between the mind and physical illness as "largely folklore,"[1] but today modern science is recognizing
the dynamic relationship between our emotions, our brain chemistry, and our physical bodies. This has created a new scientific field,
psychoneuroimmunology, which studies the relationships between the
mind (*psyche*), brain (*neuro*), and immune system (*immunology*).

There is good evidence that each and every thought, feeling,
mood, desire, and experience is accompanied by corresponding and
instantaneous changes in the brain's chemical messengers. These
messengers, which were initially discovered in the nervous system,
are now known to communicate with every other physiological system in the body. They are like chemical keys searching for the correct

lock to initiate a desired response. The "locks," which are embedded on the surface of cells, are called *receptors,* and have been identified throughout the nervous system. We have learned that the cells of the immune system also have receptors for and respond rapidly to these same chemical keys. Immune cells also *release* many of these same chemical messengers, which feed back information to the nervous system on the body's immune status.

Our mind body dialogue may sound like this:

MIND: Boy, am I tired. My boss is a real pain, my car needs a new muffler, and I think my girlfriend is interested in her fitness trainer.

BRAIN: I am reducing my production of pleasure chemicals and increasing my production and release of anxiety molecules.

IMMUNE CELL: Uh, oh. I'm feeling somewhat anxious today. What is that protein particle doing here? I'm going to sound an alarm and mobilize all my buddies to react to this invasion.

CLINICAL RESULT: Allergic reaction to pollen.

MIND: Great. Not only are my job and relationships a mess, but now my allergies are acting up.

Under different circumstances the internal conversation may go like this:

MIND: My life is really great these days. I love my job, my family life is fulfilling, and I feel that I am really in a creative phase.

BRAIN: All physiological systems are working perfectly. The endorphin factory and immune-enhancing manufacturers are at 80 percent capacity and producing life-supporting chemicals very efficiently.

IMMUNE CELL: I feel invincible today. I'm going to escort this poor little virus who has apparently lost its way and ended up in my bloodstream out of the body, pronto.

CLINICAL RESULT: No symptoms despite exposure to a cold virus.

MIND: I feel so vital. I wonder what opportunities for success and enjoyment will present themselves today.

The principal function of the immune system is discrimination, which is the ability to separate *self* from *non-self.* To our immune system, "self" is understood as something that was present during

COMMUNICATING IMMUNITY

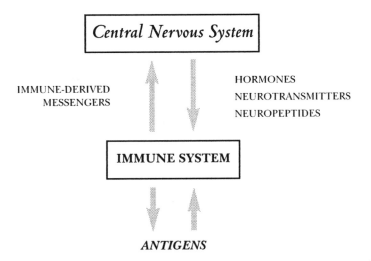

the period of our earliest development. Proteins that existed during our cellular infancy display the right "identity card." A protein, absent when our immune cells were maturing, is branded non-self, or alien.

When an alien protein enters the body, the immune cells identify it and begin a response. Part of this response includes sending information back to the nervous system, which then gives orders to regulate the body's defenses. These orders are communicated by way of the endocrine (hormonal) and autonomic (involuntary) nervous systems, which form the links between the mind and the body's immune responses.

Nervous- and Immune-System Similarities

There are many remarkable similarities between the nervous system and immune system.[2]

- They both contain a variety of highly specialized cells, which are designed for specific tasks. This specialization begins early in development, but remains adaptable even in adult life.

- Memory is an essential feature of both the nervous and immune systems. The brain, of course, has the most sophisticated ability to record and recall information, but immune cells also carry biological intelligence gained over millions of years of evolutionary experience. These biological memories are encoded in our genes. They allow us to respond to new challenges as if we've already faced and overcome them in the past.

- Both systems are designed for adaptation, which is the ability to maintain the dynamic balance known as homeostasis in an ever-changing environment. The body is constantly evaluating incoming impulses and deciding if they are potentially nourishing or potentially toxic. Both the nervous system and the immune system participate in continuous, active surveillance of the surroundings. Useful input is welcomed, while potential threats are quickly identified and avoided.

- The many diverse cells of the nervous and immune systems communicate with each other via potent chemical messengers. Many of these messengers, initially called neuropeptides, are now also known as immunomodulators. Electron microscopes have captured fascinating images of one immune cell directly releasing a chemical messenger into an immune cell of a different type. This process is almost identical to the exchange of information that takes place when a nerve cell releases a neurochemical that travels across a gap, or synaptic cleft, and communicates with a neighboring neuron.[3]

The close similarities in both form and function of the nervous and immune systems suggests that the immune system can be thought of as a circulating nervous system. Immune cells respond to our ever-changing states of mind and mood, whose fluctuations are reflected in the changing chemistry of our brain. In other words, our immune cells are constantly eavesdropping on our mind's internal dialogue.

Immune-System Components

The various components of the immune system are designed to begin a defensive response whenever something unfamiliar enters our physiological environment. A potential enemy is usually identified by a protein antigen. Each "friendly" cell carries on its surface membranes identifying proteins, which tell the immune system that they are on the home team. If a substance cannot produce the right identification, the immune system goes on alert to identify and escort the potentially unfriendly invader out of the mind body system.

Some of the specific types of cells that comprise the immune system are described below:

- The cells that recognize and alert the other immune cells to the presence of an unfamiliar visitor are known as *antigen presenting cells.* The most common of these cells, called a *macrophage,* takes in the foreign protein, breaks it down into smaller components, binds it to another protein, and then presents the processed antigen on the surface of the cell in a form that other immune cells can easily recognize.

- *T lymphocytes* acknowledge the processed antigens and respond by producing chemical messengers called *lymphokines.* These molecules carry information to other lymphocytes, exciting them to respond to the newcomer.

THE IMMUNE DEFENSE SYSTEM

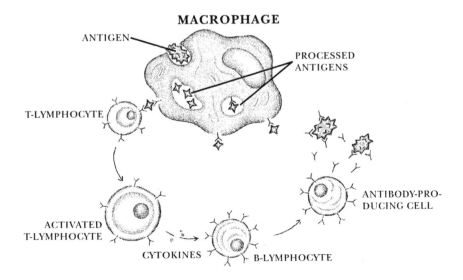

- Cells known as *B lymphocytes* produce *antibodies* to neutralize the invading cell. These antibodies are like missiles that are released from the B lymphocytes and attach to the foreigner. This may neutralize the invader or make it easier to be removed by other immune cells.

- If the invader is perceived to be potentially harmful, *cytotoxic T cells* and *natural killer cells* (*NK*) come into play. These are designed to directly attack and remove the invading organism.

When it's functioning well, the immune system is a magnificently complex and coordinated sequence of responses. But as in any complex system, there exists the potential for things to go awry.

Neuroendocrine-Immune Network

How does the body respond to stress? As discussed earlier in Chapter 5, Dr. Walter Cannon, an American physiologist in the 1930s described our response to a threatening situation as the "fight-or-flight" response.[4] When we feel danger, an alarm system is triggered, resulting in some dramatic changes in our bodies:

- Our heart speeds up and pumps more forcefully.
- We start breathing faster and more deeply to increase the oxygen in our blood.
- Our blood pressure rises to ensure adequate circulation.
- We start sweating to cool our body.
- Blood is diverted away from our gut, where we were digesting our last meal, and shunted to the muscles of our arms and legs.
- Our liver releases sugars to supply energy.
- Our adrenal glands pump out adrenaline to rev up the whole system.
- The pupils of our eyes dilate to admit more light.
- Our mind becomes hyperalert.

Hans Selye, a noted Canadian endocrinologist, took a broader view of the body's stress response in his studies of the endocrine system.[5] He described the role of the pituitary gland in the brain as it stimulates the adrenal gland to release the hormone cortisol. This steroid hormone, which enhances immune response by mobilizing white blood cells from the bone marrow, can be beneficial under conditions of acute stress but over prolonged periods its effect is to exhaust the immune system. Eventually, the thymus gland and lymph nodes throughout the body shrink, resulting in a weakened defensive response.

Not only do the nervous and immune systems communicate through hormones, but there are actually direct links between them.[6] Under an electron microscope, very fine sympathetic nerve fibers can be seen directly connecting with immune cells of the thymus gland, the bone marrow, the spleen, and various lymph nodes. Receptors for the neurotransmitters that are released by the nerve terminals have been documented on immune cells, and drugs that block the effects of these chemicals have been shown to abolish the responses.

We have evolved a remarkable system to transmit our mental and emotional states into bodily reactions. Through the mind-brain-endocrine-immune-system network we continuously monitor our internal and external environment and orchestrate a response. These changes can happen instantaneously but have effects that extend well beyond the moment of the event. Learning how to influence these consequences is a hallmark of mind body approaches.

Feedback

The pathway between the brain and immune system is bidirectional. Immune cells not only receive information from the brain, but also provide it through chemical messengers that directly communicate with the nervous system. The best studied example is interleukin-1 (IL-1), which stimulates the production of a hormone called corticotrophin releasing factor (CRF).[7] CRF is produced by the hypothalamus, which sits just below the brain, and is in continuous communication with the pituitary gland. CRF stimulates the pituitary to release adrenocorticotrophin hormone (ACTH), which in turn causes the adrenal glands to release cortisol. As we've already discussed, cortisol dampens the immune response, so IL-1 functions to prevent an overly aggressive reaction.

If you immunize an animal, electrical changes can be measured

IMMUNE FEEDBACK

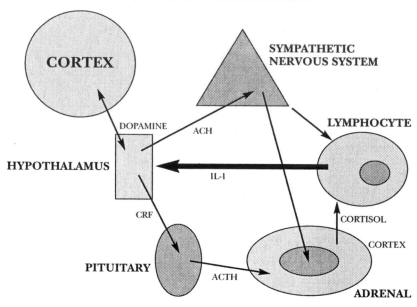

in the hypothalamus before any measurable changes are seen in the immune cells. As soon as an immune cell detects an intruder, it not only calls for help from its teammates, but immediately sends off a message to central control. The brain receives information and begins regulating the immune response at a very early stage.

Animal Studies

The field of modern psychoneuroimmunology came into being when Robert Ader, at the University of Rochester, performed an exciting experiment.[8] He exposed rats to water that was sweetened with saccharin and simultaneously injected them with cyclophosphamide. Cyclophosphamide is a potent immune suppressant that is commonly used as a cancer chemotherapy drug. It has a major side effect of causing nausea. Therefore, when the rats were given the cyclophosphamide they became severely nauseated and vomited. Over the next several days, they also showed the expected suppression in their immune function. Days later, when the rats were reexposed to the saccharin-sweetened water, they promptly vomited even though they were not given the cyclophosphamide. They had been conditioned to become nauseated in association with the sweetened water. This part was not surprising as it was an example of conditioning, not unlike Ivan Pavlov training a dog to salivate when he rang a bell.

But something else very unexpected was discovered. When the rats were exposed to the saccharin-sweetened water the second time *without* the cyclophosphamide, they again showed a marked suppression in their immune function. *The rats' immune systems had also become conditioned to be suppressed when the rats tasted saccharin-sweetened water.* Blood studies showed a reduction in antibody production and impairment in the cell-mediated responses. This was dramatic evidence that the mere expectation of an effect could create weakness in immunity. The immune cells had learned (inappropriately) that sweetened water was harmful to them.

If we can teach our immune cells to be negatively conditioned, can we teach them to respond positively? A study from Japan showed this was easy to accomplish.[9] Two groups of poor mice were stressed using random electrical shocks in a testing chamber. When they weren't being tormented, they were housed in safe enclosures that had cedar shavings on the floors of the cages. Over time, the recurrent stress caused a range of immune-function abnormalities. Later in the experiment, the stress-inducing procedure was repeated, but this time some of the animals were exposed to the aroma of the cedar shavings. Under these conditions there was a much milder effect on their immune cells. The sense of security associated with the aroma of the cedar shavings blunted the impact of stress. I find this study fascinating because aromas have been used as healing tools in many natural-medicine systems for thousands of years. As discussed in Chapter 6, aroma therapy is an integral part of Ayurveda.

Human Studies

There has been an explosion of research over the past ten years in an effort to document and understand how the immune system mirrors our emotional state—how perceptions of stress can weaken our immunity. The best way to study the effects of stress on health is to look at people who are under a lot of stress. Most people would agree that medical students fit into this category, particularly during final exams. And, if we measure their immune function at this time, they show a decline in several aspects of their cellular immunity.[10] If we rank this same group of future doctors according to their sense of loneliness, we discover that the lonelier they feel, the less they are able to resist the infection of common viruses.[11]

A groundbreaking study published a few years ago in the *New England Journal of Medicine* measured people's recent stress level and then had them sniff a dose of the virus that produces a cold. To no grandmother's surprise, the study showed that the more stressed you've been lately, the more likely you are to start coughing and sneezing soon.[12]

Loss is always attended by stress, and loss of a spouse through divorce or death is consistently ranked as one of the most stressful occurrences of life. To add insult to injury, the emotional and psychological pain of losing a mate is accompanied by major changes in our ability to cope with immune challenges. White blood cells become less capable of fighting infection after the death of a spouse, mirroring mental depression.[13] Even more than death of a spouse, divorce leads to long-term weaknesses in immune function in both men and women, reflecting the ongoing distress that accompanies the breakup of a family.[14] Caring for a spouse with Alzheimer's disease, which is very similar to watching your loved one die slowly, is also associated with a measurable fall in immunity.[15]

As would be predicted, these changes in immune function as a consequence of a major life stress result in more serious sickness. A widower's risk of developing cancer or dying from any type of illness is higher for at least ten years after the loss of his spouse.[16,17] It is accurate to say that a major loss not only hurts us emotionally, but can make us physically sick and result in early death.

Positive Interventions

I've made the case that emotional stress can harm our immunity and raise our risk for future illness. Fortunately, mind body approaches can be successful in strengthening our immune systems when we are attempting to recuperate from a major life stress, although recognition of these approaches by mainstream health care has until recently been limited.

Teaching a simple meditation technique to geriatric residents improves their immune function.[18] Their reduction in anxiety and improved sense of well being is promptly reflected in improved cellular immunity.

A similar benefit holds for people infected with the AIDS virus. Relaxation training and assertiveness exercises in people with HIV infection result in improved cellular immunity.[19] We now recognize that despite the same AIDS virus, people show a wide range of clinical expressions. Mind body approaches are inexpensive, nontoxic, and provide psychological and physical benefits.

A useful and easy means to process emotional pain is to write about it, for in the mere act of expressing it, some of the hurt can be dissipated. Undergraduate college students encouraged to write about events that were experienced as stressful or traumatic have improved immune function and make fewer visits to the campus health clinic.[20]

In his landmark book, *Anatomy of an Illness,* Norman Cousins described his personal experience with a serious rheumatic disorder.[21] Through good humor, self-empowering relationships with his physicians, and unwavering confidence in his healing abilities, he was able to overcome his illness. While watching reruns of Marx brothers movies and *Candid Camera,* his laughter sent positive messages to his immune cells, reminding them of their legitimate purpose. The culturing of a positive attitude means more than putting on a happy face. It requires being rooted in a state where panic and dismay are incapable of arising, the creation of a compelling future, and the active development of a healing environment. Reports demonstrating the positive physiological and immunological benefits of laughter are confirming that it is indeed the best medicine.[22,23]

In a widely quoted study, Dr. David Spiegel provided group support meetings for women with metastatic breast cancer.[24] He intended to prove that this simple intervention would *not* influence their life span. To his surprise, the women in the support groups not only felt their quality of life improved, but actually lived twice as long as women who did not participate in groups. Other studies have confirmed that patients receiving cancer-therapy programs that employ meditation, stress management, emotional release, and education will show improved immune function and live longer.[25,26]

I take care of many people who are simultaneously using mind body approaches along with standard cancer treatments and time and again see the benefits of an integrated approach. A retired businessman receiving radiation therapy for throat cancer who is meditating, performing daily yogic breathing exercises, and gargling with herbalized oil has so few side effects that his radiation oncology now recommends a similar program to other patients. A woman receiving chemotherapy for her breast cancer sees a dramatic reduction in her nausea during treatments and her fatigue afterward since beginning meditation, a daily massage, and using a fragrant essential oil. I recommend a complementary approach using the best of the Eastern and Western healing sciences.

Mind Body Interactions and Immunity

By discriminating between "self" and "non-self," the human immune systems can respond to a wide range of internal and external challenges. But in a sense the basis of this discrimination is quite arbitrary. Our sense of self derives from identifications that form during our developmental years. Although psychobiological development is generally held to be complete around the time of adolescence, our true nature in the realm of consciousness remains flexible throughout our lives. The consciousness-based approach suggests that new connections can be established based on spiritual experiences that transcend the limits of biology as it is usually understood. Ongoing development is always possible; experience can be interpreted and reinterpreted; and we can continue to evolve throughout life.

I have previously referred to Dr. Jonas Salk's concept of metabiological evolution in which he suggests that for humanity to endure, our human species must progress from "survival of the fittest" to "survival of the wisest."[27] Applying this idea to immunity, we can see that what is really needed is not an overtly aggressive immune system, but one that is continuously evolving. Evolution occurs when a wide repertoire of experiences is embraced and integrated into meaningful responses. Evolution is, therefore, a continual expansion of the concept of self until the self embraces the whole universe. Ultimately, nothing can threaten the fully evolved self because everything is included within it.

When the relationships between consciousness, mind, and body are integrated and harmonious, immune cells are unerringly able to discriminate potential sources of nourishment from sources of toxicity. But when basic harmony and integration are lacking, the immune system may become either too aggressive, or, conversely, it may fail to perform its defensive functions. Allergies, for example, are the result of an overactive immune response to external provocations, while autoimmune disorders such as rheumatoid arthritis and multiple sclerosis are a result of excessive reaction to internal stimuli. Infections are brought on by weak immune response to external challenges, but cancer is the result of an inadequate response to internal threats.

IMMUNE RESPONSE	INTERNAL THREAT	EXTERNAL THREAT
Excessive	Autoimmune Diseases	Allergies
Inadequate	Cancer	Infections

From a mind body perspective, allergies and autoimmune diseases are expressions of an internal dialogue of threat and alienation that results in self-destructive hostility; cancer and susceptibility to infection are immune-system expressions of internal conflicts that result in desperation and hopelessness; health, however, is a state of flexibility that integrates all challenges and experiences into a meaningful response.

An ancient Vedic expression declares, "Infinite flexibility is the secret of immortality." The stability of the body's immune system depends upon the flexibility of our responses to the challenges of daily experience. Stability is built upon a foundation of dynamic non-change in the midst of numberless swirling and chaotic influences. The essential feature of a healthy immune system is the capability to mount a dynamic response while maintaining stability and integrity.

The healing traditions of the world have always asserted the mind's influence on the body, but modern science is just beginning to understand how thoughts, feelings, and perceptual interpretations of the world can influence well being. When our lives are in balance and our internal dialogue is harmonious, our immune systems and every other aspect of our being receives the message of health.

MIND BODY PRESCRIPTION FOR IMMUNE HEALTH

1. Listen to your internal dialogue. Is it one of lamenting or blaming? Realize that you have a choice in the way that you interpret your circumstances.

2. Identify sources of toxicity in your life. Choose *one* to reduce or eliminate.

3. Spend time in nature. Stroll in the park, hike in the woods, walk by a stream.

4. Simplify your diet for two weeks (pages 165–66).

5. Perform a daily massage with the appropriate dosha-specific oil for one week (pages 103–5).

6. Take one-half ounce of aloe vera juice twice per day for two weeks.

7. The Ayurvedic herbs traditionally used to balance and nourish the immune system include amalaki (Indian gooseberry) brahmi (Indian pennywort), *hapusha* (juniper berries), katphala (bayberry), and tulsi (basil).

8. If you are having allergies:

    • Use a *neti* pot each morning and (see below) perform ghee or sesame-oil nasya several times per day for one week (see below).

    • Use agni-enhancing digestive aids such as fresh ginger, coriander, fennel, or long pepper.

9. Laugh regularly at the world and at yourself. Lighten up!

USING A NETI POT AND NASYA

A neti pot is a small container with a spout that can be gently placed in one's nostrils through which warm salt water is administered. Following the warm-water cleansing, the membranes just inside the nostrils should be lubricated with a little ghee or sesame oil. A small amount of oil is placed on a finger, gently applied into both nostrils, and then sniffed up into the nasal passages. This procedure reduces the concentration of allergens and provides some protection to the mucous membranes to reduce allergic reactions. If this is done a couple of times a day, decongestants and antihistamines may be avoided.

NETI POT

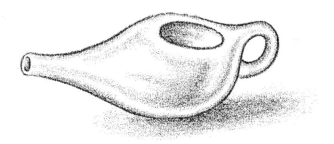

14

Mind Body Interactions in Digestive Disorders

"The belly is the counterpart of the face."

William Harvey

Mealtimes were never pleasant for as long as Joyce could remember. Angry arguments between Mom and Dad were a more consistent feature of dinner than dessert. When her parents divorced before her twelfth birthday, she actually felt some relief, but shortly thereafter, she began to have frequent episodes of cramping belly pain and bloating after meals. After an extensive medical evaluation, Joyce was given the diagnosis of irritable bowel syndrome.

Now as an adult in her late twenties, eating and eliminating continue to be problematic for her. Under stress, her bowels dictate her activity and she misses up to a week of work every month. Her digestion remains so delicate she almost never goes to a restaurant with friends.

We are all aware that our emotions influence our digestion. We lose our appetite when we're sad, get heartburn when we're under stress, or develop diarrhea before a final exam. Our language is filled with expressions like, "I have a gut feeling," "You make me sick to my stomach," or "I can't absorb what you're telling me," which reveal our intrinsic understanding of the mind body linkage. Although the relationship between emotions and digestion may appear obvious in daily life, science is just beginning to look seriously at this important connection.

Coordinating Digestion

Although the gastrointestinal (GI) tract can be visualized as a series of tubes, the transportation of food through the digestive system is far from a simple process. Muscles, nerves, and chemical messengers have to be coordinated if the GI system is to perform its essential job of extracting nourishment from the environment. Through both direct and indirect linkages, information is constantly flowing between our digestive and nervous systems.

Our gastrointestinal tract has an enteric (*enterikos* meaning "intestines" in Greek) nervous system (ENS) that is remarkably self-sufficient. This system, which can partially regulate and coordinate digestive activity independently of the brain, is a collection of nerve networks embedded in the gallbladder, the pancreas, and the walls of the digestive tract.[1] The system includes ten to one hundred million cells organized into two nerve networks: the *myenteric* (Auerbach's) plexus organizes the muscles of the gut, while the *submucosal* (Meissner's) plexus coordinates release and absorption of fluids and salts. The wisdom of our body integrates these two networks to relax and contract the intestines while absorbing the nutrients necessary for our survival. Although considered a part of our involuntary (autonomic) nervous system, the ENS is actually closer in design to our central nervous system. It contains complete reflex pathways that include sensory, associative, and motor nerves that regulate muscle tone and blood vessels, as well as secretion and absorption by the cells.

Reflex circuits between different parts of the digestive tract coordinate the sequences necessary for digestion. For example, nerve connections between the gallbladder and the small intestines assist in the release of bile at the appropriate time. This neurological connection is in addition to the gut hormones that communicate information throughout the digestive tract.

The *vagus* nerve is the main nerve from the brain to the digestive system. Its name is derived from the same root as the word *vagabond* because it wanders throughout the belly. It was traditionally viewed as mainly supplying brain input *to* the gut, but it actually contains more nerve fibers that bring information *from* the GI tract *to* the brain. The area of the nervous system that regulates the digestive tract, the *locus ceruleus* ("dark blue place"), receives extensive input from the gut and is the source of an essential neurochemical, norepi-nephrine.[2] This area has connections throughout the brain and is responsible for alertness and may also be our anxiety center. This same group of nerve cells is right next door to brain structures con-trolling heart rate and blood pressure. So this small region of the brain links our thoughts, digestion, and heart. Even from a purely anatomic viewpoint, we can see the intimate relationship between our mind and stomach. This connection between our brain and gut predisposes us to translate feelings into physical digestive symp-toms. When we are facing high levels of stress, our guts are likely to be affected.

Alternatively, when our lives are balanced and comfortable, our digestive system is able to perform its job of efficiently receiving nour-ishment from the environment and eliminating material that is not beneficial. Taking in what's nourishing and leaving behind what's not is really the function of both a healthy digestive and psychological system. It's not surprising, then, that if our mind is having trouble finding nourishment, our gut is having the same problem.

Chemical Transmitters

Chemical messengers are usually named according to the areas of the body in which they were first discovered. Transmitters first identified in the brain were called neurotransmitters, while those discovered in the digestive tract were given names reflecting their GI presence. At least two dozen peptides have been identified in the gut, represent-ing at least fifteen major peptide families.[3] Some of the common ones are listed in the table below with a few of their known functions.

GUT PEPTIDE	FUNCTION
Gastrin	Regulates gastric acid
Somatostatin	Regulates gastrin and gastric acid
Secretin	Regulates pancreatic secretions
Cholecystokinin	Regulates pancreas and gall bladder
Neurotensin	Regulates intestinal motility
Vasoactive Intestinal Peptide	Regulates motility and secretions

Peptide messengers can act in the gut in three different ways. (1) They can be released from one cell and carry a message to other cells very close by; (2) they can be released by one cell, enter the circulation, and act on other cells at a considerable distance; or (3) they can be released from a nerve cell and act locally as a neurotransmitter. It's fascinating that the same chemical code can play a different role in a different circumstance, highlighting the very fuzzy divisions between the brain, endocrine, and gastrointestinal systems.

A good example of this remarkable versatility is the hormone cholecystokinin (CCK). It was initially discovered in the cells of the small intestines, where it is released into the circulation in response to fats in the small bowel. When the gallbladder receives the message of CCK, it is stimulated to contract and release its bile salts. These bind with the fats so they can be more easily absorbed. CCK is also widely distributed in the nervous system. It is present throughout the cerebral cortex, in the brain stem, and in cells that project to the brain's limbic system, which is closely associated with emotions. CCK is also concentrated in the hypothalamus, where it plays a role in satiety and the regulation of food intake.[4] It has also been identified as a pain modulator.[5] Thus, this same messenger that governs a basic digestive function is involved with hunger and the feelings of pleasure associated with eating.

Another amazing transmitter that was originally discovered in the digestive tract is vasoactive intestinal peptide, or VIP. VIP was identified as one of the first new chemical messengers of the gastrointestinal system. It has been shown to regulate the secretions of the pancreas and intestines as well as the movement of food through the gut. Although named for its ability to regulate intestinal blood flow, this same chemical was discovered to influence the blood supply to the cardiovascular system, respiratory system, urinary system, and central nervous system.[6] VIP is widely distributed in the brain and in nerve cells throughout the GI tract. It is also found in the skin, where it can be released through massage. Early studies suggest that massage can dilate heart blood vessels, possibly as a result of VIP release. VIP also has affinity for the same receptor on immune cells that the AIDS virus uses to enter lymphocytes.

Here again, this simple protein shows us how our arbitrary divisions between components of the mind body network are scientifically inaccurate. In reality, the body is a complex web of energy and information that uses the same chemical codes of intelligence for communication throughout the physiology.

Gastrointestinal Immunity

The gastrointestinal system has been called the body's largest endocrine organ, and it may also be the largest organ of the immune system. Considering the large amount of foreign material that enters the body through our gut, it's not surprising that our immune system is standing guard there. The intestinal immune system is vast, with most immunocytes localized in discrete areas known as Peyer's patches.[7] There are direct links between the nerves of the gut and certain immune cells, particularly mast cells, which are responsible for releasing potent chemicals that activate the immune response.

This connection between the GI and immune systems may illuminate the role of stress on digestive disorders, and peptic ulcers provide a good case in point. It has recently been shown that a majority of patients with peptic-ulcer disease have a bacteria known as *Helicobacter pylori*. Although this bug makes an infectious contribution to a condition often associated with stress, it is likely that susceptibility to *Helicobacter* is influenced by our immune status and by levels of gastric-acid production. Both of these factors are affected by our emotional and psychological states. Studies show that *Helicobacter pylori* can be cultured in about three-quarters of patients with peptic ulcers, but there is a significant minority who remain uninfected.[8] I predict that future studies will reveal that the state of the immune system, which is clearly influenced by emotions, is as important in the development of an ulcer as the bacteria. The brain-gut-immune linkage may explain why some people are more predisposed to developing gastric inflammation with this infectious agent than others who are immune.

Functional Bowel Disorders

Disordered bowel function is present in almost 30 percent of our population, and almost half of all patients seen by digestive-disorder specialists are eventually diagnosed with "functional" bowel disorder.[9] It is estimated that this accounts for more than 1.5 million medical visits per year and the dispensing of more than two million medications.[10]

Functional bowel disorders comprise a spectrum of conditions in which symptoms cannot be attributed to structural problems such as cancer, tumors, or inflammation. This family of conditions includes noncardiac chest pain, non-ulcer stomach pain, simple constipation, simple diarrhea, gallbladder spasm, and irritable bowel syndrome (IBS).

IBS is the term most commonly applied to patients with digestive complaints who show no structural abnormalities when evaluated by the usual gastrointestinal diagnostic procedures. Despite its prevalence, the standard contemporary definition of IBS—"a disordered bowel habit, with or without abdominal pain, without organic explanation and of unknown etiology"—highlights our lack of understanding of this condition.[11] Patients with IBS generally have a host of symptoms, primarily but not exclusively localized to the GI system. Common symptoms include: abdominal pain relieved with elimination; altered stool frequency and consistency; passage of mucus; and frequent feelings of bloating or abdominal distention.

Electrophysiologic studies show that patients with IBS tend to have abnormal intestinal motility.[12] Functional bowel studies show that people with diarrhea have too many fast contractions while people with constipation have too few. Stool moves through the colon faster in patients with IBS than in people with normal bowel function. But despite these changes in the motility of the intestines, symptoms of bloating or pain are not clearly associated with times of altered bowel activity.

The most consistent finding in patients with functional bowel disorder is their increased sensitivity to pressure and distention within their gut.[13] People with IBS can often detect very subtle volume changes throughout the digestive system. If a balloon is inflated in the colon of patients with IBS, for example, they will detect it at a much lower level of pressure than the average person. They will also report discomfort that includes both the belly and the lower back. They also show more sensitivity to distention of their esophagus and stomach.

Yet, people with IBS are *not* wimps. They are not *generally* hypersensitive to pain. If tested for their tolerance to annoying electrical shocks or to cold, their responses are the same as everyone else's.[14] They simply have a diminished ability to filter sensations coming from their gut. Subtle impulses, below the level of perception in most people, cause conscious discomfort in people with irritable bowel syndrome. And in addition to feeling uncomfortable, IBS patients respond with irregular intestinal contractions, resulting sometimes in diarrhea, and at other times in constipation.

Beyond their GI symptoms, people with IBS frequently have other health concerns; fatigue, chronic pain, fibromyalgia, and non-cardiac chest pain are common. There may also be psychological problems, including frequent anxiety, hostility, phobia, and para-noia.[15] Some of these derive from the stress of dealing with a chronic illness; others reflect the underlying imbalance in the mind body network.

Making It Better

Medical therapy for IBS has generally been useless, though not worthless. An evaluation for this condition usually includes both X-ray and endoscopic studies at a cost of several thousand dollars. In the vast majority of people, a structural problem is ruled out and the label of irritable bowel syndrome is applied. Medical treatment is usu-ally symptomatic, but, because they tend to be sensitive to drugs, IBS patients often discontinue prescribed medications upon finding the side effects intolerable. A recent report reviewed forty-three studies on the drug therapy for irritable bowel syndrome.[16] They looked at drugs to reduce spasm, anticholinergic drugs to slow motility, bulk-forming agents to equalize pressure, opiates to relieve pain, and anti-depressants and tranquilizers to treat the associated psychological symptoms. The author concluded that "not a single study offers con-vincing evidence that any [drug] therapy is effective." An interesting feature of these studies was the recognition of improvement in almost 50 percent of patients *not* receiving drug therapy, presumably as a result of a *placebo* effect.

On the other hand, several studies have demonstrated the value of hypnotherapy and relaxation training in people with functional bowel disorders. The most successful approaches are often the sim-plest. Patients are first taught to enter a relaxed state and then instructed to place their hands and attention on their bellies, invoking a sense of warmth. Then they are guided to imagine a healthy and relaxed functioning of the smooth muscles of their intestines.

Studies show that if you have typical IBS and practice this technique, you have an excellent chance of getting substantial relief from your symptoms within a short time with lasting benefits even after a year and a half.[17,18] If you have been suffering for many years and have atypical symptoms or more long-standing anxiety and depression, there is still a good chance of some benefit from this simple procedure.

In an important study from England, people with refractory irritable bowel syndrome participated in four forty-minute hypnotherapy sessions over a couple of months.[19] Almost half of the people improved and a third had almost complete relief! These were patients who had previously failed to respond to any other medical therapy. They were taught relaxation in groups of eight, making this approach undeniably the most cost-effective treatment for this condition. Combining relaxation techniques with supportive psychological therapy to identify and reduce negative thinking patterns improves both digestive and psychological symptoms.

Mind Body Interactions in Digestion

Our gastrointestinal system is truly remarkable. Through it we ingest energy and information from the environment to create both our physical form and the energy we need to support our activities. This may be the most convincing expression of the Vedic understanding that the environment is our extended body. Nature has packaged her biological energy and information in the form of food containing the basic substrates needed to create and replenish our cells; through the process of digestion, basic codes of intelligence are exchanged between our individual and our environmental physical sheaths. Ayurveda describes the physical body as *anna maya kosha,* which means "the layer made out of food." In its essence, our body really is the intelligence carried on our DNA molecules wrapped in food.

The ability to digest fully the experiences presented to us at any moment is the key to good health. When we are able to extract the nourishment we need and leave the rest behind, we create balance and integrity in mind and body. Under ideal circumstances this beautiful and dynamic process occurs spontaneously. When the mind is balanced and integrated, our appetites are strong and appropriate. Our gastrointestinal system receives healthy messages from our brain and is able to extract the elements necessary for maintaining structure and energy.

There is constant communication between our mind and gut via the nervous system. As a result of this exchange our mental state is reflected in our gut. When our emotional and psychological state is turbulent, the GI system mirrors this. One of the earliest physical expressions of emotional distress is a change in our appetite. Our loss of hunger reflects our lack of enthusiasm for any new input from the environment while our physiology attempts to process a hurtful experience. Emotional upset can also be associated with an increase in appetite, as we seek solace for our wounded feelings in food. In both cases, imbalance in our emotional body is mirrored in our digestive state.

From an Ayurvedic perspective, any attempt to create balance in the emotional body through food will be met with very limited success, because the true problems and solutions must be approached at subtler levels. Our physical sheath is the most condensed manifestation of consciousness, and therefore the most gross. Our emotional sheath exists at a subtler level, and has the capacity to influence the physical body more readily than the reverse. The ultimate healing potential is found at the level of consciousness, because everything that we create has its origins in the field of pure potentiality, beyond the many layers of our bodies, our emotions, our thoughts, and our beliefs.

We have several tools available to restore our digestive power to its natural state so that we can supply our energy and physical needs. We first need to believe at a fundamental level that we are deserving of nourishment and are not deserving of toxicity. This is true on every level of our existence—environmental, physical, and emotional. We need to assess honestly those aspects of our life that are not providing the sustenance we deserve and take steps to change them. The messages from our body are gifts that help us identify what needs to change in our life. Listening to our body—listening to our *gut*—allows us to tune into our innate intelligence, which can guide us along the path of greater well being.

Eating with awareness is great practice for living with awareness. When we are fully present while enjoying a meal, we efficiently extract the available nutrition and spontaneously avoid consuming that which is toxic. The Body Intelligence Techniques are cues to bring us back to present-moment awareness.

If you are having symptoms of digestive imbalance—heartburn, bloating, discomfort—use attention and intention to reestablish balance. After a quiet meditation, localize your attention to your alimentary system and visualize comfortable, smooth, effortless, balanced digestion. Eating and digesting are such primordial processes that simply remembering how natural they are can improve their function.

Use nature's gifts to enliven healthy digestion. Enhance digestive power with spices that stimulate our metabolic fire—pepper, ginger, asafetida, wild celery seeds, cardamom, cayenne, and cloves. Simplify your diet when your digestion is delicate, pay attention to your appetite, and make certain your elimination is regular, using gentle, natural agents to restore balance when necessary.

Like the skin, the digestive tract is an area of junction between perceptions of self and non-self. When our awareness is established in the unity value of life, we view the environment as a source of nutrition—a quantum soup from which we can receive sustenance whenever we need it. But if our awareness is fixated on notions of boundaries and separation, the environment will be perceived as alien, a source of threat, and we will be distrustful of the nourishment it provides even as we seek it. Healing digestive disorders takes place when we expand awareness of our universality. From this vantage point, we can understand and experience the Vedic expression that describes food consumption as "Brahman eating Brahman"—the unmanifest field of pure awareness nourishing itself. When this state of consciousness is our internal reference point, the possibility of indigestion does not arise.

MIND BODY PRESCRIPTION
FOR DIGESTIVE HEALTH

1. Follow the Body Intelligence Techniques at every meal.

2. Follow your dosha-specific dietary recommendations.

3. Pay attention to your appetite level and only eat when you are really hungry, stopping when you are comfortably full.

4. Eat an occasional meal in silence.

5. If your digestion is delicate, follow the ama-pacifying program for a couple of weeks.

6. If your appetite is weak, eat a mixture of fresh grated ginger, lemon juice, and rock salt to stimulate the agnis (one-half teaspoon fresh ginger, one-half teaspoon lemon juice, a pinch of salt) one half hour before meals.

7. If you tend to get heartburn after meals, chew a quarter teaspoon of roasted fennel seeds or a pinch of fresh coriander leaves.

8. To decrease gas or bloating, add cinnamon, cardamom, and bay to your cooking.

9. Ayurvedic herbs traditionally used to enhance appetite and digestion include sunthi (ginger), *maricha* (black pepper), pippali (long pepper), and ajwan (wild celery seeds).

10. Ayurvedic herbs traditionally used to quiet excessive digestive fire include shatavari (Indian asparagus), amalaki (Indian gooseberry), and Yasti madhu (licorice).

11. Ayurvedic herbs traditionally used to enhance absorption include jatiphala (nutmeg), haritaki (Chebulic myrobalan), and *musta* (nut grass).

12. Celebrate eating! Don't strain.

15

Mind Body Interactions
in Diabetes

"Sweet, sweet, sweet poison for the age's tooth."

William Shakespeare

Connie was nine years old when she was diagnosed with diabetes. After recovering from the initial shock, and with the loving support of her family and pediatrician, she learned to adapt to her illness. Throughout her teenage years, her blood sugars were kept under good control and she considered her condition more of a nuisance than a disease.

This changed when she started her freshman year in college. It was the first time she had lived away from her family and she found herself frequently feeling anxious. She was keeping up in her classes but was having trouble sticking to her diet. She adjusted her insulin to her erratic eating habits but was having much wider fluctuations in her blood sugars than ever before.

Because she had been snacking while cramming for a midsemester exam, she gave herself an extra dose of insulin before going to bed. The next thing Connie knew she was waking up in the local emergency room being told she had had a seizure due to very low blood sugar.

If during our evolution we had had unlimited access to nourishment, we may not have needed to develop insulin. This remarkable hormone, released when the bloodstream is filled with sugar, moves the basic energy currency of the body into the cells of our tissues and into our liver for storage. Insulin enables us to save carbohydrate packets of energy to be used in leaner times. If we do not produce enough insulin or if despite its presence our cells do not heed its call, sugar molecules overflow from the bloodstream into the urine. We call this real or apparent lack of insulin *diabetes mellitus*.

Approximately twelve million Americans suffer from this illness.[1] The disease is a major cause of disability, including blindness, kidney failure, and nerve damage. It raises the risk of blood-vessel disease throughout the body, including the brain and heart. And, the treatment of diabetes carries a high price tag, estimated at over ten billion dollars each year.[2]

We now know that the complications of diabetes are directly related to high levels of blood sugar. Recent studies have demonstrated that precise control of glucose levels approaching normal can reduce the complications of diabetes.[3] Achieving this control is not easy and requires close monitoring and regulation of blood sugar, diet, and activity.

Although diabetes is primarily a problem of insulin production or responsivity, the regulation of blood sugar is influenced by a dynamic interplay between mind, activity, food, and biochemistry. Besides insulin, other hormones are also involved in blood-sugar regulation, including glucagon and growth hormone. Both of these are often present at high levels in diabetics. Glucagon, which, like insulin, is secreted by the pancreas, elevates blood sugar by causing the breakdown of the complex carbohydrate glycogen into simple sugars. Growth hormone raises blood sugar by antagonizing insulin.

Insulin is a versatile messenger. Within the brain it is an important neurotransmitter, influencing appetite, hunger, and satiety.[4] It is found in the cerebrospinal fluid and receptors for it have been identified throughout the central nervous system.[5] In addition to its role in eating behavior, insulin has been shown to influence the maturation of nerve cells.

There is a close relationship between insulin, blood sugar, and our emotions. Stress causes the release of adrenaline and cortisol, which have a direct effect on blood sugar and other sugar-regulating hormones. In the initial phase of a stressful challenge, our sympathetic nervous system stimulates the release of stress hormones, which raise blood-sugar levels so our vital organs are assured of available fuel. People with diabetes, however, cannot readily tolerate this sugar challenge because of their impaired production of or insensitivity to insulin.

Stressful events may be a precipitating factor for diabetes in animals or people at risk. For example, certain types of overweight mice will show high blood sugars when put in a stressful environment.[6] When rats who have had most of their insulin cells removed are restrained in a tight space, most show elevated blood sugars and almost one in seven will develop permanent diabetes.[7]

The Native American Pima Indians of Arizona have the highest incidence of diabetes of any ethnic group. Among this culture, men and women are considerably heavier than the average American, and almost 60 percent eventually develop diabetes. When Pimas who have not yet manifested diabetes are subjected to a time-pressured mental math test, more than three out of four will have a rise in blood sugar, compared to only one of eight Caucasians.[8]

Too Sweet

We generally categorize diabetes into two groups. Type I diabetes is characterized by an actual insulin deficiency. Because it occurs in children and adolescents, Type I is called juvenile-onset diabetes, but it can occur at any age. The exact cause of the condition is not clear, but it seems to be an autoimmune disorder that may occur after a viral insult in a person genetically predisposed.

Type I diabetes patients show symptoms of insulin deficiency, including polyuria, polydipsia, and polyphagia—they urinate a great deal, they drink large volumes of water, and they eat a lot—yet they still lose weight. Sushruta, a great Ayurvedic rishi who lived four thousand years ago, described Type I diabetes in a very lyrical way: "Drinking, but always thirsty, eating, but always hungry, the poor patient watches his flesh melt away in a stream of sugary urine."[9]

In Type II diabetes there is no deficiency of insulin—in fact, there may be excessive amounts of it in the blood—but Type II patients are insulin resistant. Their receptor sites do not respond adequately to the circulating insulin. Most Type II diabetes occurs after middle age, although in American Indians Type II diabetes is found among the young.

Type II diabetes patients are usually overweight. Treatment

becomes much more effective when weight is reduced. Type II diabetes, therefore, is best controlled through diet, weight loss, and exercise. The behavior-modification approaches of mind body medicine are often most effective with Type II patients.

Stress and Diabetes

People with diabetes often have difficulty maintaining blood-sugar control during periods of psychological or physiological stress. Both anxiety and stressful life events can raise blood-glucose levels, insulin requirements, and glycosylated (sugar-bound) hemoglobin levels, reflecting poorer diabetic control.[10,11,12] In addition to direct effects, people under stress often neglect their eating habits and ignore the need for exercise. In diabetic patients this can worsen the existing condition and possibly precipitate a latent illness.

People facing chronic illness develop a variety of coping styles. Children with diabetes often use avoidant coping strategies such as wishful thinking or detachment, which result in poorer control.[13,14] By identifying a person's response to life stresses, including the stress

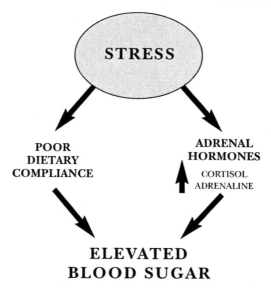

STRESS AND BLOOD SUGAR

STRESS

POOR DIETARY COMPLIANCE

ADRENAL HORMONES
CORTISOL ADRENALINE

ELEVATED BLOOD SUGAR

of dealing with a chronic disease, and teaching the skills to cope more effectively, we can help improve diabetic control.

If we feel that our behavior has no relationship to what is happening to us, we learn to feel helpless. Children with diabetes often wish that with good self-care behavior they can eliminate their disease. When they find that there is not such a simple and direct relationship, they begin to lose optimism that their efforts really influence the outcome of their illness. This creates a negative cycle wherein their feelings of helplessness lead to poorer control resulting in more frustration and helplessness.[15]

Depression is often a feature of both Type I and Type II diabetes and interferes with adherence to diet and medication. In juvenile-onset diabetes, there is an increased incidence of bulimia (self-induced vomiting) and anorexia.[16] Abrupt weight changes associated with these eating disorders can be a nightmare for patients, families, and doctors trying to achieve some semblance of stability.

The feedback loop between the stress of dealing with a chronic disease and control of the disease is apparent in people with diabetes. Life stresses, including the stress of having diabetes, result in hormonal changes that worsen blood-sugar control. The emotional distress of having diabetes influences how well people take care of themselves and this influences control of the diabetes. The recognition of this relationship between mind and metabolism has motivated the search for stress-reducing approaches to improve diabetic management.

Help

Over the past several years mind body techniques have been used as complementary therapy for patients with diabetes mellitus. Many, but not all, reports have demonstrated the benefits of relaxation and biofeedback training in helping to stabilize blood sugars. Studies in small groups of people with diabetes show that a stress-management program with relaxation training can improve average blood-sugar levels, improve stability, and reduce insulin requirements.[17,18,19] Episodes of insulin-related hypoglycemia (excessively *low* blood sugar) can also be reduced.[20]

Although it would be nice to think that specific mind body approaches, including relaxation techniques and biofeedback, are consistently beneficial in diabetes, this complex disease does not surrender so easily to science. Even from the same institution, studies can yield puzzling results. At Duke University, an initial report showed that training people in a relaxation program could improve their blood-sugar control and reduce their stress-hormone levels.[21] But, a later report on biofeedback-assisted relaxation could not find a difference between the trainees and controls—they both improved.[22] One way to interpret this is that simply in the process of putting their attention on the desire to have better diabetic control, there was some improvement independent of any particular technique. Future efforts will be directed at finding the best ways to enhance the power of attention in this illness. It may be different for different people.

Kids with Diabetes

Children with insulin-dependent diabetes are forced to face serious physical and emotional challenges. Concerns expressed by adults with diabetes are magnified in youths, who have to be ever vigilant and responsible. Children are concerned about how they are perceived by their peers and often have control issues with their parents. Mind body approaches in adolescents can improve their ability to cope with the stresses of diabetes.[23] Larger studies will be needed to determine if stress-management programs in children also improve blood-sugar control.

Relaxation and Circulation

Blood-vessel complications of diabetes are associated with major suffering and shortened survival. When blood vessels are damaged there is a real risk of skin ulcers and limb amputation. Since circulation is influenced by stress, it would make sense that influencing blood flow through relaxation training could help in diabetes. Using biofeedback-assisted relaxation training, people with diabetes can learn to increase their skin temperature and improve blood flow to their limbs.[24] Some people can increase blood flow to their legs by almost 50 percent just by listening to relaxation tapes that encourage the feeling of warmth and heaviness.[25] Learning to relax and let the blood flow can speed up the healing of skin ulcers in people with diabetes.[26]

Mind Body Interactions in Diabetes

Dealing with a chronic illness such as diabetes is taxing to the body, mind, and emotions. The intimate relationship between our mental experience of the world and the neurochemical and hormonal changes in our bodies can be tapped to utilize mind body approaches in a complementary manner for diabetes. In our experience, people with Type I diabetes have not been able to eliminate their need for insulin, but have often demonstrated more stable control using mind body approaches. In addition, the stress-reducing benefits of restful-alertness techniques improve the quality of life of those with diabetes.

Obesity is frequently an issue in Type II diabetes, which has proven to be an extremely challenging problem for Western medicine. Regardless of the approach, the vast majority of patients respond only temporarily before regaining their weight.[27]

From an Ayurvedic perspective, obesity is most often a hypo-metabolic or Kapha disorder. From this viewpoint, treatment includes a vigorous exercise program and a diet that reduces foods with sweet, sour, and salty tastes. Body Intelligence Techniques (BITS) can help to develop awareness of internal signals, and to avoid such common problems as eating when one is not really hungry or past the point of satiety. Mind body approaches encourage overweight people to develop a better awareness of their internal signals of hunger and satisfaction and not to confuse emotional needs with nutritional ones.

Occasionally, people with substantial Vata imbalances will become obese as they attempt to pacify their anxiety and agitation with food. They feed their anxieties through food: Whenever they feel restless, they eat something. For these people we recommend a Kapha-pacifying diet but a Vata-pacifying lifestyle.

When we are aware of our internal signals of hunger and satiety, we no longer attempt to fulfill our emotional needs by eating. To create this level of awareness, it is important to take time for silence each day in the form of meditation. This diminishes stress and improves integration between our mind and body. Taking a meal in silence is another very useful technique that helps us get in touch with our internal signals of hunger and fullness and ensures that we take in only the most nourishing foods.

From an Ayurvedic perspective, Type I diabetes is a Vata disorder.

Patients are often hypermetabolic, have a tendency to lose weight, and frequently suffer from anxiety or depression. When this is the case, we recommend Vata-balancing exercise and diet programs. Vata-pacifying music, aroma, massage therapy, and yoga are also helpful in treating Type I diabetes.

Type II diabetes, in contrast, is a Kapha disorder. Recommended treatment includes a Kapha-pacifying diet that emphasizes pungent, bitter, and astringent tastes. In correct balance, these can stimulate metabolism and reduce blood sugar. Ayurvedic herbs such as neem (*Azadiracta indica*) and *mehasringi* (*Gymnesyl sylvestre*) are also useful for enhancing sugar metabolism, as is a type of squash called bitter gourd, which is available in oriental groceries. Patients who use these natural substances should closely monitor their blood sugars and make appropriate adjustments in their diabetic medications in partnership with their physicians.

Kapha exercises and a Kapha-pacifying program of sensory modulation through sound, touch, sight, taste, and smell are all recommended for Type II diabetes. Vigorous Ayurvedic breathing exercises such as Kapalabhati (forceful exhalation) and Bhastrika (forceful inhalation and exhalation) are also of value, as they are designed to stimulate metabolic activity.

Although biofeedback-assisted relaxation training is not universally successful, it can be particularly useful when people with diabetes recognize a relationship between their life stresses and elevated blood sugars. Learning to activate the restful-alertness response can have wide-ranging benefits for people facing diabetes.

Facing an illness such as diabetes is a genuine challenge. Fortunately, we are seeing important advances in the scientific understanding and treatment of this problem, resulting in improved quality of life for people with diabetes. Contacting deeper levels of silence and stability through complementary mind body approaches can add real value to the lives of people with diabetes.

MIND BODY PRESCRIPTION
FOR PEOPLE FACING DIABETES

1. Follow the Ideal Daily Routine as closely as possible.

2. Practice meditation daily.

3. Practice body awareness—check in regularly with the physical sensations in your body.

4. Use the BITS at every meal.

5. If you tend to be overweight, follow the Kapha-pacifying diet and routine.

6. If you tend to be thin, follow the light Vata-pacifying diet and the Vata-pacifying routine.

7. Favor bitter herbs and vegetables that have a blood-purifying effect. Commonly available bitter culinary herbs include turmeric, cilantro, fenugreek, and rosemary.

8. Ayurvedic herbs traditionally useful in stabilizing metabolism include neem (*Azadiracta indica*), guggulu (*Commiphora mukul*), and mehasringi (*Gymnesyl sylvestre*).

9. Whenever you make any changes in diet or activity, carefully monitor your blood sugars and work closely with your diabetes doctor.

16

Mind Body Interactions in Heart Disease

"If you should take the human heart and listen to it, it would be like listening to a seashell; you would hear in it the hollow murmur of the infinite ocean to which it belongs."

Chapin

John, a forty-nine-year-old hard-driving advertising executive, felt trapped. The excitement he used to feel while working on a new account had been missing for years. Despite a large house, luxury automobile, and a profitable stock portfolio, he felt restless, perpetually frustrated and unfulfilled. He frequently lost his temper and blamed his wife's lack of understanding for the deterioration in their relationship. Frequent business trips kept him away from home half the month and he felt his kids were growing up without him. Although his family physician had escalated his warnings, John was too busy to exercise and continued to smoke a pack of cigarettes per day.

Last Monday morning, while racing to a high-pressure sales presentation, John suddenly felt a tightness in his chest and couldn't catch his breath. He was able to drive himself to the nearest emergency room, where he was admitted to the coronary-care unit with an acute heart attack.

Most of us are not surprised when we hear stories like this one. Deep in our human psyche we carry the understanding that our heart is more than a circulatory pump. Our language interweaves the experience of emotions with the beating drum in our chest.

We use expressions such as "heartbroken" to describe our feelings when we are grieving a loss. When we are filled with happiness, we say that "our hearts are overflowing with joy." The mind body approach acknowledges and uses this intimacy between our state of mind and our heart to create the optimal environment for cardiac fitness.

The Problem

Cardiovascular disease is the epidemic of our modern age. If you live in the Western world, there is an excellent chance that you will eventually develop heart disease and even die from it. The statistics are staggering:

- At least 1.5 million Americans will have heart attacks this year and over 500,000 people will die as a result. Over 40 percent of all deaths are attributable to cardiovascular diseases each year.
- Forty-five percent of heart attacks occur in people under the age of 65.[1]
- At least 300,000 Americans this year will undergo coronary-artery bypass surgery at a cost of over seven billion dollars.[2]

The media is regularly reminding us of the major conventional risk factors for coronary heart disease (CHD), which are: smoking, hypertension, high cholesterol, family history, diabetes, and obesity. These factors were initially identified in the Framingham, Massachusetts, studies, first reported in the early fifties.[3] Other than family history, we can modify each of these risk factors through our choices. Smoking-cessation programs report variable short- and long-term success rates, but if you are able to stop, your risk of a heart attack may be reduced by half in just one year.[4] Lifestyle choice can moderate other risk factors as well. For example: Meditation and relaxation techniques can lower blood pressure, and in some cases can reduce or eliminate the need for medication;[5] reducing your dietary intake of saturated fats can lower your cholesterol level;[6] obesity and adult-onset diabetes mellitus can be influenced by appropriate diet and exercise programs.[7]

The Risk Beneath the Surface

Although the major coronary risk factors are clearly important, we have learned that they are definitely not the whole picture. Some disappointing studies suggested that even if you are able to reduce smoking, blood pressure, and cholesterol, you may only minimally lower your risk of heart disease and may actually increase the chance of dying from other causes.[8] In fact, even with fairly similar patterns of risk factors, there are dramatic differences in the risk of heart disease in different cultures. Some studies have shown that Europeans have half the rate of coronary events as Americans, and people living in Hawaii have some protection against heart disease that continental Americans lack.[9,10] It seems to be more than just not having to shovel snow from the driveway each winter.

As it became apparent that the standard risk factors did not completely explain the incidence of heart disease, studies on the role of personality and behavior began in earnest. These led to the recognition that certain personality characteristics are present in a high percentage of heart patients.[11] People at high risk for heart disease tend to perceive their environments as threatening battlefields, requiring intense competitiveness in order to survive. This hostile interpretation of life doubles our risk for a heart attack, even if none of the other usual risk factors are present. The meaning is clear: Our minds and emotions influence the physical well being of our hearts.

Mind Heart Linkages

William Harvey, the seventeenth-century physiologist, created the first description of the circulatory system in the Western medical tradition. Harvey elegantly portrayed the mind heart connection when he wrote, "Every affection of the mind that is attended with either pain or pleasure, hope or fear, is the cause of an agitation whose influence extends to the heart."[12]

The mind and the heart are both directly and indirectly linked. Direct connections exist through the autonomic (involuntary) nervous system, which can influence heart rate and rhythm as well as blood pressure. If we perceive a circumstance as threatening, our blood pressure rises and our heart beats faster. If you tend to see your environment as hostile you are more likely to show an overactive cardiovascular response to annoyances.[13] If you feel aggravated much of the time you are priming your heart to overreact to challenges with aggravation and aggression.

Indirectly, mental states such as frustration or anger influence our cardiovascular system through the release of stress hormones such as adrenaline and noradrenaline. These activating chemicals can cause the tiny blood-clotting cells known as *platelets* to clump together.[14] One might say that these "jittery" platelets huddle together in fright, activating the clotting cascade and cutting off the supply of nourishing blood to the heart. Over time, the chronic effects of stress play an important role in the development and acceleration of atherosclerosis, or hardening of the arteries.[15]

Personality and Heart Disease

The association between stress and cardiac disease dates to antiquity. The ancient physician Celsus wrote in A.D. 30 that ". . . fear and anger and any other state of the mind may often be apt to excite the pulse."[16] References to fainting and death as a result of a powerful emotional encounter are described in Ayurvedic texts dating back four thousand years. The great physician sage Charaka said, "One who wants to protect the heart . . . should avoid particularly the causes of the affliction of mind . . . and make efforts for serenity."[17]

In modern times, Drs. Friedman and Rosenman identified a cluster of characteristics that predisposed people to coronary artery disease. These traits were:

- hard-driving
- competitive and hurried
- need for recognition and advancement
- under constant deadline pressure
- presence of a hyper mental and physical state

These characteristics were labeled *Type A Behavioral Pattern* (TABP), implying a strong need for perfection by those who displayed these traits. People displaying this pattern seemed to be much more vulnerable to coronary heart disease, independent of other risk factors. A study of over three thousand middle-aged men without known heart disease indicated that men with type A traits developed coronary artery disease *twice as often* as those who did not have these characteristics (type B).[18]

Efforts by other researchers to replicate these findings met with contradictory results.[19,20] An extensive seven-year effort from the University of Texas could *not* confirm a definite connection between type A behavior and the risk of heart disease.[21] These reports raised questions of whether *specific* aspects of the type A pattern might put a person more directly at risk. The answer surfaced that the essential personality feature that puts us at greatest risk for heart disease is not competitiveness or the need to succeed, but rather, *hostility.*

If you score high on a hostility test you have a much greater chance of showing serious narrowing in your heart vessels than someone who has a low hostility score.[22] You are also more likely to have a heart attack and will probably not live as long as your more relaxed friends.[23]

The news is worse if you are a doctor or a lawyer with hostility as part of your nature. A twenty-five-year study of physicians showed that if you carry a lot of hostility you have a six-times-higher risk of dying than if you take life a little easier.[24] If you are an attorney and score high on a hostility test, you have a 20 percent chance of dying by age fifty compared to your more mellow lawyer colleagues, who have only a 4 percent mortality risk.[25]

Within the category of hostility, three even more specific traits have been identified as correlating with the risk of heart disease: *cynicism,* an underlying negative belief that other people are inherently unworthy, deceitful, and selfish; *hostile affect,* in which the emotions of irritability, impatience, and loathing are dominant; and *aggressive responding,* in which anger and aggressiveness are considered reasonable and justifiable ways of responding to life's challenges.[26]

People who view others as frequent sources of mistreatment, frustration, and aggravation—and therefore as untrustworthy—are at much higher risk for both coronary heart disease and other life-threatening illnesses.[27,28] Although other components of the Type A Behavioral Pattern, including intensity and hurriedness, do not show up as independent risk factors, people who score high on hostility tests often display these traits as well.

ARE YOU HOSTILE?

Check off the statements below that describe your tendencies.

1. ___ I often suspect that I am carrying more than my fair share when facing a task that requires many people's input.

2. ___ When I can't find something, I suspect that someone took it without my permission.

3. ___ If someone rapidly becomes prosperous, I suspect that they achieved their wealth unethically.

4. ___ I feel annoyed when someone sits down in front of me at a movie theater.

5. ___ I become frustrated when another customer at a department store is conversing with a clerk whose attention I'm seeking.

6. ___ I become irritated when minor mishaps occur.

7. ___ If someone criticizes me, I respond by pointing out their faults.

8. ___ I notice myself clenching my fists when I am frustrated.

9. ___ When others disappoint me, I quickly label them as stupid or incompetent.

10. ___ I often vent my anger and feel better only to discover that I have hurt other people's feelings.

11. ___ I ascribe manipulative motivations to other people, suspecting they have a secret agenda to take advantage of me.

12. ___ I resent people who want my attention when I have other things to do.

If you checked off:

    0–2 items, you have fairly low hostility

    3–5 items, you have moderate hostility

    6–8 items, you have high hostility

    > 8 items, you have a seriously high hostility level

Several recent studies have provided even further evidence of the role of stress and hostility on the heart. At the Mayo Clinic, people discharged from a coronary-care unit after either a heart attack or an anginal episode took tests to determine their level of psychological distress. Those who were the most distressed had the highest risk of subsequent serious cardiac problems and spent more than four times as much money than the relatively nondistressed patients.[29] Another Mayo Clinic report showed that people who scored high on hostility tests had a much higher rate of reblocking their heart blood vessels after they had been opened by angioplasty than those with low hostility scores.[30]

Our understanding of what happens when people get heart attacks has been going through a revolution of the past few years. We are learning that most attacks are not due to gradual closure of a blood vessel like a progressively plugged plumbing drain. Rather, most catastrophic coronary events are due to sudden clotting of a mildly narrowed blood vessel.[31] It seems that the standard risk factors, such as smoking, high cholesterol, and high blood pressure, predispose the inner lining of the heart blood vessels to damage. Inflammation at the site of these vulnerable arteries can incite blood clotting, leading to sudden blockage of blood flow. High levels of stress hormones are known to trigger the clotting cascade, partially explaining how stress and hostility can lead to heart attacks. Although we do not yet entirely understand the mechanisms at work, the message is clear: *Hostility is bad for your heart.*

Reducing Hostility

Among hostile people, even the memory of a stressful circumstance can trigger an excessive response, but the *expression* of anger appears to cause the greatest changes in heart rate and blood pressure. Although some hostility-reducing techniques encourage verbal and physical "acting-out" of anger, this may not be the best approach in patients at risk for heart disease. Other interventions, including meditation, noncompetitive forms of exercise, laughter, music therapy, acquiring pets, and taking up spiritual pursuits, are likely to be safer and more effective.

We have found that *identifying* the nature of anger, *witnessing* the emotion, and then *releasing* it can be an effective technique for extinguishing this emotion. The first step is to ask, "What am I feeling now?" Once the feeling of anger is recognized, shift your awareness and witness your agitated internal dialogue and the sensations in your body. The very act of witnessing your feelings allows them to fade.

Once the strong negative emotion begins to dissipate, ask, "Where are the seeds of my hostility? What is the basis of the anxiety and fear that causes me to react in anger?" This is important, because no matter how justifiable the expression of hostility may seem in a particular circumstance, the effects of anger are always harmful to the heart.

Then reward yourself by finding some healthy and enjoyable physical outlet for the strong feeling, such as brisk walking, riding a bike, swimming, or dancing. This allows your body to work through the energy created without harming yourself or others.

Relationships and the Heart

Nourishing, intimate relationships are an essential aspect of good health. A loving family and close friends can prevent illness and improve chances of recovery if illness does occur. Alternatively, the stress of losing social support through divorce, death of a spouse, or loss of a job has been shown to harm your health.

There are many different forms of social support including marriage, friends and family, religious affiliations, and group associations. A large study from Alameda, California, showed that people with close relationships and social ties have half the deaths from all causes compared to those without a nourishing social-support system.[32]

Support can be as simple as a phone call. If a compassionate nurse checks in by a monthly telephone call with men who have recently suffered a heart attack, the death rate can be reduced by half over the first year.[33] Surely, this is a cost-effective intervention, but very few cardiac programs offer such a service.

A caring, loving spouse or confidant can truly be life-saving after a heart attack. Studies from around the world have shown that your risk for recurrent chest pain, heart attack, and death is cut almost in half if you have someone to support you emotionally after suffering heart damage.[34,35,36] An atmosphere of love and caring reduces mental stress and stabilizes your nervous system. Our health-care system and society need to provide sensitive and caring environments for heart-disease patients, starting with our coronary-care units. It is clear that a safe and loving experience can reduce the risk for further heart attacks and is at least as important as interventions directed at smoking, exercise, or diet.

Work Stress / Work Satisfaction

Most of us spend at least a third of our waking hours on the job, so it's not surprising that our level of accomplishment, appreciation, and meaningful communication with co-workers directly influences our mental and physical well being. Work provides much more than a source of income; it offers a social network that can be either nourishing or toxic.

Simply by inquiring, "Do you like your job?" or "Are you happy in your job?" it's possible to determine whether a person is at risk for heart disease. Reports from Sweden have shown a correlation between high levels of job stress and elevated blood pressure, heart disease, and death.[37,38] It seems that the most stress-producing circumstance is when there is a high demand for output with little influence on how to accomplish the task.[39,40] Programs that allow workers to improve the quality of their time on the job can improve health, morale, and productivity.

Studies on the incidence of heart attacks have disclosed a quite fascinating statistic: In our society, more people die on Monday morning at nine A.M. than at any other time![41,42,43] This extraordinary fact must be unique to the human species, for surely no other animal knows the difference between Monday and Tuesday. Most of us have had that sinking feeling when, after a long, relaxing weekend or vacation, we have to gear up to return to a stressful job. The power of thoughts and feelings is immense, and can be the difference between life and death.

Through the Stomach to the Heart

The relationship between high serum cholesterol and heart disease is well established, and the benefits of a low-fat, low-cholesterol diet are generally accepted. Several studies have supported the favorable effects of reducing dietary animal fat on cholesterol levels and cardiovascular disease. One of the earliest was the Leiden Intervention

Trial, completed in 1981, which showed that people who followed a vegetarian diet not only dropped their cholesterol level but also showed a stabilization in their coronary artery disease.[44]

Dean Ornish's Lifestyle Heart Trial has received a lot of attention since he showed that a comprehensive heart-disease program that included smoking cessation, a vegetarian diet, meditation, moderate aerobic exercise, and group support could actually *reverse* coronary artery narrowing.[45] Those who followed the program lost weight, lowered their cholesterol levels, and reduced their blood pressure. Of greatest significance was the evidence of improved blood flow to the hearts of people following the program, showing for the first time that coronary artery disease could be reversed without drugs or surgery.

From a mind body perspective, there are many reasons to suspect that reducing your intake of red meat can have health benefits. If hostility plays a role in heart disease, reducing the intake of food derived from killing reduces hostile input on a subtle level of consciousness. From a planetary perspective, red meat is costly in terms of grain and water.[46]

There are clear health benefits of reducing red meat and increasing the proportion of fruits, vegetables, and other foods high in antioxidants. In a recent French study, participants who suffered heart attacks were counseled to follow a diet containing more breads, green vegetables, fruits, and fish, while reducing their intake of meat, butter, and cream.[47] The diet groups experienced fewer fatal and nonfatal heart attacks. Diets rich in the antioxidant vitamins C and E seem to confer the greatest protection against heart disease, as demonstrated in a Finnish study of five thousand men in which the risk of a heart attack was cut in half.[48] In people with very high cholesterol levels who require medication, the combination of a primarily vegetarian diet plus a cholesterol-lowering drug provides the greatest benefit in reducing coronary artery narrowing and the risk of heart disease.[49]

How We Eat

For more than thirty years, research has shown that cholesterol levels are not fixed, but fluctuate in response to states of mind. During times of stress, for instance, cholesterol levels rise.[50] Cholesterol levels in first-year medical students, for example, were found to range from a mean of 205 milligrams at low-stress times to 226 milligrams at the time of the final anatomy exam.[51]

In the population as a whole, wide variations in cholesterol levels occur from week to week and year to year, *independent* of diet. One of the most interesting reports in this area was published in the journal *Science* during 1980.[52] Investigators at Ohio State University were studying cholesterol metabolism in rabbits, because these animals develop atherosclerosis (hardening of the arteries) similarly to humans. The researchers wanted to learn whether the type of care given to the rabbits would influence levels of cholesterol and fat deposits in their blood. Some of the rabbits were treated routinely while others received loving and compassionate attention. In the latter group the attendant regularly played with the bunnies, talking to and cuddling them several times per day. Both groups were fed the same high-cholesterol diet for six weeks.

At the conclusion of this study, the lovingly treated rabbits showed reduced cholesterol levels and less than half the number of fatty deposits in their major blood vessels compared to the control group. If these findings are relevant to us, we've learned something very important from this study: Our interaction with our environment has a real influence on how we metabolize our food. Rabbits treated compassionately were able to metabolize cholesterol in a way that was less harmful to their health.

This fascinating experiment reveals a great opportunity for avoiding and reversing heart disease by adjusting our relationship with the environment and with the people around us. While it may be true that you are what you eat, you are not only what you eat. According to Ayurveda, the human body is the end product of the sum total of the experiences taken in through *all* the senses, including sound, touch, sight, taste, and smell.

Mind Body Interactions in Heart Disease

Heart disease is the leading cause of death in our civilization. The major risk factors of this epidemic have been identified and most can be modified through changes in interpretations and behavior. The means for accomplishing these changes, however, must be made available. People smoke because they do not know how to access an alternative nontoxic source of satisfaction. High blood pressure, in part, results from an ongoing perception of the world as a hostile environment. Elevated blood cholesterol derives from excessive intake of animal fats and from altered metabolism, which is influenced by stress levels. Hostility is the expression of an internal dialogue of cynical mistrust. Lack of social support and job satisfaction reflect alienation from the community and failure to recognize one's own inherent creativity.

Mind body approaches can influence each of these risk components. Meditation can provide us with access to an inner field of comfort that is independent of external props. Stress reduction through yoga and exercise can normalize blood pressure and reduce harmful reactivity to challenging situations.

Eating healthy foods—and doing so with focused awareness—can influence our body's metabolism. According to Ayurveda, eating is a holy experience in which energy and information from the environment are converted to life energy. If we eat when our mind is settled, all the sights, tastes, smells, and textures of the meal can be fully experienced. This can have a profound effect on the way food is metabolized.

In the area of job satisfaction, the Ayurvedic perspective offers the beautiful concept of *dharma*. Dharma is the state of being in which one's purpose in life is fully expressed. When we are in dharma, we are in tune with our higher self and spontaneously serve others, while expressing our unique talents. If these ideas could be incorporated into our culture's definition of job satisfaction, there would be a fundamental transformation in the way we regard work. The concept of dharma holds that there is no one in this universe who has the exact talent that you have; everyone possesses a unique ability and a unique way of expressing it, and our task is to discover what that is. Once this has been accomplished, work becomes a way of making a real contribution to the world.

Dean Ornish's landmark study showed that regression of coronary artery disease took place among people who practiced yoga and meditation, eliminated tobacco, and followed a vegetarian diet. From the Ayurvedic perspective, all of these changes in lifestyle are effective because they provide nourishment and encourage the elimination of toxicity from the mind body physiology. Stress, and the cardiovascular dangers associated with it, results from encountering toxins in our environment. These toxins may be in food or water, but they can also exist in a relationship or a job. All mind body approaches—meditation, yoga, diet, intimate relationships, massage, herbs—are simply ways of reducing and eliminating the harmful effects of toxins from all areas of our life.

In his book *Travels*, the popular writer Michael Crichton describes a fascinating discovery made while a medical student at Harvard.[53] During his rotation on the cardiac service, he asked patients, "Why did you have a heart attack?" Everyone had an answer, and it was not that his cholesterol level was too high or that he didn't exercise enough. The responses were personal and meaningful. One man said he got a promotion but his wife didn't want to move. Another said his wife was planning to leave him. Most responses expressed deep distress over relationships, children, or jobs. Crichton wrote, "What I was seeing was that their explanations made sense from the standpoint of the whole organism, as a kind of physical acting-out. These patients were telling me stories of events that had affected their hearts in a metaphysical sense. They were telling me love stories. Sad love stories, which had pained their hearts. Their wives and families and bosses didn't care for them. Their hearts were attacked. And pretty soon, their hearts were *literally* attacked."

Ultimately, the keys to the prevention and treatment of heart disease are waiting for us in the field of consciousness. In the West, awareness, intelligence, and discrimination have been localized in the brain, but in Eastern thought there is such a thing as "heart intelligence." This is the recognition of an inherent intelligence that can be accessed through attention to sensations in the physiology.

Whenever a choice needs to be made in any area of life, the body provides a message of either comfort or discomfort, and for most of us the message is felt in the heart. Simply by honoring this heart intelligence, we can effortlessly avoid toxic substances, foods, and relationships, and we can begin to eliminate heart disease. Consciousness, the field of pure potentiality, can become our creative and loving internal ground state, and from this vantage point we can experience the world as a source of unlimited opportunity for health and for joy.

MIND BODY PRESCRIPTION FOR A HEALTHY HEART

1. Practice meditation twice daily, for twenty to thirty minutes in the morning before you begin your day, and again in the evening before dinner. Allow your mind body system to experience the state of restful alertness regularly.

2. Perform a daily oil massage with the appropriate dosha-specific oil.

3. Begin practicing gentle yoga with breathing awareness. Set aside ten to fifteen minutes each day for this purpose.

4. Reduce your intake of animal fat while increasing your consumption of fresh fruits, vegetables, and whole grains. Follow the Body Intelligence Techniques (BITS), and supplement your diet with Ayurvedic herbs traditionally used to balance and nourish the circulatory system. These include guggulu (Indian gum myrrh) and arjuna (Arjuna myrobalan).

5. Think of ways to make your work more creative and interesting. An unsatisfying job is one of the most important elements of the depression and stress associated with cardiovascular disease.

6. Assess your personal and professional relationships. Enjoy and cultivate those that are essentially nourishing; eliminate those that are toxic.

7. If you are smoking, do so with total awareness. This means do nothing else but pay attention to your physical sensations from the moment the urge arises to the time you put out the butt. Have the intention to release this habit.

8. With your physician's approval, begin an exercise program that gradually increases your level of physical activity. In the first month, for example, you might aim to increase your pulse level 25 percent above resting rate for the duration of your exercise period. In the second month, increase your activity until your pulse is 50 percent above resting rate. Finally, try for twenty to thirty minutes of exercise, three times per week, at 75 percent of your maximum heart rate.

9. Spend a few minutes each day doing something for the pure enjoyment of it. You may want to take a walk in the park,

listen to music, or play a game with your children. But regardless of how you spend this time, let the activity be its own reward. Let go of the belief that everything you do must achieve a goal or serve a purpose.

10. Identify elements of anger and hostility that you carry in your heart and have the intention to release them. This doesn't mean you should try to transform yourself into a saintly personality overnight. Just let yourself become aware of the anger you may be feeling, and remind yourself that it's something you want to let go.

11. Notice any circumstances that trigger a stress response. Listen to your internal dialogue to discover whether your reaction to a situation raises or lowers your stress level. Pay special attention to any moments when you've responded to only a partial picture of the triggering situation, and later discovered that your reaction was inappropriate.

17

Mind Body Interactions
in Cancer

"Each patient carries his own doctor inside him . . .
We are at our best when we give the doctor who resides
within each patient a chance to go to work."

Albert Schweitzer

Tom had been a steady beer drinker since high school. When he got to
college, he would limit himself to a few beers per day during the week,
but could easily go through three or four cases on the weekend. This con-
tinued until he reached age thirty, when his wife threatened to leave him
and his doctor warned that his liver would fail if he continued drinking.
With the help of Alcoholics Anonymous, Tom remained dry for the next five
years.

Then tragedy struck. His wife was killed instantly in an automobile
accident. When six months after his misfortune Tom began to lose weight,
his friends suspected that he had started drinking again. But this was not
the explanation. When he finally saw his doctor for worsening belly pain,
the condition had gone too far. Tom was diagnosed with liver cancer that
had already spread.

Cancer is all around us. It is a rare person whose life has not been
touched in some way by this dreaded disease. It's the scourge of our
modern age, creating pain and suffering for those afflicted and for
their families and loved ones.

Although our medical establishment is vigorously addressing
this problem, each day three thousand more people in the United
States are diagnosed with cancer, and more than fourteen hundred

people die. It kills more Americans than any other illness besides heart disease.[1]

What's particularly frightening is that despite all of our efforts to date, the percentage of cancer-related deaths is rising, as is the overall incidence. Among men, malignant melanoma, bladder, and lung cancers are diagnosed more frequently. Prostate cancer is increasing so dramatically that current estimates predict that one out of every ten men will develop prostate cancer by the age of eighty-five.[2] For women, breast cancer is really an epidemic in this country, with almost one out of nine women developing a breast malignancy by the time they are eighty-five years old.[3]

In addition to its enormous cost in physical and emotional suffering, cancer has a staggering economic impact. The cost of cancer rose from $2.5 billion in 1985 to more than $100 billion in 1990, and all evidence points to this trend continuing.[4,5]

In view of these overwhelming numbers, it is not surprising that people are seeking alternative cancer care. It is estimated that between 10 percent and 50 percent of all people with cancer are using some form of unconventional or nontraditional approach to treating their illness.[6] The fact that almost $4 billion per year is spent on these approaches suggests that important human needs are not being met by standard cancer treatments.[7] I believe that mind body interventions have an important role to play in the treatment of people facing cancer.

Studies on Stress, the Immune System, and Cancer

The relationship between life stress and cancer has long been suspected. As reviewed in Chapter 8, prolonged stress in laboratory animals raises cortisol levels, which results in lower numbers of white cells and shrinkage of lymph tissue throughout the body. These changes increase the risk of infection and cancer.[8]

There are many common life situations that create stress and potentially weaken immunity. If you crowd animals together and limit their access to food, they will show a much higher percentage of tumors when infected with a virus than their relatives housed in more luxurious accommodations.[9]

Just the stress of traveling can weaken our immune defenses. During long-distance airplane trips the air and food are less than optimal, the crowding and immobility make us irritable, and our bio-rhythms are disrupted. In an experiment designed to test the effects of travel stress, mice were separated into two groups and shipped cross-country by airplane. Upon arrival, one group was immediately injected with lymphosarcoma tumor cells, while the other group was allowed to relax for several weeks before the tumor cells were implanted. The stressed mice that were immediately injected with cancer cells had a 100 percent mortality rate, while the mice that were allowed time to rest had a much lower death rate.[10]

We've learned that we can condition an animal's immune sys-tem to fail if we associate a stimulus such as saccharin water with ad-ministration of an immune-suppressing drug like cyclophosphamide. After initial exposure, just the taste of the sweetener can cause white blood cell counts to fall.[11]

A similar situation for people with cancer is known as anticipa-tory nausea and vomiting (ANV). Some people have the misfortune of developing very strong reactions to chemotherapy. They associate the medical environment, including the people who administer the drugs, with the symptoms of nausea. When due for chemotherapy, they may become ill just by thinking about the treatment. In these patients, immune suppression also occurs as a result of condition-ing.[12] Even before the chemotherapy is given, their immune systems act as if they have been poisoned. Fortunately, we now have very pow-erful antinausea drugs available that work well for most people. At The Chopra Center, we have also found that meditation, breathing exercises, and herbal teas made with aromatic spices can reduce the nausea associated with cancer therapy.

The Role of the Mind in the Development of Cancer

Depressed people have a higher risk of cancer. People who have recently divorced or lost a spouse show impaired immune function and an increased risk of serious illness, including cancer.[13,14,15] When prolonged depression occurs after the death of a loved one, the risk of developing and dying from cancer is increased for twenty years after the loss.[16]

Do certain personality characteristics predispose someone to cancer? Although this question has been raised for many years the answer remains hazy. A British study looked at women undergoing

breast biopsies, and reviewed their personality traits prior to determining whether or not there was cancer. The results suggested that
women found to have a malignancy were less able to express anger
openly.[17] The idea of a "cancer-prone" (type C) personality style was
raised. A type C person presumably suppressed her emotions, and
some reports suggested that this trait correlated with poorer outcome.[18,19,20] Other studies, however, failed to detect a consistent relationship between personality characteristics and the tendency to
develop cancer or influence the outcome of patients with cancer.[21,22]
This type of research is very difficult to perform because there are
many confounding factors. Although the scientific relationship between personality traits and cancer risk is not well established, it is
safe to say from a mind body perspective that honest, nonblaming
emotional expression is healthy.

Behavioral Choices

Unhealthy lifestyle choices account for up to half of all cancer
deaths,[23] and smoking alone accounts for over 30 percent of these.[24]
In addition, dietary factors contribute to more than a third of cancer
deaths. A relationship between diet and cancer has been shown in
malignancies of the esophagus, stomach, pancreas, liver, colon,
breast, prostate, lung, kidney, and bladder.[25] The high fiber content
of a primarily vegetarian diet reduces the concentration of certain
bile acids that have been implicated in tumor growth.[26] Seventh-Day
Adventists, who do not smoke, drink minimal alcohol, use caffeine
moderately, and favor vegetarianism, have notably lower rates of both
lung and digestive-tract cancers.[27]

There is now abundant evidence that our response to stress,
general emotional state, and nutrition can influence our risk of
developing cancer. It's common sense that changing these basic
aspects of our behavior can reduce our risks and improve our health.
In view of the harshness and limited efficacy of modern treatments
for cancer, it's essential that we pay real attention to preventing it
through lifestyle changes.

Mind Body Interactions in the Response to Cancer

There is no doubt that loving emotional support improves the *quality* of life in people with cancer. We know that people who participate in supportive group therapy and learn relaxation and meditation techniques report an improvement in their mood, feel more empowered with their illness, have better relationships, miss less work, have less sleep disturbance, require less pain and antinausea medications, and are more compliant with their treatments.[28–32]

Do these improvements in *quality* of life increase the *quantity* of life? The answer seems to be yes. Women with breast cancer and a close social-support network live longer and have a lower risk of relapse than women who are more emotionally isolated.[33] Just daily contact with a supportive friend or family member is one of the most important components associated with longer survival. Dr. F. Fawzy's work with melanoma patients at UCLA showed that a short-term intervention with emotional counseling and education improves immune status and results in fewer recurrences and longer survival.[34,35] Participants in this program only receive one session a week for six weeks, showing that even a relatively brief intervention can be successful with people at a critical time in their lives.

Is the improvement in survival in people receiving emotional support simply due to better compliance with the cancer treatments? A study of people with leukemia showed that although those receiving supportive counseling did follow their treatment recommendations more closely, their improved survival was independent of compliance.[36]

Dr. David Spiegel's work from Stanford generates hope and excitement by showing that weekly support-group meetings for women with breast cancer not only reduce their need for pain medication while improving overall well being, but also result in a doubling of survival time.[37,38] If a new chemotherapy drug could produce this effect, physicians would be guilty of malpractice if they failed to employ it—yet only a very limited number of oncology centers have integrated this cost-effective approach into their protocols. We have been so pharmaceutically oriented that nondrug approaches to health have only recently received serious attention. Fortunately, the National Cancer Institute has taken an interest in this area and is funding studies in an attempt to replicate these findings.

Ayurveda and Cancer

The materialistically based medical model views cancer as a result of a structural change in the genes of a cell, resulting in unrestrained growth. Treatments based on this material model include surgery, radiation, and chemotherapy. These approaches are recognized to carry serious and potentially life-threatening side effects, but the considerable toxicity of treatment is justified by improved rates of remission and survival. Damage to healthy tissues is considered a necessary and acceptable price of waging war on cancer cells.

Indeed, warfare is a common image for much of Western medicine's approach to cancer treatment. The nature of the disease is such that even the most detached clinicians and researchers are drawn to think of cancer in metaphorical terms. The illness has been described in terms of battles and massacres, has been compared to the Holocaust and to a barbarian invasion. But Ayurveda characteristically chooses a less bellicose terminology. From an Ayurvedic viewpoint, cancer cells are elements of the mind body system that have lost their memory of wholeness, so that the patterns of intelligence that maintain healthy boundaries in the physiology have become distorted and fragmented. The renegade cells, having forgotten their true purpose in life, become insensitive to the needs of others. In their egotism to expand their territory of influence, they destroy their environment and eventually destroy themselves.

According to Ayurveda, cancer results from a breakdown of self-referral. Owing to accumulations of stress and its resulting toxicity, cells forget their true purpose for existence. Having lost their connection with wholeness, they are cut off from the flow of biological intelligence. These malnourished cells mutate into cancer cells.

From the consciousness-based perspective, then, cancer is viewed as a distortion in the field of intelligence. It is the result of imbalance and toxicity in the continuum of physical environment, body, mind, and spirit. The mind body goal is to eliminate toxins and restore balance. This is accomplished through detoxification procedures and nourishing approaches designed to activate healing impulses and reduce stress throughout the field of consciousness.

In scientific terms, stress is defined as that which causes us to lose our physical or psychological equilibrium. In Ayurveda, stress is defined as that which interferes with the spontaneous flow of nature's intelligence in the human physiology as it moves from unmanifest to manifest. When this flow of intelligence is accompanied by self-referral, there is energy, vitality, creativity, and harmonious order. Self-referral is the state of awareness in which the self is never overshadowed by the object of experience. Self-referral can apply to the life of the body as a whole, but it applies equally to the life of a single cell. A cell—functioning with the memory of wholeness, never overshadowed by its fragmented experience—is a healthy, cancer-free cell.

Memory of wholeness at the cellular level includes three components that are also crucial to health and happiness in general. First, the cell must remember its higher function, which is to maintain the integrity and harmony of the whole organism. Second, it must express its unique talents, whether it be the secretion of hydrochloric acid or acting as a pacemaker for the heart. Finally, it must constantly have one question in its awareness: "How can I serve?"

Stress, which is the perception of threat, interferes with one or more components of the memory of wholeness. A cell that maintains self-referral does not allow threat to overshadow its purpose, known in Ayurveda as dharma. A cancer cell is a renegade cell that has lost its memory, or *smriti*. Having lost its smriti, it has lost its dharma—and having lost its dharma, it makes karmically incorrect choices. Healing therefore must restore smriti, or memory. More specifically, healing is the process that restores the memory of wholeness.

All perception of threat is experienced as fear. Fear is the basic disrupter of the spontaneous, effortless, frictionless flow of nature's intelligence in its self-referral mode. And the ultimate fear is always the fear of death; every other source of fear—the loss of a job, the end of a relationship—is just the fear of mortality in disguise. All day-to-day fears and anxieties are really quantified fears of mortality. Only by becoming intimate with the immortal realm within can we see mortality as quantified immortality.

From the consciousness perspective, a totally self-referred being is completely without fear, including the fear of mortality. The uncertainty of the unknown is no longer feared, but embraced. This cannot occur through psychological effort. It can only occur through a spiritual experience in which a person connects with that component of himself or herself that is beyond mortality. It is for this reason that I do not encourage visualizations that set up more conflict in the mind and body. Some behavioral cancer programs teach patients to envision their cancer cells as deformed invaders and their immune cells as PacMan-like creatures gobbling them up. I have found it more useful to envision cancer cells as shadowy beings that are best reminded of their true purpose by bringing in light. If you are facing cancer, try this simple guided meditation after you have performed a quieting meditation technique for at least ten minutes.

How do we translate these lofty healing concepts into a practical program for someone facing cancer? At The Chopra Center we immerse people in a healing environment that supports their inner exploration of wholeness. When people arrive, they are taught primordial sound meditation so they can have a direct experience of their deeper, more expanded consciousness, beyond the anxieties and worries that have been gripping them. Patients are encouraged to safely express the emotions they have been carrying about their illness, including their worst fears. We emphasize recapturing integration between mind and body through yoga and yogic breathing exercises. Classes on healthy nutrition from food as well as all the five senses are provided. Each day our guests receive panchakarma detoxification therapies to encourage the release of deep-rooted stresses. Instructions in purification and rejuvenation procedures that can be used at home are provided so that the momentum gained can continue.

The treatment of people with cancer is always a delicate balancing act. As a physician, I want to support hope and optimism, while not denying the life-threatening nature of the illness. I want them to embrace the self-empowering mind body approaches but not abandon potentially helpful medical interventions. I want my patients to assume their responsibility as active partners in their treatment but do not want them to feel guilty that they created their disease. I want them to have the intent of regaining their vibrant individuality while believing that the ultimate possibility of healing lies in surrendering to their universal, spiritual nature.

From an Ayurvedic perspective, cancer is invariably a tridoshic

HEALING VISUALIZATION

Sit comfortably, close your eyes and take a deep breath. Now, slowly exhale, allowing the tension in your chest, shoulders, and abdomen to release. Innocently observing your breath, allow each exhalation to take you to a quieter, more comfortable, more relaxed state. Release the tension, the tightness, the weight of your body with each breath.

Now imagine that you are in a beautiful, serene natural environment. The air is warm, the sun is shining, the sky is clear, and the ground is covered with soft, sweetly fragrant grass. Find a comfortable spot and lie down in the grass, allowing the earth to cradle you, and feel the soothing sun on your body. Enjoy this moment of peace and serenity.

Now envision your body as a glowing cocoon of golden light. See and feel the life force radiating within and around you. Now notice the area of your body that is unwell. See the ailing cells as shadowy beings that have lost their way. They have forgotten their dharma, their purpose in life, and in their effort to gain attention, they have gone beyond their healthy boundaries.

Now imagine that a warm, pure, healing light is gradually glowing brighter in your heart. Allow it to radiate comfort, peace, and love throughout your entire body, encompassing every cell. As the soothing, healing light fills your being, direct its luminescence to the area of illness. Allow the purifying light to illuminate the shadows hiding there and watch them melt away. Observe the clearing of darkness as the healing energy suffuses the tissues, bringing lightness and clarity.

Allow the nourishing energy of the environment—the pure air, the nurturing earth, the luminous sun—to infuse your being, purifying and nourishing your body, mind, and soul. Release the resistance, release the pain, release the fear. In the light and warmth of your healing awareness, and with the wisdom of Nature, the memory of wholeness is rekindled.

disease associated with the accumulation of ama. Agni is weakened, ama has accumulated, the subtle circulatory channels are blocked, and ojas cannot sufficiently support immunity. Ayurvedic treatment seeks to eliminate accumulated toxicity, strengthen digestive power, and supply nourishment to the tissues. If the patient can tolerate a vigorous detoxification, this is the recommended first step. Because the purification treatments are somewhat depleting, however, a debilitated cancer patient may not be able to tolerate intensive detoxification. Therefore, the focus may at times be on replenishing and supporting the person, rather than on trying to clear the deeper impurities.

Over this past week, I have seen three people with cancer. A thirty-year-old woman completed her treatment for Hodgkin's lymphoma two years ago and is probably cured of her illness. Her goal is to rebuild her energy and learn how to live a healthier life. An elderly man with metastatic lung cancer was told by his doctors that he has only a few months to live. He is hoping for a miracle but understands that our primary focus is on improving his quality of life in his remaining days. My third patient, a forty-year-old mother of two, recently learned she has breast cancer and is scheduled to begin a course of chemotherapy. She wants the tools to minimize the side effects of her treatment and help her with the stress of facing her disease.

There are similarities and differences in the approaches to each person's problems. For the lady with treated lymphoma, the focus is primarily on helping her get on with her life. She will learn how to promote her health and embrace a lifestyle that supports mind body balance. For the man with widespread cancer, we will help him walk the delicate line between hope and surrender, encouraging him to embrace and release his fears while focusing on living each day with awareness. For the woman facing a course of cancer therapy, we will encourage her to create grounding associations using the five senses so that she can work with, rather than against, the powerful drugs she will receive.

In my experience, patients facing a life-threatening illness such as cancer can re-create health only when they release their attachment to the idea of being cured, and when they surrender to the inner field of wholeness, eternity, and spirit. Only in this surrendering does the rare spontaneous remission manifest. But surrender should in no way be confused with resignation, hopelessness, and helplessness. Surrender to the spirit is actually an experience of the infinite and eternal. Immersion in spirit provides the experiential knowledge of immortality.

The recovery of health, of wholeness, is the experience of dynamic non-change in the midst of inevitable, eternal change. When a person is facing death, complete surrender to spirit is a rare phenomenon, and therefore remissions are rare. In caring for patients with cancer, every attempt should be made to create the opportunity for a real spiritual experience totally outside the context of their disease. Ultimately, this must occur in the field of silence. When the field of pure potentiality and all possibilities becomes the internal reference point, profound changes can occur in mind and body. The mental script changes from fear and anxiety to comfort and confidence. Having tapped into spirit, the message being conveyed from mind to body is one of wholeness. Because the mind body connection is real, the quality of our conscious attention profoundly influences every cell in the body. When the mind is fearless and identified with eternity, every cell will reflect this state of health.

Creating a Healing Environment

In addition to the obvious clinical issues raised by the presence of a serious illness, cancer causes severe disruptions of the patient's lifestyle even on the most basic everyday level. Work routines, time spent with family, exercise, and even opportunities to relax must be suddenly and severely cut back or eliminated in order to deal with the many pressing concerns of this life-threatening illness. Compared to cancer, everything else is relegated to a distant second place, because cancer is a full-time job.

Cancer's power to preoccupy the patient is obvious and unavoidable, but from an Ayurvedic point of view this is also an important obstacle to the process of recovery. By riveting our attention on the details of treatment and other concerns raised by the disease, cancer distances us from our inner selves. It can cause the spiritual dimension of life to seem irrelevant to the pressing issues of treatment and cure. Yet Ayurveda teaches that our spirituality is absolutely fundamental to recovery from cancer. It's crucial, therefore, to recognize the preoccupying nature of cancer as yet another sign of the illness, and one that it's very important to counter.

I've associated the phenomenon of spontaneous remission from cancer with a spiritual experience that takes place outside the context of the illness. While this connection may not be documented by research studies, it has been my experience that patients who have been able to overcome the preoccupations of the disease have substantially benefited. According to Ayurvedic teaching, daily meditation is the most effective means of accessing the spiritual self. For the cancer patient, setting aside time to meditate may present a challenge, and, at least initially, the restful awareness of meditation itself may also seem difficult amid all the mental static generated by the illness. But, again, Ayurveda teaches us to regard meditation as a fundamental element in the cancer recovery process, and one that will greatly reward commitment of time and concentration.

Once meditation becomes part of a cancer patient's daily routine, he or she will enjoy this opportunity to experience silence and restful attention. As a supplement to meditation, try also to spend some time each day outdoors in a natural environment. These activities are more than just enjoyable. They are an important part of the return to wholeness that recovery from cancer represents.

Cleansing and Rejuvenating Techniques

Ayurveda describes cancer as arising out of toxicity in the body, mind, and spirit—but, as I've emphasized throughout this book, these elements are seen as inseparable by mind body medicine. Just as meditation will benefit the physical self through the spirit, there are some simple but powerful Ayurvedic techniques for cleansing and rejuvenating the physical self.

A daily oil massage, for example, draws toxins from the body while toning and restoring tissues at the same time. You can perform the massage yourself or have a friend or family member help you. If possible, try also to have a professional massage at least once a week.

Drinking warm water and ginger tea throughout the day is

another traditional method of cleansing the system. This technique has benefits for everything from weight control to dealing with cancer. Within the limits of comfort, try to keep the water as warm or as hot as possible. A good way to do this is to keep a thermos with you, and sip water throughout the day. If you drink at least one cupful each hour, you'll soon feel the purifying effects throughout your body.

It's also important to move your bowels at least once a day. Constipation is a common side effect of cancer treatments, particularly narcotic pain medications, and from a mind body perspective this works against the need to reduce toxicity in the system. Drinking warm water can also provide benefits in this area, but commercial laxatives should be discouraged. Eating fresh fruit and well-cooked fresh vegetables will also help.

Herbal supplements can help reduce the toxic conditions that are the ground state of cancer. Ayurvedic herbs traditionally used for detoxification include kumari (aloe vera), neem (Persian lilac), and guggulu (Indian gum myrrh). The Western herbs echinacea and goldenseal have similar purifying properties. Rejuvenating herbs include amalaki (Indian gooseberry), ashwagandha (winter cherry), shatavari (Indian asparagus), and bala (country mallow).

Reducing Treatment-Related Stress

Receiving chemotherapy or radiation can be stressful both physically and emotionally. Fortunately, stress can be diminished by associating pleasant sensory experiences with times of comfortable relaxation and then using the sensory cue when facing a more stressful situation. Try using rose, sandalwood, jasmine, or other pleasing aromas during your daily meditations, and then keeping a bit of these scents with you during your treatments.

Broadening Your Perspective

I've emphasized the limiting influence cancer can have on contact with our spiritual nature, or even with the simple pleasures of daily life. While your daily meditation sessions can be very helpful in avoiding this effect, it can also be very therapeutic to share your thoughts

MIND BODY PRESCRIPTION
FOR PEOPLE FACING CANCER

1. Practice meditation on a daily basis.

2. Spend time in silence in natural environments on a daily basis.

3. Follow an ama-reducing diet, emphasizing fresh vegetables, fruits, and whole grains.

4. Drink plenty of water each day.

5. Make certain that you are eliminating your bowels at least once daily.

6. Perform a daily oil massage, and if possible get a professional massage at least once per week.

7. Ayurvedic herbs traditionally used for detoxification include: kumari (aloe vera), neem (Persian lilac), and guggulu (Indian gum myrrh). The Western herbs echinacea and goldenseal have similar purifying properties.

8. Ayurvedic herbs traditionally used for rejuvenation include: amalaki (Indian gooseberry), ashwagandha (winter cherry), shatavari (Indian asparagus), and bala (country mallow).

9. If you are undergoing cancer treatments, associate a pleasing aroma (for example, rose, sandalwood, jasmine) with your meditations. Keep the scent with you throughout your treatments.

10. If you are having a problem with nausea, try chewing on fresh ginger root, whole cloves, or cinnamon sticks.

11. Although the scientific data is still limited, discuss with your oncologist the timing of chemotherapy to maximize the effects of the drugs on the cancer cells and minimize the side effects on normal cells.

12. Talk about, write about, express, and share your feelings with your family, friends, and health providers.

13. Surround yourself with nourishing music, sights, and smells.

14. Read spiritual literature.

15. Watch comedies . . . laugh!

and feelings with family, friends, and caregivers. Or, just write them down or record them for your own benefit. Reading spiritually oriented literature, listening to music, looking at beautiful things, and even just laughing out loud can all help you get outside the boundaries of the cancer experience. And this can have very real benefits for your recovery.

18

Mind Body Interactions in Reproduction and Pregnancy

"Your children are not your children. They are the sons and daughters of Life's longing for itself."

Kahlil Gibran

Like most married couples, Barbara and Alex assumed that children would be a part of their lives. Although Barbara's menstrual cycles had been occasionally irregular, she never considered that she would have trouble getting pregnant when she was ready to have children.

After trying unsuccessfully to conceive for a year, Barbara and Alex went to an infertility clinic for evaluation. A complete examination failed to identify a problem with either Barbara or Alex. They were recommended to chart her monthly cycles and have sex only on peak ovulation days.

Making a baby soon became a job. The pressure of having sex on specific days, the hope turning to despair every month when Barbara's period arrived, and the mounting sense of frustration, failure, and self-doubt began to erode their marriage and Alex moved out of the house.

After a three-month trial separation, they met for a romantic reconciliation weekend in Sedona. Three weeks later, Barbara's urine tested positive on a home pregnancy test.

The impulse to reproduce ourselves is structured within our genes. After meeting our needs for air, water, and food, the desire to procreate is probably the next to arise. Biologists will tell us that the essential purpose of life is to pass our genetic inheritance down to the next generation. With the instinct to have children so intrinsically hardwired into our minds and bodies, it is easy to understand that when a couple that desires offspring has problems with fertility, it can be agonizing to body, mind, and soul. Although difficulty having children usually has a physical basis, there is increasing recognition that stress can contribute *to* as well as result *from* infertility.

Conceiving, carrying, and giving birth to a baby involve all aspects of our physiology, but the mind, the brain, and the endocrine system are especially important. The close relationship that exists among these three elements has a profound impact on the reproductive capacities of both men and women.

It is estimated that almost ten million couples in the United States have a problem with fertility. In almost 500,000 couples, a thorough evaluation fails to reveal any "organic" cause for infertility. These cases are sometimes labeled unexplained infertility and are the most likely to benefit from mind body approaches.

Nerves and Hormones

We have spoken earlier of the hypothalamus and its influence on the emotions. It is closely connected with the limbic system, which is involved in our basic life-sustaining behaviors including feeding, fighting, fleeing, and sexual attraction. The hypothalamus is most concerned with visceral, involuntary, and hormonal functions and is intimately tied into our moods and feelings. Nerve cells in both the limbic system and the hypothalamus not only have an influence on the regulation of sex hormones involved in reproduction but also have been shown to have a high concentration of receptors for these hormones.[1] Thus, these parts of the brain modulate reproductive hormones and are also sensitive to their feedback.

The pituitary gland lies below the hypothalamus at the base of the brain, where it receives chemical messengers that regulate the release of the hormones important in fertility. The chemical messengers from the hypothalamus govern the release of two main reproductive hormones from the pituitary—follicle-stimulating hormone (FSH) and luteinizing hormone (LH). In women, these chemicals are responsible for the maturation of the ovum and the preparation of the uterus for implantation after fertilization occurs. In men, these hormones regulate the production of sperm and the release of the male hormone testosterone. FSH is secreted in increasing amounts during the first two weeks of the menstrual cycle, where it functions to stimulate maturity of the ovum. Around midcycle, LH appears in greater concentrations, which stimulates the ovary to release the mature egg into the fallopian tube. This process of ovulation depends not just on the right amounts of the various hormones, but also on their rising and falling in a very delicate, precisely coordinated sequence.

Stress and Fertility

Many kinds of stress can disrupt hormonal communication between the brain, the pituitary, and the ovary, interfering with both the maturation of an egg and the ovulation process. The neurochemical changes that occur when we are under stress can alter the ordered release of hormones that regulate the maturation and release of an egg. Concentrations of many of our important chemical messengers

STRESS AND FERTILITY

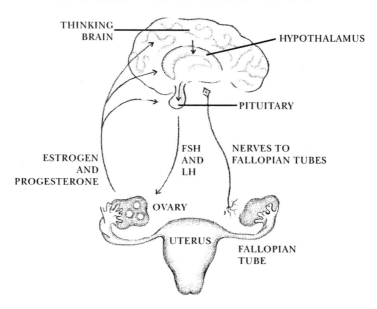

involved in reproduction (norepinephrine, epinephrine, dopamine, prolactin, and the endorphins) have all been shown to change under different emotional states.[2] Direct links also exist between the brain and the reproductive tract, with nerve fibers directly connecting with both the fallopian tubes and the uterus.[3] Both the sympathetic and parasympathetic branches of the autonomic nervous system influence the ovary's ability to produce healthy eggs and hormones.[4] For example, when a woman is under stress, spasms occur in both the fallopian tubes and the uterus, which can interfere with movement and implantation of a fertilized egg.[5]

Infertility may result from altered regulation of pituitary hormones, or from abnormal nervous-system influences on the ovaries and fallopian tubes. Stress can make us less fertile, and the resultant failure to conceive can create further stress, resulting in a vicious cycle. Women who are unable to conceive often experience a loss of self-esteem, depression, anger, and anxiety over disappointing their partner; men may begin to feel guilty, resulting in relationship problems and reduced sexual activity.[6] Sexual enjoyment often diminishes, as the focus becomes making a baby instead of making love. All of this reinforces the cycle of stress and infertility.

Both physical and emotional stress have been reported to influence male fertility. Sperm counts, motility, and structure can all be altered under stress.[7,8,9] In addition, other problems including impotence and difficulties with ejaculation have all been associated with emotional distress in men.[10]

In both men and women under stress, sleep cycles are commonly disturbed. Sleep deprivation and insomnia have been shown to alter the daily rhythms of several hormones involved in reproduction and fertility.[11] The sleep disturbances associated with stressful events may also contribute to infertility.

Our thoughts are powerful. Studies have shown that just our expectations of how good a parent we will be can influence fertility.[12] Women who have doubts about their ability to be good mothers have more difficulty getting pregnant than those who can imagine themselves as good mothers. If you are a man and are fearful or apprehensive about having a child, you may be less likely to father one.

Mind Body Therapies for Infertility

Science has not expended a lot of effort looking into the possibility that stress-reducing programs may influence fertility. What we know to date is that in couples with unexplained infertility, programs to reduce anxiety improve the rate of pregnancy. In an early report, over 50 percent of couples learning to relax became pregnant over three months versus none of the controls.[13]

Stress-management programs can reduce depression, anxiety, anger, and fatigue, all of which are commonly part of the lives of people struggling with infertility.[14] It seems that as these negative emotions diminish, the chance of becoming pregnant increases.

Feelings of social isolation can be a sad side effect of infertility. Support groups can be helpful in establishing a sense of community with other people who understand the anguish of not being able to have children. Couples who attend support groups feel less depressed, anxious, and hostile and find themselves less obsessive about child-bearing.[15] And, in what seems to be a common theme in mind body medicine research, improving quality of life leads to an improvement in the underlying problem. A University of Massachusetts Medical School study showed that 71 percent of infertile couples participating in support groups conceived versus 25 percent for those who did not participate.[16]

Stress-management programs are not the cure for infertility, but mind body approaches focusing on decreasing anxiety and increasing relaxation can be cost-effective ways to help couples with unexplained infertility. Reducing stress through the restful-alertness response may help normalize menstrual cycles, improve the health of both egg and sperm, and increase the likelihood of fertilization and implantation. In addition, helping couples to reduce their stress will improve the quality of their relationships and their lives.

Stress and Pregnancy

There is a positive correlation between birth defects and unwanted pregnancies. Women who want to have an abortion but are denied have a higher rate of babies born with abnormalities.[17] A sad but fascinating study from Scandinavia showed that the offspring of women who are widowed during pregnancy have more health and behavior problems as adults than those whose fathers died shortly after their birth.[18] The severe stress experienced during pregnancy by the mom is experienced and metabolized by the fetus, resulting in real difficulties later in life.

Intrauterine Experience

According to Ayurveda, consciousness arrives early in fetal development and the ability to perceive changes in the environment is present long before birth. Western science is learning that we are amazingly capable of perception while we are developing in our watery wombs.[19,20]

- Hearing: The first indication of a developing acoustic apparatus is seen in human embryos as soon as twenty-two days of development. By the seventh week, the precursors of the three small middle-ear bones are fairly well developed.
- Vestibular: The organs to perceive changes in position begin to differentiate by the fifth week and are fairly well developed by the fourteenth week.
- Touch: Spinal and peripheral sensory nerves capable of responding to pressure, pain, and temperature are present by the seventh week of fetal development.
- Sight: The lens, retina, and optic nerves are present by six weeks. The visual apparatus is well developed by eight weeks.
- Taste: Taste buds are present by eight weeks and appear developmentally mature by twelve weeks of gestation.
- Smell: The olfactory components appear by six weeks. Smell receptors and nerves are present by ten weeks.

Sound Before Birth

In the Gospel According to Saint Luke (1:44), Elizabeth exclaims to Mary, "The moment that the sound of your greeting came to my ears, the babe in my womb leaped for joy." Many studies have shown that we can and do perceive sounds while in the womb. As a fetus, we will adapt to a specific sound after just a few trials.[21] If you play a beautiful piece of music by Debussy at a time when a mother feels relaxed, playing the same piece at other times can soothe an agitated infant.[22] Similarly, we do *not* appreciate loud sounds when we are in the womb. For example, it has been shown that pregnant women living close to an airport have lower levels of growth-promoting hormones and smaller newborns compared to a control group.[23,24]

These scientific reports support the Ayurvedic position that the baby hears the many sounds of the mother's body—her heartbeat, her voice, and even the sounds that the mother herself hears. On some level, all the sounds that the mother perceives are also heard by the baby. Beyond helping to develop our hearing apparatus, sounds are important in creating the nerve networks of our developing brains.

The sound of our mother's heartbeat is a constant accompaniment throughout our stay in the womb, and we remember how changes in this beating correlate with our sensations. If after birth, infants are provided with a recording of heart sounds at 72 beats per minute, they become calm and relaxed. If, on the other hand, a recording of a heart rate of 120 beats per minute is played, newborns become restless and agitated. We learn *in utero* to associate a rapid heartbeat in Mother with discomfort and distress.

Amazing studies in animals are relevant. Unhatched chicks can hear and respond to the sounds of the mother hen and distinguish their mom from others.[25] If recordings of the mother bird are played to an unhatched chick, there is an increase in mouth movements; if, however, calls of another bird are played, the unhatched chick shows a rise in heart rate, suggesting the perception of stress. During normal development, a bird embryo hears sounds in its environment that allow its brain to recognize bird calls after birth. If those sounds are not present at the earliest stages of development, there is an abnormal response to them later.

Sounds also enhance the synchronicity of hatching.[26] One might expect the various eggs in a brood to hatch over a period of hours or even days, but in fact, eggs kept together in a nest under natural conditions all hatch at about the same time. Eggs kept separated in incubators, however, show a much wider spread of hatch times. Sounds made by chicks preparing to hatch are heard by their siblings while still in the egg, resulting in synchronization. The ability to arrive and stay together confers an evolutionary advantage, by allowing them to huddle together for warmth in the cool night air and perhaps by confusing predators with their random, jerky movements. Hearing how conscious of their environment even unborn birds are makes it harder to enjoy an omelet!

Human intrauterine life enjoys a full range of sensory experiences, and these experiences can have an effect on childhood development. The unborn child is capable of perceiving its mother's voice, responding to music, perhaps even discriminating languages.[27] The possibilities of enriching the prenatal life of a child are unlimited. The nickname a mother calls her unborn child, the music she listens to, the language she speaks, even the fairy tales she reads may all be influencing the personality of the developing child. The remarkable abilities of a fetus need to be recognized and acknowledged by every potential parent.[28]

Becoming Human

Just eight weeks after conception, we move in fairly sophisticated ways in response to prodding.[29] By the time we are only a half-inch in length, we show fairly complex movements alternating with periods of rest.[30] By about twelve weeks we show primitive facial movement, and by sixteen weeks we can grimace, smile, and squint. At twenty-four weeks we respond to minor changes in sound, and have already developed a surprisingly sophisticated sensitivity to taste. Our swallowing rate increases if a sweet solution is placed in the amniotic fluid and decreases if an unpleasant-tasting substance, such as iodine, is given.[31] With modern ultrasound, a fetus can actually be seen to grimace if something doesn't taste very good.

Even though our eyes remain closed, as a fetus we will show a response to bright light as early as the sixteenth week *in utero.* Our heart rate speeds up and we will turn our head away from the light.[32] At twenty-eight weeks, our neuronal circuits are fairly well developed, brain waves can be recorded, and we are going through some primitive sleeping and waking cycles.[33]

Our fetal ability to perceive the environment has profound implications. If, as a result of stress, the mother releases hormones that cross the placental barrier, the fetus experiences the same physiological effects that its mother is undergoing. If the mother is a smoker, an unborn baby's heart rate will react when she inhales the nicotine, and eventually, even just showing a cigarette to the mother results in the same effect on the fetal heart.[34] The fetus anticipates the toxic experience about to occur. From a mind body perspective, we could say that a mother's internal dialogue influences the release of circulating hormones, which cause changes in both mother's and baby's physiology.

Nourishing the Unborn Child

I believe that the environment provided for our unborn children is as important as the one after they are born. Acknowledging that the womb is potentially rich with experiences, we at The Chopra Center for Well Being have developed a prenatal program for creating the most nourishing possible intrauterine environment. Mothers participating in the program are encouraged to:

- Learn and practice primordial sound meditation, to elicit the restful-alertness response.
- Listen to beautiful, soothing instrumental music, lullabies, and chanting.
- Choose and use a nickname for the unborn child.
- Read aloud poetry, fairy tales, and myths that express the highest values of human culture.
- Practice yoga postures and breathing exercises specific to pregnancy to create physical flexibility and vitality.
- Perform a daily Ayurvedic massage, which stimulates the release of life-enhancing peptides and growth factors.
- Eat a balanced, prana-rich diet with full awareness.
- Use natural approaches to cope with common pregnancy concerns: ginger for morning sickness, yoga for back discomfort, warm milk with cardamom and nutmeg for insomnia, massage for swollen feet.
- Learn healthy ways to communicate with their partners so the unborn child perceives the world as a safe and nurturing place.

Diet

Diet during pregnancy should focus on Kapha-enhancing foods, which should be as nourishing and as fresh as possible. Dairy products and calcium-rich foods should be especially encouraged. Because the mother is providing the substrates for the development of her child's body, Kapha foods rich in carbohydrates and protein are extremely important. Sweet tastes should be favored, but all six tastes should be part of each meal. To ensure smooth elimination, plenty of fresh fruits and vegetables should be eaten, and about two weeks before delivery the mother should begin adding extra oil to her diet to increase the level of oleation in the system.

Because digestion often becomes delicate, particularly during the later months of pregnancy, follow the Body Intelligence Techniques. The pregnant mom should always eat in a settled environment and honor her appetite, maintaining her awareness that she is feeding her child when she is feeding herself.

Although Ayurveda does not generally encourage vitamins, an expectant mother should rigorously follow all recommendations from her health-care provider, particularly in regard to the need for additional folic acid.

A Healthy Delivery and Postpartum Period

For the delivery itself, Ayurveda advocates performing a soothing genital massage with sesame, almond, olive, or coconut oil beginning about four weeks before the anticipated birth. This softens the tissues around the vaginal opening, and Ayurvedic physicians in India report a reduction in episiotomies and vaginal tears.

During the birthing process, we recommend breathing exercises based on yogic principles. At the onset of each contraction a deep and slow cleansing breath is taken in and released through the nose. During mild-to-moderate contractions, paced rhythmic breathing is encouraged. During the intense contractions of transition, when the cervix is completing its dilation, a blowing breath is used. This involves forcefully exhaling through the lips as if blowing out a candle.

The use of music, massage, pictures, and pleasing scents are encouraged during delivery to engage the senses and focus Mom's attention. The birth partner is essential, serving to ground the mother, pace her in the breathing exercises, and provide the much-needed support.

We recommend that immediately after birth the newborn infant be placed on the mother's chest, where the familiar heartbeat can be heard. The lights should not be overly bright and the sounds should be soothing. If possible, playing the lullabies or chants that were played during the pregnancy is ideal. Over the next several days, a gentle, warm oil massage on the baby will provide comfort and promote growth. We recommend the use of natural nut or seed oils rather than those that are mineral based. Almond or coconut are usually well tolerated by the newborn's gentle skin.

Ayurvedic approaches during the postpartum period can reduce the likelihood of depression, which is often related to interrupted sleep; the stressful experience of being a new mother; and the sudden fall in brain opioids and other hormones, which occurs soon after giving birth. Naturally occurring pain-relieving chemicals can be increased through massage, exercise, and meditation. A healthy social-support network is also crucial. If the mother is nourished on all levels, she will be able to provide the best nourishment for her infant.

It is particularly important to follow a Vata-pacifying program for at least the first six weeks after delivery, for the process of giving birth is imbalancing to the component of Vata (Apana) that is responsible for moving the baby through the birth canal. To the extent possible, mothers should attempt to get enough rest, eat a balanced meal, take time to meditate, and perform a daily oil massage. Meditating while breast feeding can be beneficial for both mother and child. By following an Ayurvedically balanced diet, the mother can ensure that her breast milk provides optimal nourishment for the growing baby.

A healthy environment uses all the sensory modalities—sound, touch, sight, taste, and smell—to provide nourishment for newborn children. We want to ensure that their transition into the world is secure and nurturing and starts them off on the smoothest path toward realizing their full potential.

Mind Body Interaction in Reproduction and Pregnancy

Our genetic information, coded in our DNA, carries the memories of millions of years of evolutionary experience. Living beings are created from the information wrapped in the patterns of our genes. One of nature's prime forces is the impulse to continue the life cycle by passing the biological intelligence on to the next generation. Human beings have the longest child-rearing period of any species, and for most couples, having children and raising a family is a primary reason for making a commitment to a relationship.

When a couple who wants to raise a family has difficulty conceiving a child, their anxieties and fears over their potential loss are reflected in physiological responses that potentiate their problems of fertility. To the extent that infertility concerns are functional, as opposed to anatomic, mind body approaches can be useful in reducing stress and improving the chances for conception.

Once conception has occurred, two localized fields of consciousness share the same psychophysiological system for the nine months of pregnancy. Whatever the mother breathes, baby breathes; whatever mother eats, baby eats; whatever mother experiences, baby experiences. Therefore, during the pregnancy, mother should treat herself with the same love, care, and concern that she will treat her child.

Once the new soul arrives in the world, the nurturing that was provided before and during pregnancy is continued into the neonatal period and beyond. We have the opportunity to create a generation of human beings who express the highest values of life and health by providing them with the knowledge and experience of consciousness as the ground state of existence. For them, the "new paradigm" will be the prevalent worldview. We believe there is a real possibility for creating a positive shift in consciousness on this planet. Magical beginnings create enchanted lives.

The Infinitely Extended Family

When we speak of our own children as separate from someone else's, we are of course making a very understandable distinction. But it's also useful to acknowledge the sense in which all children are "ours," and in which the entire human species is really one enormous family. From this perspective, the route taken to parenthood is much less significant than the love and wisdom we share with the children who come into our care. Adoption, artificial insemination, surrogate motherhood, these are all to be celebrated along with natural conception as perfectly wonderful ways of forming a family. Nature's deepest intention is that every child who comes into the world should have loving parents, regardless of how those parents are acquired.

MIND BODY PRESCRIPTION
FOR A HEALTHY PREGNANCY

1. Treat your unborn child as if she/he were experiencing whatever you are experiencing.
2. Take time for silence each day in meditation and nature.
3. Pay careful attention to your diet, eating nourishing prana-rich food.
4. Perform a daily oil massage. During the month prior to delivery, gently massage the perineal region (area between the vagina and rectum) with sesame, almond, olive, or coconut oil. Work the oil into the tissues and gently stretch the inner opening to the vagina.
5. Choose a nickname for your unborn child and talk to her/him regularly.
6. Listen to beautiful, soothing music. Read stories and poetry that are beautiful and elevating to the soul.
7. Eliminate all toxins (substances, food, air, emotions) from your life.
8. Try fresh ginger root, cloves, or cinnamon to relieve morning sickness.
9. Practice yoga and breathing exercises designed for pregnancy.

19

Mind Body Interactions in Women's Health— Menstruation and Menopause

"Age cannot wither her, nor custom stale
Her infinite variety . . ."

William Shakespeare,
Antony and Cleopatra

The paradigm shift that is taking us into the next millennium can be described as an awakening of an inner goddess, a female perspective that has been suppressed or ignored since the days of the Roman Empire. Now the linear, logical, analytical, goal-oriented, win-lose orientation that has dominated modern Western consciousness, and that has been identified with male modes of thought and feeling, is undergoing a transformation. We are beginning to recognize that intuition, synergy, process, context, and relationship are essential if we are to be complete as human beings.

When we first recognized this psychological and cultural shift, it was described in terms of a left brain/right brain orientation. But we can also see this evolutionary change as a recognition and embracing of our feminine nature. According to psychoanalyst Carl Jung, each of us carries both primordial male and female archetypes within our psyche and that intimacy with our inner woman and inner man is the key to love, wisdom, and personal empowerment. It is also the basis of well being, for health is really *wholeness,* and it requires that we embrace every aspect of our nature.

Our expanding awareness of the feminine is transforming all aspects of life. As we collectively acknowledge the value of a more global, unifying, integrative vision, the goddess within our collective psyche is empowered to express herself in social, political, and economic spheres. The changing role of women is transforming relationships, families, organizations, and society.

Many of the changes we are seeing in health care derive from the new wisdom the goddess is bestowing upon us. As women regain their power in the many arenas of life, the model of a patient as a passive, unquestioning recipient of medical care becomes untenable. People who see themselves as important, powerful, and wise beings want to be active partners in creating their own health. Although it is natural to regress in the presence of a physician, we do not need to surrender all authority completely. Questioning and challenging are qualities of intelligent beings, and the empowerment of women in all decisions relevant to their lives and health is having effects throughout health-care. Research indicates that female patients consider good rapport and positive relationships with health-care providers to be extremely important. As women become more assertive in asking for what they want, the mechanical approach that has characterized health care must change to meet their needs.

Masculine / Feminine

What do *masculine* and *feminine* really mean? What distinguishes one from the other? Although poets, scientists, and philosophers have been exploring this question since the story of Adam and Eve in the Old Testament, I suggest that the fundamental and essential difference between our male and female nature can be described in one word: *rhythm*.

The male psyche is deeply imbued with the quest. The male principle in us sets a goal and pursues it unrelentingly, whether it's the purchase of a new car, achieving a high position in an organization, reaching a certain financial status, or winning the heart of a lover.

The zero-sum, win-lose tools of male consciousness are designed for intense focus on achieving specific aims, and this approach has been phenomenally successful in our achieving the major material accomplishments of the past century. We have developed self-powered vehicles, global communication networks, spaceships capable of exploring other worlds, and major medical breakthroughs that have substantially changed the way we treat disease. But anxiety and alien-ation, disruption of family and community bonds, and the loss of connection to nature have accompanied our technological advances. None of us wants to relinquish our automobiles, cellular phones, and ATM machines, but we are also beginning to recognize that these things alone can never bring us lasting happiness.

The linear, male-consciousness approach has not been intrinsi-cally wrong, but it is seriously incomplete. Conquest and achieve-ment have been our reasons for being, and human history over the last two millennia has been the chronicle of this paradigm. When we've achieved a goal, we've set our sights on another. But the goals we've set have been in the external world rather than in our own hearts, and the path we've chosen has been a straight line pointed outward, rather than a circle leading back to ourselves.

Our feminine nature is intrinsically entwined with the cyclical rhythms of life. In fact, our concept of time is closely interwoven with a woman's cycle. The word for womb in Greek, *metra,* is derived from the same word for measurement, *meter,* which is also the origin of the words *mother* and *time.* Feminine time, however, is not the same as linear time, since the former is *self-referral.* It can be observed in the passage of seasons, in the ebb and flow of the tides, and in the phases of the moon—each acts out a cyclical return. Until recently, our patriarchal society has substantially denied the power of nature's goddesses, and the price for this repudiation has been great. As we embrace our holistic, intuitive nature, we naturally become more attuned to our connection to Mother Earth and our responsibility for her well being. Whether we are genetically male or female, embrac-ing both aspects of our nature creates health.

Implications for Health Care

One consequence of our predominantly male viewpoint has been the medicalization of women's health issues. Pregnancy and menopause, and even menstruation to a degree, have become medical issues requiring pharmacological interventions to "keep them running smoothly" or to "fix them" despite the fact that women have been moving through these cycles of life without drugs for millions of years. Once again, we see a well-intentioned medical system dedicated to relieving suffering, but relying only upon a limited, expensive, and frequently invasive therapeutic repertoire. In contrast, it has been our experience that complementary mind body approaches to menopause and premenstrual syndrome can be very beneficial, in both relieving symptoms and as tools to enhance mind body integration in women. As women recapture balance, rhythm, and harmony within themselves, the world benefits.

Premenstrual Syndrome (PMS)

Christine received very little direct talk about sex as an adolescent girl. Her young mother, divorced soon after the birth of her third child, was perpetually exhausted from single-handedly raising Christine and her two older brothers while working full time.

At age twelve, as her body began to show the changes of developing into a woman, Christine received predominantly negative messages from her mother about sex and reproduction. When she had her first real period, her mother described it as "the curse" and warned her not to get into the same mess that she was in. As a junior in high school, Christine began to have distressing cramping, migraine headaches, and mood swings as her menstrual time approached. As a result, she regularly missed several days of school each month. This pattern continued after she graduated and entered the workplace, limiting her ability to advance in her job.

At age thirty-three, following the death of her mother from ovarian cancer, Christine decided she was going to take charge of her life and began counseling sessions. This led to her visiting us at The Chopra Center, where she learned to meditate, eat healthier, follow a more balanced daily routine, begin regular exercise, and reduce her use of caffeine and alcohol. When I saw her after she'd followed this program for several months, she was a much more comfortable and confident woman, had lost ten pounds, and had only missed two days of work over the past three months.

The menstrual cycle links women to the rhythms of the natural world. According to Ayurveda, effortless menstruation is one of the four key fundamentals to good health, along with strong digestion, regular elimination, and restful sleep. When menstruation is smooth and natural, it is a sign that a woman's mind and body are integrated in a healthy way. But distress and discomfort in a woman's monthly cycle is evidence of an underlying imbalance in her mind body continuum. The fact that so many women in the Western world are troubled with PMS, therefore, should raise a red flag of concern about women's experience in our society. It should cause us to question how women are regarded, and how they regard themselves.

PMS affects women of all ages, with several studies suggesting that almost a third of childbearing females have distressing-to-disabling symptoms prior to their menstrual periods.[1] There are over 150 disturbing mental, physical, or behavioral symptoms associated with PMS, including anxiety, mood swings, irritability, headaches, breast tenderness, bloating, fatigue, increased appetite with food cravings, sleep changes, and memory and concentration problems. The hallmark of PMS is the repetitive presence of symptoms during the week prior to the menstrual period, which subside once menstrual flow begins. Well over half of all women have some of the symptoms associated with PMS, although they are usually not severe enough to interfere with normal activities. But even if her symptoms are not severe enough for a woman to stay in bed or miss work, the mind body interventions recommended in this chapter can still be very beneficial.

The Magnificent Menstrual Cycle

Before delving deeper into what is known about the cause and treatment of premenstrual syndrome, I'd like to review the extraordinary choreography that regulates a normal menstrual cycle. The brain, hypothalamus, pituitary gland, ovary, and uterus are harmoniously integrated to ripen an egg for fertilization and prepare the womb for implantation. Although I briefly discussed this process in Chapter 18, on reproduction, I'll go a little deeper here. This detail is well justified, for the normal menstrual cycle is a beautiful expression of nature's intelligence. A close consideration of the cycle can help us not only to understand it intellectually, but to minimize its potential for causing distress in women's lives.

Cells in the hypothalamus, the nervous and hormonal center at the base of the brain, secrete pulses of a chemical messenger that stimulates the pituitary gland to release two hormones, luteinizing hormone (LH) and follicle-stimulating hormone (FSH). These two protein messengers enter into the bloodstream until they reach the ovary. Here, egg cells are stimulated to ripen and, in the process, produce estrogen, which stimulates the lining of the uterus to prepare for a fertilized egg. The process starts on the first day of menstruation so that by Day 14, the egg is ready for release and ovulation occurs.

After the egg is released, the cells that surrounded it in the ovary begin making another hormone, progesterone, which further prepares the womb's lining. What follows next depends on whether a sperm reaches the ripe egg and fertilizes it. If fertilization occurs, the egg floats down the fallopian tube and eventually finds its way into the uterus, where it becomes embedded into the lining and begins to receive nourishment to support the development of a fetus. If a sperm does not reach the egg, the cells in the ovary stop making estrogen and progesterone, the lining of the uterus is released, and menstrual flow begins.

There are many other hormones and chemical messengers that also play roles in this elegant, though complicated, dance (Table 1). All of these codes of intelligence have widespread effects, not only on the ovary and uterus, but also on many aspects of the brain. Therefore, it is not surprising that subtle imbalances in this process can lead to distressing psychological and physical symptoms. Other factors that influence the normal cycling include emotional stress, level of physical activity, and nutritional status, all of which have important roles to play in premenstrual syndrome.

TABLE 1: PRIMARY MENSTRUAL-CYCLE CHEMICAL MESSENGERS

MESSENGER MOLECULE	PRODUCED IN THE . . .
Gondatrophin-releasing hormone (GnRH)	Hypothalamus
Follicle-stimulating hormone (FSH)	Pituitary gland
Luteinizing hormone (LH)	Pituitary gland
Estrogen	Ovary
Progesterone	Ovary

SECONDARY MENSTRUAL-CYCLE CHEMICAL MESSENGERS

MESSENGER MOLECULE	PRODUCED IN THE . . .
Prolactin	Pituitary gland
Thyroid hormone	Pituitary gland
Melatonin	Pineal gland
Serotonin	Brain, platelets, digestive tract
Endorphins	Brain, hypothalamus
Prostaglandins	Diffusely
Insulin	Pancreas
Adrenal hormones	Adrenal gland

Proposed Causes of PMS

It is safe to say that despite intensive efforts to understand PMS scientifically, there is no clear and widely accepted explanation. Several studies have suggested that women with PMS have different patterns of estrogen and progesterone secretion, but no consistent findings have emerged.[2,3] Theories have proposed that there may be either a deficiency or an excess of certain prostaglandins involved in pain regulations. Evening primrose oil, which contains about 10 percent of an essential fatty acid, γ-linoleic acid, has been shown in some trials to reduce premenstrual breast pain, possibly because it leads to an increase in an important prostaglandin.[4] Antiinflammatory medications such as naproxen block other prostaglandins and have been partially successful in treating headaches, abdominal cramps, and back pain.[5]

A low vitamin B_6 level has also been suggested as a cause for PMS symptoms, and although several studies have shown B_6 supplementation to be of benefit, others have failed to confirm its value.[6-9] Vitamin B_6 plays an important role in serotonin production and many researchers have sought to explain the mood and appetite changes in terms of altered serotonin metabolism.[10,11] Although it is clear that several medications that affect serotonin in the brain can improve aspects of PMS, the precise role this important chemical messenger plays remains to be clarified.[12,13]

It is becoming obvious that looking at PMS from a localized perspective may yield interesting findings but is unlikely to give us a specific reason for a woman's monthly discomfort. I am firmly convinced that the reason we have not been able to find the medical scientific explanation for premenstrual syndrome is simple: *It is not a disease.* The extremes of emotional and physical symptoms in women with PMS represent imbalances in a normal and natural hormonal tide, which, when ignored, lead to greater imbalances. Studies attempting to define the characteristics of women with PMS show that they have higher life-stress levels, lower self-esteem, and carry more anger and guilt.[14,15] This understanding opens up the possibility for a more holistic approach to this common problem, one that integrates spirit, mind, body, and environment.

Standard Treatment Approaches

A vast array of medical interventions has been tried in women with premenstrual syndrome, generally directed to a specific physical or emotional symptom. To offset water retention, diuretics are prescribed. To reduce abdominal cramping, migraine headaches, and musculoskeletal pain, pain-relieving medicines, particularly anti-inflammatory drugs, are used. For the mood changes, irritability, and depression, almost every psychoactive medicine has been tried, including those used to treat depression, anxiety, epilepsy, and blood pressure. Oral birth-control pills, estrogen, and progesterone all have their proponents, although the enthusiasm for these remedies seems to outweigh the scientifically demonstrated benefits.[16–19]

Mind Body Approaches to PMS

Diet: A variety of nonpharmacological interventions can be helpful to lessen the symptoms of PMS. Dietary recommendations are widely suggested although most have not been fully evaluated scientifically. There is some support for reducing the intake of refined sugars and favoring a low-fat, high complex-carbohydrate diet.[20,21] These simple dietary changes seem to stabilize mood swings and reduce breast tenderness. Eliminating caffeine-containing beverages (cola, coffee, and tea) can be helpful in reducing anxiety, tension, and insomnia.[22] Although some women try to self-medicate with alcohol and other mood-altering drugs, there is often a substantial price to pay in terms of the severe agitation and irritability that follows.

Nutritional Supplements: Several nutritional supplements have been used in PMS for symptomatic benefit. As noted earlier, vitamin B_6, or pyridoxine, has been helpful in reducing symptoms of PMS, but in fairly high dosages of two hundred to five hundred milligrams per day.[23] The recommended daily B_6 requirement is only two milligrams per day, and at the higher doses used, nerve damage is a real risk. Trying B_6 in doses of fifty to one hundred milligrams a day during the second half of your menstrual cycle for several months is a reasonable approach, but discontinue using it if it is not clearly helping or you notice any tingling or numbness in your hands or feet.

Vitamin E, calcium, and magnesium all have their proponents. Vitamin E in doses of four hundred international units daily has been shown to produce modest benefits with minimal side effects.[24] One gram per day of calcium can reduce both psychological and physical symptoms of PMS, including irritability, depression, bloating, and backaches.[25] Magnesium supplementation can improve mood and reduce bloating but it takes several months before women notice any benefit.[26]

Although it is instructive to identify various specific nutritional elements that have been shown to produce some relief in PMS, I don't believe that this type of approach alone reflects a real shift in perspective. Focusing on one or another vitamin or mineral perpetuates the "magic-bullet" mentality, which anticipates the entire problem disappearing if we only discover the one substance that is missing. Nutritional intervention under an integrated mind body approach focuses on the overall quality of food, the way it is prepared, and the environment in which it is eaten. It has been my experience that when we are prepared to look at our overall life patterns and make nourishing choices, the need for specific nutritional manipulations often evaporates.

Group-Therapy and Cognitive-Behavioral Approaches: Developing a deeper understanding of the nature of premenstrual syndrome, clearing emotional toxicity, and learning ways to enhance mind body integration can improve the quality of life in women dealing with this condition. Many women who received negative messages about their sexuality as children later develop PMS, and an agonizingly high number experienced sexual abuse.[27] As adults, many of these women continue to have negative feelings about sex, menstruation, and reproduction along with anxiety, depression, and low self-esteem.[28] Efforts to address the emotional pain and anger these women carry through group-therapy sessions have not received a lot of scientific scrutiny, but there is some evidence that women in support groups benefit from sharing their experiences with others facing similar issues.[29]

Biofeedback, relaxation techniques, stress-management programs, and meditation are sometimes collectively lumped together as cognitive-behavioral therapies. Several reports using one or more of these therapies have shown that both emotional and physical symptoms of PMS can be lessened, with less depression and a reduction in negative thoughts. Relaxation techniques have been useful in reducing premenstrual muscle tension and stabilizing mood variability, while programs designed to lessen anxiety and more effectively manage anger have proven valuable.[30,31,32] In our experience, combining meditation techniques that offer the opportunity to quiet the mind with emotional processing programs that teach effective ways to cope with stress and address issues of repressed pain and anger provides the greatest benefit.

An important component of any effective behavioral program for women with PMS is exercise. Regular aerobic exercise has many benefits, including reduced fluid retention, less breast tenderness, and improved emotional states.[33,34] The good news for those not used to being physically active is that even a low-intensity exercise program can provide substantial benefit in reducing PMS symptoms.[35]

Ayurvedic Perspective on Premenstrual Syndrome

The Ayurvedic framework provides valuable insights into the nature and treatment of PMS. With its emphasis on alignment with natural rhythm as the basis of health, Ayurveda views PMS as an imbalance, rather than as a disease. The goal then is to identify the source of imbalance, reduce any toxicity, and provide nourishment to the reproductive system.

Premenstrual syndrome may reflect imbalance in any of the three doshas, Vata, Pitta, or Kapha. Anxiety, depression, moodiness, and cramping pain reflect an imbalance in Vata dosha. Irritability, anger, hot flashes, and migraine headaches represent imbalances in Pitta dosha. Water retention, bloating, heaviness, weight gain, fatigue, and breast swelling are manifestations of imbalanced Kapha. When two or more doshas are prominently disturbed, it is a sign of ama accumulation, most likely due to accumulated emotional toxicity, poor diet, and a disrupted daily routine. Both general and specific Ayurvedic interventions can be helpful, depending upon which dosha is most predominantly aggravated. Learning to entrain with natural rhythms is key to healthy menstruation.

Ayurvedic Program for PMS

The most important component of our PMS program involves setting aside time each day for silence in meditation. The centering and stress-reduction benefits of meditation can immediately begin to reestablish balance. Focus on creating an ideal daily routine, getting to bed before eleven P.M., and awakening around sunrise. This helps to harmonize your internal rhythmic pacemakers with natural cycles.

Look carefully at your diet and eliminate anything that is not nutritive. This includes obvious substances such as alcohol, tobacco, and caffeine, and it is also important to increase prana-rich foods, particularly fresh fruits and vegetables along with whole grains. Favor those tastes that are pacifying to the most-aggravated dosha. If pain, mood swings, and insomnia are prominent, favor heavier, warm foods that pacify Vata. If irritability, agitation, and hot flashes are troublesome, reduce spicy, sour, and salty foods, which aggravate Pitta. If swelling and bloating are a problem, favor lighter, warm, Kapha-pacifying foods.

Pacifying aroma therapy, soothing music, and a daily oil massage can help to stimulate your internal pharmacy of pain relievers and mood stabilizers. Take extra rest during the second half of your menstrual cycle and minimize activities as much as possible on the first day or two of your period.

Several specific herbal nutritional substances have been traditionally used in Ayurveda to balance the female reproductive system. One-half ounce of aloe vera juice is a useful and inexpensive female tonic that can be taken throughout the month. Indian asparagus (*Asparagus racemosus*), known as shatavari in Sanskrit, is the primary Ayurvedic female rejuvenative. One to three grams taken with warm milk at bedtime is soothing and nourishing to the reproductive tract. Angelica root has been used in both Chinese and Ayurvedic pharmacopocias for thousands of years. Known as *dong quai* in Chinese and *choraka* in Sanskrit, this herb promotes normal menstruation and combines well with shatavari. Another useful female tonic is musta, or nut grass (*Cyperus rotundus*). It has been used traditionally to relieve congestion and promote easy menstrual flow. One-half to one gram of both angelica and musta two to three times per day is the usual dose to balance and nourish the female organs.

If irritability is a major problem, Ayurveda recommends taking a purgative at midcycle to reduce Pitta accumulation. Take a table-spoon of ghee herbalized with grated ginger root and licorice for a few days before using an herbal laxative such as senna or castor oil. Adjust the dose so that you have a few loose bowel movements and eat lightly for a few days before and after the cathartic is taken. If mood swings and anxiety are troublesome, be certain to perform a daily oil massage with special attention to your head and neck. Pre-pare warm milk before bed with saffron or cardamom to pacify aggra-vated Vata, and use soothing aroma therapy with rose, bergamot, patchouli, sandalwood, or ylang-ylang. If congestion is a major con-cern, reducing your intake of salty foods and adding wild celery seeds (ajwan), cinnamon, mint, and fennel to your diet will help to reduce excess fluid.

Regular physical activity is entirely consistent with an Ayurvedic approach. Daily yoga postures can be helpful in reducing back pain and abdominal congestion. Aerobic exercises three times per week for twenty to thirty minutes increase endorphins and help stabilize emotions.

A simple remedy for abdominal cramping and tension is mas-saging castor oil onto the belly, covering the abdomen with a thin cot-ton or linen towel and applying a hot-water bottle or heating pad. Soaking in a hot bath to which dried ginger, chamomile, comfrey, or lavender has been added, along with a teaspoon of almond oil and a few drops of essential aroma oil, can be very soothing. Use all five senses to balance mind and body, particularly in the week prior to your period.

Mind, Body, and the Rhythms of Women

As the new paradigm of health permeates all aspects of our life, we will see both men and women changing. Times of transformation are challenging, often requiring us to look at basic aspects of our life in a new light. Our reproductive rhythms remind us that our apparent ability to isolate ourselves technologically from nature is an illusion. We are dynamic living beings inextricably interwoven into the rhythms and cycles of nature. When we are healthy, our fundamental rhythms are harmonious, and when they are not, it is a signal from our innermost being that we need to look at what we are not paying attention to in our lives.

Modern women face unprecedented challenges. In addition to the traditional role of mother and homemaker, most women are now also in the workplace, seeking fulfillment through achievements in the world. But there is little recognition of a woman's natural rhythms in the marketplace, and therefore there is conflict between a woman's inner wisdom and the world's outer demands. Even today, in remote parts of the world, when a woman's monthly flow begins, she retires to a designated location, which may be a straw mat or a separate hut, and remains there for several days. One could certainly argue that this constitutes a form of exclusion, and perhaps even oppression. On the other hand, is it reasonable or fair simply to ignore the important physiological changes that take place in a woman's body each month? Perhaps there is something to be said for withdrawing from the everyday routine while menstruation takes place. And perhaps the widespread incidence of PMS in Western society is an expression of physical and spiritual dissatisfaction, or even anger, at our current view of the monthly cycle and how it should best be dealt with.

Although nature flows in tides of rest and activity, we are just beginning again to consciously appreciate the cyclical dance of the universe. As women collectively embrace the many facets of their nature, healing on individual, community, and planetary levels will unfold.

Menopause

Mrs. Roseman's husband died of a heart attack a year ago. At age fifty-six, she was not ready to abandon her hope for a new life and new love, and despite the fact that she had gone through a very smooth menopause almost eight years earlier, she asked her gynecologist if she could begin hormone replacement. At first, she liked that her breasts were fuller and her vaginal dryness relieved, but after several months, she was troubled by breast tenderness and irregular bleeding. Despite reductions in her doses of estrogen and the addition of progesterone, she continued to feel uncomfortable with her choice and discontinued her hormone-replacement therapy.

Seeking a more natural approach, she began meditating regularly, increased her dietary intake of legumes, whole grains, and fresh vegetables, added a daily calcium supplement, and started exercising regularly with a personal fitness trainer. When she saw her physician nine months later, her cholesterol level was perfect, her bone-density test showed minimal signs of osteoporosis, and she felt genuinely healthier than she had in years.

A girl reaching puberty has between 200,000 and 300,000 potential eggs in her ovaries. Each month, many of these ovarian follicles are activated but only one ripens into a mature egg that is released for possible fertilization. Over a woman's forty or so childbearing years, only about five hundred eggs fully develop. As her ovaries exhaust their supply of eggs, a woman transitions into menopause—a pause in her monthly cycling.

Menopause is rich in psychological, physical, and cultural symbolism. A woman can look at "the change" as an end to her productive years or as the beginning of a new freedom of expression. She can see the shifts in her body as a loss of her youthfulness or a blossoming of her feminine divinity. Her role in the community can be seen as a dependent liability or as a valuable wisdom resource. The uncertainty of menopause is an opportunity to tap into the field of infinite possibility and create something new and vital.

The debate in the medical community continues as to whether menopause is more appropriately viewed as a normal physiological process or as a disease. Although the tendency in the Western world is to view menopause, like birth, as needing medical intervention, this is not universally true. In Japan, for example, over one-half of women experience menopause as relatively uneventful. A symptom such as hot flashes, which most American women anticipate as inevitable, is relatively uncommon in Japanese menopausal women.[36] Known as *konecki* in Japanese, menopause is considered as a natural life-cycle transition that includes both men and women, with each sex experiencing it differently based upon their biological constitution.[37]

From the mind body perspective, the goal is to facilitate this time of change with as much awareness as possible, with a focus on enhancing balance and eliminating unnecessary obstacles to a smooth transition.

Menopausal Symptoms

Hot flashes, emotional distress, bone weakness, and an increased risk of heart disease are the most common concerns of women facing menopause. Hot flashes and psychological imbalance create immediate distress, whereas osteoporosis (weak bones) and heart disease are longer-term problems. Vaginal dryness, a reduced sex drive, and skin changes are also frequent health issues in menopausal women.

Hot flashes are one expression of a generalized instability in the vascular system of many menopausal women. Flushing of the face, neck, and chest is most common with episodes lasting several minutes. Sudden sweating during the day or at night, nausea, heart palpitations, and headaches are other common manifestations of vasomotor instability. Hot flashes are more likely in women who have had surgical removal of their ovaries and in women who are thin. Without treatment, hot flashes may persist for a year but a small percentage of women will have symptoms that go on for several years. Alcoholic beverages and pungent, spicy foods often precipitate the symptoms.

Cells throughout the nervous system are affected by circulating estrogen, which may explain why some women undergoing menopause have changes in mood and memory. The steroid hormones, including estrogen, work by entering the nucleus of a cell and influencing the activation of certain genes. Receptors for estrogen are present in the pituitary gland, hypothalamus, and emotional part of the brain (the limbic system), so it is not surprising that women with less available estrogen report changes in their moods and memory.

Osteoporosis, or bone weakness, is a serious concern for postmenopausal women. Well over a million osteoporosis-related bone fractures occur each year in the United States at a considerable physical, emotional, and financial cost to society. Estrogen lack plays an important role in the development of bone loss, which occurs at about 2 percent per year for the first five years of menopause and then decreases to about 1 percent per year thereafter. One of the most useful ways to determine the strength of one's bones is through a bone-densitometry test, most of which use special X-ray equipment to measure bone mass. In addition to estrogen loss, physical activity level, dietary calcium and vitamin D, daily caffeine intake, smoking, and alcohol consumption all affect the strength of our bones and the risk of fractures.

Estrogen has widespread effects on the cardiovascular system, influencing our heart, blood vessels, circulating blood cells, and serum lipids. The risk of cardiovascular diseases rises in menopausal women. Heart attacks are reduced in women who take estrogen-replacement therapy, but it does not seem to lessen the risk of stroke.

Hormone Replacement Therapy (HRT) and Medical Management of Menopause

Modern women have definite choices about how to perceive menopause and what course to pursue. At The Chopra Center, I see women with a wide range of beliefs regarding medical management of menopause, and despite my own opinions, I am committed to honoring each woman's choice. Some women strongly feel that any medical intervention is a sign of failure and are committed to a totally natural approach. Other women do not want their lives disrupted by disturbing symptoms and gratefully take medications that can alleviate their distress. Most fall somewhere in between, wishing to minimize or eliminate the need for drugs but not wanting to tolerate present or future health concerns. As a physician, I believe it is my role to provide education about available choices so that people can make responsible decisions. I don't believe that there is one right approach for everyone.

Many of the distressing symptoms of menopause promptly respond to hormone-replacement therapy, but several studies have shown that less than 50 percent of women continue using estrogen two years after starting it due to uncomfortable side effects or psychological concerns.[38,39,40] Despite this, it is clear that most, if not all, of the major health issues of menopause can be impacted by medications; however, as is true with every drug, there are benefits and risks that need to be weighed.

Hot flashes, experienced by more than two-thirds of American women, respond almost universally to estrogen-replacement therapy within a few weeks of treatment. The other symptoms of vasomotor instability, including nausea, vomiting, dizziness, and sweating, also improve on HRT. Progesterone therapy has also been used in women with a history of breast cancer with some benefit. Other medicines, such as clonidine, usually used in hypertension, have been used to stabilize the vascular system but have a wider range of potential side effects, limiting the usefulness.

Estrogen-replacement therapy has been clearly shown to arrest bone loss and reduce the chances of fracturing a hip or wrist.[41,42] Recent studies have suggested that the combination of continuous low-dose estrogen with progesterone can improve bone mineral density without causing the vaginal bleeding common when estrogen is used alone.[43] Other agents, such as calcitonin, flouride, and the biophosphonates, are used to slow or reverse bone loss but most physicians consider estrogen to be the treatment of choice in menopausal women.

Many studies have shown that women who take estrogen replacement are at a lower risk for heart disease.[44] Cardiovascular disease currently accounts for over a third of all deaths in women, and estrogen therapy has been shown to reduce it by about half. Estrogen replacement's benefit on heart disease, as on every other symptom of menopause, rapidly diminishes as soon as hormone replacement is discontinued; therefore, lifelong usage must be anticipated if this route is taken.

Risks and Side Effects of Estrogen Replacement

Although today's medical standard of care recommends HRT for women going through menopause, there are well-recognized complications of its usage. Vaginal bleeding is one of the more disturbing side effects of estrogen alone or in combination with progesterone and may be seen in over half of women receiving treatment. Low continuous doses of progesterone may substantially reduce this problem but this requires the long-term use of two drugs. Breast tenderness and swelling is a common concern of women taking estrogen and may occur at very low doses. Reducing estrogen intake to the point of eliminating this symptom may also eliminate HRT's potential benefit to the bone and heart.

Of greater concern than the annoying symptoms of bleeding and breast tenderness is the potential risk of uterine and breast cancer. In studies of large groups of women, those taking estrogen alone do show a substantial increase in the risk of cancer of the uterus. Abnormal changes in the endometrium, the rich inner lining of the womb, are common in women on estrogen. Although the risk is reduced in women who take progesterone along with estrogen, it is still higher than in those who receive no hormone at all.[45]

Most reports have also found a relationship between HRT and breast cancer. The increased risk of breast cancer seems to be greater in women who have been on estrogen for at least five years. Those who get breast cancer while on estrogen seem to have less malignant disease and better survival. It has been suggested that estrogen doesn't actually trigger cancer but simply accelerates the development so that it is discovered at an earlier stage. This is not an argument that is easily accepted.

With all the information that is becoming available on menopause, it is easy to become confused. The right choices are not crystal clear, so there is room for personal opinion in this area. If we accept that there are some benefits to estrogen replacement but are not certain if the risks outweigh them, an important question becomes, what are the alternatives?

There are alternatives, but they must be presented along with a number of caveats. If you are willing to commit time and effort to exercise at least three times a week, if you are able to ensure that you are getting adequate calcium intake, if you are certain that your diet is rich with natural sources of estrogen, and if regular monitoring of your bone density does not reveal any signs of ongoing osteoporosis, then natural approaches to hormone replacement are a reasonable alternative.

Natural Alternatives to Reduce the Symptoms and Health Risks Associated with Menopause

If you are going or have gone through menopause, there are several things you can do to improve your well being. Although there is good reason to believe that many of these natural approaches can reduce symptoms and potential complications of menopause, few of them have been systematically compared to HRT and no long-term studies are available. Whether or not you are planning to take estrogen, these approaches will benefit your health.

Diet: Calcium and Vitamin D are the building blocks of healthy bones. Ideally, young women should be building strong skeletons long before they complete their reproductive years. A woman usually attains her maximum bone mass by her mid-twenties, or by thirty at the latest. Calcium intake during childhood and early adulthood, therefore, is crucial for building a skeletal foundation that can withstand the changes that occur later in life.

Doses of one thousand milligrams of daily calcium have been shown to significantly decrease the rate of bone loss, and calcium supplementation can actually increase the bone mineral density in the lumbar spine.[46] Eight ounces of milk, a cup of yogurt, or one to two cups of dark green leafy vegetables or broccoli all supply about three hundred milligrams of calcium per serving, so three to four servings per day should provide the necessary amount.

Studies from around the world suggest that hip fractures are more common in cultures where there is high animal-protein intake. It has been proposed that the high protein load increases the amount of acid the body needs to dispose of, resulting in a breakdown of the bone, which is used to buffer the acid.[47] Although there have not been studies suggesting that reducing animal fat improves bone strength, this may be another good reason to favor a vegetarian diet in addition to its clear benefit for the heart.

Reducing consumption of caffeine, alcohol, and excessive salt can all play a role in improving bone strength and reducing the risk of fractures.[48] Stopping smoking is also an important step toward cardiovascular and skeletal health.

Exercise: Exercise and fitness training are important components of a healthy lifestyle and have been clearly shown to reduce the complications of menopause. Strength-training exercises, performed twice a week for a year, can improve bone density and muscle mass, reducing the risk of falls and the likelihood of fractures.[49] The benefits of regular exercise on cardiovascular health are widely known, yet more than 50 percent of Americans continue to follow very sedentary lifestyles.

Natural Estrogens: Many commonly available fruits and vegetables contain natural estrogens, known as phytoestrogens. Soybean-derived foods such as tofu and miso are the richest source of plant-derived estrogens, which are also found in smaller quantities in almonds, apples, beets, cabbage, carrots, cashews, cherries, corn, cucumbers, rice, squash, and yams. Studies of the dietary habits of women in different countries have shown that there is often a good correlation between reduced symptoms of menopause and increased amounts of dietary estrogens. One study reported a better than hundredfold superiority of phytoestrogens in the diet of Japanese women compared to women in the United States and Finland, mostly due to the Japanese women's greater consumption of soy foods.[50]

For thousands of years, beans and legumes were our principal source of protein, and it appears that over the centuries the human body evolved an ability to convert the estrogen chemicals of plants into useful biological agents. In addition to providing a natural source of hormones, the phytoestrogens seem to provide protection against a wide range of cancers.[51] The full physiological effect of these natural estrogens is still being clarified, but there is reason to hope that increasing our consumption of flaxseed flour, lentils, chickpeas, soybeans, kidney beans, oat bran, and kelp can diminish the need for hormonal drugs and reduce the risk of a variety of cancers.

Ayurvedic Perspectives on Menopause

Ayurveda teaches that blood (*Rakta dhatu*) is a major site of Pitta in the physiology. Throughout a woman's menstruating years, she has the ability to eliminate this accumulated Pitta through her monthly blood flow. Because men do not have this capability, they more frequently develop Pitta-aggravated health concerns such as stomach ulcers and heart disease, as well as Pitta emotional imbalances such as chronic anger and aggressiveness. As women go through menopause and are no longer able to eliminate Pitta, they too begin to develop manifestations of Pitta imbalance. In menopausal women, hot flashes are the most acute expression of this tendency. The increased risk of heart disease in postmenopausal women is also a manifestation of greater susceptibility to Pitta imbalance.

The loss of the menstrual elimination mode also leads to increased Vata imbalance in women undergoing menopause. The consequences of rising Vata include bone weakness (too much air, not enough earth), dry vaginal tissues, and mood instability.

Interventions designed to pacify Pitta and Vata can improve emotional balance and physical well being in menopausal women. If she finds that hot flashes and irritability are problematic, a woman should follow a Pitta-pacifying diet that includes reduced pungent, sour, and salty foods. The diet should include cooling spices such as fennel and coriander, as well as Pitta-pacifying herbs such as sandalwood, saffron, musta, shatavari, and manjishta. Aloe vera juice, one-half ounce twice daily, is cooling and balancing to the female reproductive tract. When the symptoms of Vata imbalance are a concern, warmer, heavier Vata-pacifying foods including heated milk, herbalized with saffron or cardamom, can be beneficial. In general, maintaining a regular daily routine and eliminating all potential sources of toxicity are vitally important.

Aroma therapy, using balancing essential oils and daily massage, can also contribute to a smooth transition through menopause. To pacify Vata, ginger, rose, sandalwood, and vetiver are useful. For Pitta pacification, include clary sage, mint, sandalwood, and rose. For the bloating and heaviness of Kapha, use juniper, sage, and geranium.

Creating a Golden Transition

Change is almost always challenging, but it also creates opportunities for evolution. A charming lady in her sixties recently told me she had learned that we don't really solve our personal problems—we simply outgrow them. Menopause is a time of change and challenge, but it is not a disease. It is an opportunity to transition into a new phase of balance, purpose, and knowledge. The wisdom of a woman passing beyond her reproductive years may be the most valuable asset she has ever had. By deepening her understanding of her femininity and its connection to the earth and nature, a woman can teach her family and community members to honor their deeper selves.

Fortunately, today's women have many options in how to approach menopause, and each option has its benefits. Listen to the inner wisdom of your body for guidance in navigating this transitional time. Know that the key to a successful menopause is not found in the presence or absence of hormone-replacement therapy, or in any other medical procedure. Rather, it derives from learning more about yourself as you tap into the primordial wisdom that permeates every cell and atom of your being.

MIND BODY PRESCRIPTION FOR WOMEN'S HEALTH

1. Honor your natural rhythms and pay attention to the signals your body is sending you. Take rest when you need it, particularly on the first day of your period.

2. Take time in silence every day and consciously connect with the beauty and wisdom of nature.

3. Focus attention on getting to bed before eleven P.M. and awakening around sunrise.

4. Eat foods rich in phytoestrogens, including legumes, fresh fruits, vegetables, and soy-derived protein sources such as tofu.

5. Ensure that you receive adequate calcium intake (at least one thousand milligrams) each day.

6. Perform a daily oil massage. As your menstrual time approaches, spend extra time gently massaging your breasts and your lower abdomen.

7. Perform regular exercise to improve strength, flexibility, and aerobic capacity.

8. Try drinking aloe vera juice, one-half ounce twice daily.

9. If you are having difficulties with your periods or are going through menopause, try shatavari, one gram twice daily in warm milk.

10. Avoid the intake of any substance that does not provide nourishment to your body, mind, or soul.

11. Culture loving relationships that treat you with honor and respect.

20

Mind Body Interactions in Fatigue and Chronic Pain

"Be impeccable and you'll have the energy
to reach the place of silent knowledge."

Don Juan
(to Carlos Castaneda)

Carol used to think of herself as a person with abundant energy. But, after her second child, she found it increasingly difficult to get herself going in the mornings. Initially, her doctor told her that it was normal to be tired with two young children, but she found herself having more and more trouble getting through each day. Despite naps in both the morning and the afternoon, she always felt run-down.

When her youngest child was ten months old, Carol developed a bad flu with high fevers and muscle aches. Although the spiking fevers subsided over two weeks, she continued to feel generalized achiness throughout her body. She was also concerned because her concentration and memory seemed impaired. When her fatigue and discomfort did not abate over several more months, she was referred to an infectious-disease specialist. Other than mildly elevated titers to Epstein-Barr virus, no specific infectious or rheumatic disease could be identified. In essence, she was told that there was no medical explanation for her problem and no specific therapy was available.

Chronic pain and chronic fatigue are two sides of the same coin. Dealing with chronic pain is a drain on life's energy, and the reduced vitality of people with chronic fatigue is invariably accompanied by emotional and physical distress. Both conditions include constellations of symptoms that afflict virtually everyone who is suffering from fatigue or pain, and in this society that includes millions of individuals.

Chronic Fatigue

Fatigue is a prevalent malaise in contemporary America. It may be the most common reason that people go to see their doctors. More than 20 percent of adults surveyed at medical clinics describe fatigue as a major problem, and the complaint is responsible for more than ten million office visits each year.[1,2] Fatigue is a disabling feature of the lives of millions of Americans, and is one of the most elusive complaints for a doctor to evaluate—only rarely can a definite cause be isolated. The inability of medical science to explain its cause rationally and our incapacity to document its presence objectively adds frustration and a sense of invalidation to people whose lives are limited by fatigue.

There may occasionally be a clear-cut, treatable medical explanation for fatigue, such as anemia, a thyroid problem, hepatitis, diabetes, mononucleosis, kidney problems, or another chronic health disorder, but for the overwhelming majority of people who complain of chronic fatigue, no specific physical cause can be discovered. This lack of a good explanation may be one of the most important characteristics of the disease.

FATIGUE OF THE PAST

Chronic fatigue is not a new phenomenon. In the nineteenth century, a very common condition was known as *neurasthenia,* or nervous depletion. Its definition as "a condition of nervous exhaustion, characterized by undue fatigue on slightest exertion, both physical and mental," sounds a lot like a modern description of chronic fatigue.[3] Depression, headache, and digestive disturbances were commonly present, but there was always a big discrepancy between the person's disability and any findings on examination.

Nineteenth-century medical authorities often blamed neurasthenia on the fast-paced society of the time. The rise of technology with wireless communication, steam-powered engines, the ready availability of newspapers, and pressure for women to be educated put unprecedented demands on citizens of the day, leading to severe depletion of their energy reserves.[4] One can only imagine what previous-century authorities would have thought of today's fax machines, cellular phones, and expressway traffic—but their original emphasis on stress as a factor in chronic fatigue has much in common with the current views of both conventional and mind body medicine.

Treatments in the past, as today, covered a gamut of options. When stimulant drugs became available, they were offered to the fatigued patient, who invariably could not tolerate their side effects.[5] Based upon a model of inadequate nerve energy, electrical-stimulation therapy was used, but only temporary benefits were reported.[6] Since neurasthenia was equivalent to nervous exhaustion, the solution that became popular toward the end of the 1800s was the "rest cure." People left their usual environment to spend time in a facility that focused on rest, diet, and massage. Although many people reported benefit from these programs, there was a backlash from the established medical community of the day that there were no scientifically valid explanations for these approaches and that any value was solely the result of suggestion.[7] Not only did rest facilities fade out by the early 1900s, but the condition, neurasthenia, itself became discredited. The history of this process is a fascinating demonstration of how, when scientific medicine cannot objectively characterize a problem, we tend to belittle it and the people who are suffering with it. This is in contrast to the Ayurvedic model, which suggests that diseases can be expressed at subtler levels without definite laboratory abnormalities and can be helped with mind body approaches.

FATIGUE OF THE PRESENT

Over the years, a variety of terms has been applied to this elusive condition that affects so many people. A "diagnosis" is applied based upon one or another feature of the syndrome. Some of these labels have included hypoglycemia, candidiasis, food allergy, chemical sensitivity, and most recently, chronic Epstein-Barr virus (EBV) syndrome.

Attention on the Epstein-Barr virus was based upon reports from the mid-1980s, in which people with fatigue, difficulty concentrating, sleep disturbances, and swollen glands had elevated antibodies to the virus that causes infectious mononucleosis in their blood.[8,9]

A few years later, some people with fatigue living near Lake Tahoe were also reported to have evidence suggesting an ongoing infection with the EBV.[10,11] More extensive and detailed studies, however, failed to confirm a specific role for the Epstein-Barr virus, but did suggest a possible general disturbance in immunity.[12,13,14] To eliminate the suggestion that the EBV was responsible, the new name of Chronic Fatigue Syndrome (CFS) was coined.

Even the national Centers for Disease Control (CDC) got into the picture by convening a consensus conference and defining major and minor criteria for making the diagnosis of CFS.[15] But, despite many excellent scientists' best efforts, the picture of chronic fatigue remains murky, with recent reports suggesting that the definitions really don't define the spectrum of fatigue very well.[16,17]

Recent studies have shed faint light on this common but mysterious problem. It seems that people with CFS have difficulty maintaining normal blood pressure in an upright position, suggesting some imbalance in their autonomic nervous systems. When treated with medicines that stabilize blood pressure, about half of patients substantially improve.[18] Brain-imaging studies have not shown consistent structural problems but have suggested that there is lowered blood flow in the deep brain areas associated with alertness and autonomic nervous system control.[19]

I believe that we have problems trying to pin down this common health concern because chronic fatigue is not so much the presence of a disease as it is the disappearance of certain essential elements of good health. People with fatigue have been taxed to their breaking point so that their physical, intellectual, and emotional energy are severely spent or entirely lacking. The problem persists because we have been unable to help people directly access their natural reservoir of energy.

Prior to their illness, most people with chronic fatigue see themselves as extremely busy people, with many combining intense careers with child rearing and rigorous exercise programs.[20] Some were spending up to eighty hours each week at their jobs. Then, for many, a major stress such as serious injury, divorce, job loss, or death of a relative or close friend caused an abrupt change in their life. They had a sense of being overwhelmed by obligations and commitments, with feelings of loneliness and isolation. Most people believe that their stress was an instigating factor in a chain reaction that included a weakened immune system and susceptibility to infection.

The disability from chronic fatigue ranges from subjective feelings of everyday tiredness to an inability to carry on many normal daily activities. Severe chronic fatigue may affect up to a quarter of a million Americans who may need to sleep twelve hours per day and still struggle with memory problems, generalized pain, and difficulty concentrating.

EFFORTS TO ENERGIZE

About the most positive things we can say about therapy for chronic fatigue is that "many have tried." Almost every "anti" drug has been suggested over the past ten years. Antiviral, antibacterial, antifungal, antidepressant, antianxiety and anti-inflammatory medicines have all had their supporters, but consistent and lasting benefit has been hard to confirm.[21-24] In response to the idea that chronic fatigue represents a deficiency of something, immunoglobulin injections, fatty acids, and vitamins and minerals have all been administered, with many people reporting short-term benefits that fade over time.[25, 26, 27]

Recent reports have begun to acknowledge the value of mind body approaches in people with CFS. In a study of almost three hundred people followed for eighteen months, only 3 percent reported complete recovery, with another 15 percent showing some improvement.[28] Those who improved were more likely to believe that they were able to influence some control over their health. A report of sixty patients from England found that almost three-quarters of people who participated in cognitive-behavioral therapy improved compared to only a quarter of patients receiving standard medical treatment. These patients were taught about the role of psychological and social factors and encouraged to gradually modify their rest and activity patterns.[29]

Alternative therapeutic interventions have also been used, including homeopathy, acupuncture, yoga, hypnosis, and herbs.[30,31] Each of these approaches has its champions and yet all seem vulnerable when critically scrutinized. Studies on comprehensive mind body approaches have been lacking and are needed, but I have been encouraged by preliminary results in our patients.

Carol had been "mourning" the loss of her health. She was increasingly incapacitated by fatigue, disturbed sleep patterns, diffuse pain, and an irritable bowel. She felt she was on a downward physical and mental spiral, stating, "The joy in my life had died." She had seen many physicians, psychiatrists, and therapists with over twenty medications prescribed for her. She was unable to work and her marriage was deteriorating. She was terribly frustrated over her inability to care for her six-year-old daughter adequately.

After almost a year in which she spent most of her day in bed, she began a comprehensive program of daily meditation, yoga, and graded exercise. She began to eat fresh, primarily vegetarian, foods and followed the Body Intelligence Techniques. She performed a daily home oil massage and used simple herbal rasayanas.

After two months, she was only requiring a short nap each day and had resumed her responsibilities caring for her child. By seven months, she had much greater endurance, a drastic reduction in her pain, and was happy to be alive. She felt that she had regained a sense of empowerment in her life through the direct experience of her inner healer.

From my perspective, chronic fatigue is the expression of a disintegration between consciousness, mind, body, and environment. Since nature is an unlimited reservoir of energy, it is paradoxical that we, as creatures of nature, can chronically be out of energy. I believe that the key to eliminating fatigue lies in reestablishing a connection between ourselves and our natural sources of energy—not so much to nature in the sense of streams, mountains, and forests, although contact with these rejuvenating environments is very beneficial, but rather to the natural ocean of energy that is within all of us. Mind body medicine teaches that we can reconnect to our unbounded field of pure potentiality and receive the unlimited energy and nourishment we seek.

Chronic Pain

The physical sensation of a pinprick or of touching a hot iron seems easy enough to understand. This is acute pain, and it occurs when a message travels along nerve fibers from the site of the injury to receptors in our brain. In most cases the pain subsides after a moment or

two. It has served its purpose, which was to get our attention immediately, to make us stop whatever we were doing, and to teach us not
to do it again.

But sometimes the pain persists. It may continue long after what
would normally be expected, and even seemingly minor muscle
strains or back injuries can give rise to pain that lasts for years. This is
chronic pain, and like chronic fatigue it often exists without any iden-
tifiable medical cause. Despite the absence of an organic cause, however, chronic pain sufferers characteristically visit long successions of
doctors and ingest a wide variety of drugs in search of relief.

Mind body medicine, however, suggests that chronic pain develops out of our failure to be fully present and attentive when the pain
first occurred. The lesson that the pain was trying to teach has not
gotten through, so it must continue until that lesson has been
learned. All too often, however, this mechanism is not understood.
Instead of recognizing pain's message, there is only resentment
against the continuing discomfort and a persistent refusal to change.

What is the solution? One of the most important steps we can
take toward gaining control of chronic pain is to assume responsibility for what we are feeling. This includes both the physical and
emotional components of the pain, which usually become indistin-
guishable in the mind of the sufferer.

PAIN AND SUFFERING

When people describe their chronic pain, they usually use expressions such as, "Pain makes my life miserable," "Pain takes away my
energy," "Pain makes me irritable and angry," or, "Pain changes my
whole outlook on life."[32] It is rare that pain is only described in terms
of a physical sensation. In chronic pain, the physical sensation has
been allowed to expand its influence to include every aspect of existence. Until this expansion is controlled and reversed, pain will continue to be a problem.

This does not mean that we should deny the existence of
chronic pain, or try to ignore it. On the contrary, mind body medicine urges us to focus attention directly on the source of pain, to
embrace the message. This conscious monitoring or witnessing of
pain can be done mentally, but it can also be very useful to keep track
of pain in writing, noting how you feel at various times of the day

together with influences that seem to cause the pain to diminish or to grow worse. Witnessing and assuming responsibility for physical pain is analogous to the witnessing of painful emotions that is discussed in Chapter 12. When pain of any kind occurs, the goal must be to recognize the sensation for what it really is as well as for what it is not. In this way we can begin learning from pain instead of merely suffering from it.

We may discover, for example, that pain is alleviated by light exercise such as walking or swimming, or that it worsens when we are tired or hungry. Appropriate lifestyle changes that not only relieve the pain, but also eliminate the behaviors that caused it in the first place, can then be made.

RELIEVING PAIN

There is good evidence that mind body techniques, including meditation, can be effective in dealing with chronic pain. Researchers at the University of Massachusetts Medical Center have been teaching mindfulness meditation to chronic-pain sufferers.[33,34] In the witnessing process, people are able to distinguish the actual primary pain sensations as they occur from moment to moment and their responses to them. By the end of meditation training almost three-quarters of women and over half of men experience significant improvement both in their self-evaluations and in clinical assessments by physicians. These improvements take the form of increased capacity to stand, sit, and walk, as well as improved appearance and mood.

MULTIDISCIPLINARY APPROACHES TO PAIN

A complementary approach to care is most apparent in multidisciplinary pain centers. In perhaps no other area of modern health care is there the level of acceptance of the importance of physical, psychological, social, and even spiritual components to a problem. Physicians, psychologists, physical therapists, social workers, vocational and rehabilitation counselors, and clergy may all participate in the process of helping a person move out of the darkness of chronic pain into the light of physical and emotional relief.

Nonpharmacological approaches are often important components of a comprehensive pain-management program. Hypnotherapy and biofeedback have been used with good success to reduce the intensity of pain and allow tolerance of a wider range of movements and behaviors.[35,36] A panel of pain experts convened by the National Institutes of Health recently published a consensus paper in which they reported there was strong evidence for the use of relaxation techniques and hypnosis and moderate evidence for the use of cognitive-behavioral techniques and biofeedback in the treatment of people with chronic pain.[37] This amounts to a "stamp of approval" from the health-care establishment.

Acupuncture for pain was recommended by Sir William Osler in 1904,[38] but it did not gain widespread attention until President Nixon's trip to China in the early 1970s. A number of studies over the past twenty years have attested to the value of acupuncture therapy in the treatment of pain conditions. Overall, insertion of needles into traditional acupuncture points is effective in 60 percent to 75 percent of people with pain.[39] This is in comparison to about a 50 percent success rate if "sham" acupuncture is used and 30 percent relief in control patients without skin penetration. Sham acupuncture means the insertion of needles into areas of the body held traditionally to be ineffective. Scientific theories attempt to explain acupuncture's efficacy by the "gate theory," in which nerve impulses from needle stimulation arrive at the spinal cord and block the transmission of painful impulses. With the discovery of our endorphins, acupuncture has been suggested to stimulate the release of our natural pain relievers.

The traditional Oriental medical view is that pain is the result of blocked vital force, or *chi*. Acupuncture unblocks the circulatory channels or *meridians*, enabling the energy to reestablish its healthy flow throughout the body. Regardless of which paradigm one uses to view the world, we are increasingly recognizing the potential value in ancient healing traditions.

MIND BODY INTERACTIONS IN FATIGUE AND CHRONIC PAIN

We are bundles of energy and information. When we have unimpeded access to the field of pure potentiality, we have a connection to the source of the energy of the universe. But when we carry accumulated toxins in our minds and in our bodies, access to the wellspring of life energy is blocked. Dissolving these blockages requires awareness and understanding along with healthier lifestyle choices.

The inciting stress or injury becomes less important as time goes by. Regardless of whether the acute event was due to a ruptured disc, a whiplash injury, or surgery (in chronic pain), or a divorce, job loss, or viral infection (in chronic fatigue), over time the effect on a person's life is similar. It becomes the focus of attention and is a constant reminder of what is *not* possible to accomplish or enjoy in life. But even in people with chronic pain or fatigue, there are moments or even days when the distress is less. While engrossed in an exhilarating novel or movie, watching an exciting sports event, talking with friends, or making love, the problem temporarily moves out of the forefront of awareness. This shows us that it is not just the physical process that is causing the disability, but more importantly the power of our attention. This is where the approaches of mind body medicine can make their contributions. We can learn to change our relationship to the source of the pain and fatigue through meditation, yoga, and massage. We can create new associations using aroma and sound therapies. We can release the emotional and physical toxins that limit our intrinsic flexibility, which is essential for healthy change.

Whenever we meet with obstacles while trying to fulfill our desires, we feel tired and depleted. In this diminished state, our immune system reflects our exhaustion and functions less effectively. We become vulnerable to incidents that can give rise to pain, both emotionally and physically, and these incidents can occur at the cellular level or on the gross level of the physical body. In other words, if we lose touch with the field of pure potentiality, we are at increased risk for everything from a fight with a spouse to an automobile accident to a bacterial infection. We must re-create our selves each day by tapping into the source of creativity within our own awareness. It is the realm of pure energy and joy where fatigue and pain cannot exist.

MIND BODY PRESCRIPTION FOR ENERGY AND COMFORT

1. Tap into your inner source of energy and joy each day through meditation.

2. Regularly spend time in nature.

3. Practice yoga breathing exercises and postures to increase flexibility and mobilize energy in your body.

4. Identify and eliminate toxins (substances, food, emotions) from your life. Look for suppressed anger and seek to identify and release it.

5. Try acupuncture and/or biofeedback to disrupt the pain cycle temporarily.

6. Perform a daily oil massage to stimulate natural pain-relieving chemicals, and receive professional massages.

7. Find opportunities to laugh and be childlike.

8. Follow an ama-pacifying program for a couple of weeks, then focus on nourishing yourself with *sattvic* foods and herbal rasayanas.

9. If fatigue is prominent, the Ayurvedic herbs traditionally used to nourish the physiology include ashwagandha (winter cherry), bala (country mallow), shatavari (Indian asparagus), and Chavan prash (Indian gooseberry jam).

10. If chronic pain is prominent, the Ayurvedic herbs traditionally used to balance the nervous system include guggulu (Indian gum myrrh), brahmi (Indian pennywort), and *Boswellia* (Indian olibanum—related to frankincense).

Epilogue

Celebrating Life, Transcending Death

"Death, your servant is at my door;
He has crossed the unknown sea
And brought your call to my home.
The night is dark and my heart is fearful,
Yet I will take up the lamp, open my gate,
And bow to him my welcome."

Rabindranath Tagore

"I always knew that everyone dies," the writer William Saroyan remarked during the final hours of his life, "but I really thought there would be an exception in my case." There is a humorous intention here, of course, but I suspect Saroyan's wit reveals feelings regarding death that many of us share. During our daily lives, most of us naturally begin to think that our concerns are more important than those of other people. If my car gets a flat tire and I'm late for an appointment, the inconvenience seems of much greater significance than an earthquake in Fiji, though I may keep this hierarchy of values to myself. I too secretly believe that I'm "exceptional" in the sense that Saroyan meant, and if I sometimes lie in bed at night and find my thoughts scanning forward to the moment when my life will end, any unease about this lasts for only a second or two. I carry the belief that I'll live to a ripe old age and then effortlessly transition into my next phase. I can't remember ever not existing and I can't really imagine not existing at some point in the future. Can you?

Yet somehow, at the same time, I know that "David Simon" will not exist for more than another sixty years. I am just a parenthesis in eternity. We all have this dual nature: We are immortal, invulnerable gods and, paradoxically, tiny insects waiting to be crushed by the heavy foot of eternity. Somewhere between those extreme visions is a mature awareness informing us that someday our lives will end, and that the world will really go on very much as before. (But in my case it will first completely shut down for ten days.)

This paradox of simultaneously being an immortal spirit and a skin-encapsulated ego is the ultimate challenge of life and the basis of all anxiety and fear. Freud said that neurosis is the inability to tolerate ambivalence, so until we have reached a state of absolute enlightenment, all of us are, at least, a little neurotic as we seek to reconcile these apparent polarities.

During a prolonged meditation course I remember having the experience of transcending timebound, localized awareness and thinking, *I now know that I am a spiritual being in complete union with all other beings. I am neither above nor below anyone because we are all expressions of universal intelligence—we are all manifestations of God. I have finally gone beyond my ego.* And then, a little voice arose in my otherwise serene awareness: *You know, there are not a lot of people around who really know this.* I started laughing at myself, realizing that even as I was surrendering to my egoless state, my ego was doing its job of judging and comparing me to others. This is the nature of individuality while we are striving to establish our universality.

What do we really know about death? We think of it, we may even speak of it sometimes, but we can really only talk around the subject of death rather than about it. Hamlet calls death "the undiscovered country"—and how can we describe a landscape that lies off the edges of our maps and beyond the reaches of our telescopes?

For most of us, only one fact is certain about death, and for the greater part of our lives this fact has considerably more reality than the knowledge that someday we will indeed die. *Fear* is that one certain fact: We know that we're afraid of death. But, again, what do we really fear from something we understand so little about? Since we don't know the source of our fear except in the most vaguely conceptual way, how can we hope to deal with it or get beyond it or somehow bring that fear to an end?

In this area, a physician can really claim no more expertise than anyone else. Although I've witnessed hundreds of people die, I do not believe any of us can fully grasp the significance of death until we are imminently facing it. I am proceeding with a high degree of humility in addressing the subject of our mortality and the fear that attends it. I will suggest, however, that our fears about death can be separated into two categories. It's certainly true that *nobody knows what's going to happen,* and this sense of the baleful unknown would seem to be a primary expression of our fear of mortality. But, as I suggested above, how can we be afraid of something of which we know nothing? Freud approached this question in discussing children's fear of the dark, and concluded that children are really afraid of what they think might be in the dark, rather than of the darkness itself. But whatever we may believe that eternal darkness holds, each of us is going to face it alone—and I believe that this utterly solitary quality of the death experience is one of the most important sources of our fear.

As my friend and Ayurvedic teacher, Sunil Joshi, once eloquently expressed to me, life can be seen as a sort of arc. It begins with our existence as pure spirit, in which we have formed no attachment to any of the diverse beings and objects that fill the physical world. Conception, birth, and later development can be seen as a process of engagement with these worldly "furnishings." This is the phenomenon of ego development, and we can watch it take place in children. At first, but only for a little while, the whole notion of possession or the relative value of objects is outside a child's consciousness. A diamond means no more than a rhinestone to an infant, and a cardboard box can be as much fun as a Mercedes-Benz. Rather quickly, though, the ego begins to assert itself, so that a three-year-old can be as possessive and willful about what's "mine" and "yours" as any adult can. There are still intermittent periods of egoless play for a toddler, but consciousness is really developing in the direction of engagement with the world and with assimilating the value system of the family and of society. Gradually a young person's focus sharpens, and he or she learns that some things are more valuable than others . . . that some objects are beautiful and some are not . . . and that some people are lovable but many aren't. When the English poet William Wordsworth wrote, "Though nothing can bring back the hour/Of splendor in the grass, of glory in the flower," he was referring explicitly to the loss of our childhood capacity to find supreme beauty and joy even in the most commonplace things.

This process of ego engagement, of bonding and sometimes binding ourselves to the people and things in the world around us, must eventually confront the fact that it cannot continue forever. Especially when we contemplate our mortality, we must recognize that our ties to the material world are going to be severed someday, and that this is going to take place whether we resist it or not. Ayurveda, like every other spiritual tradition, counsels us to create a state of awareness in which we realize we are in this world, but not of this world. This cultured detachment allows us to participate in the adventure of living while always being alert to the transitory nature of everything we experience in the world. Meditation is the most important Ayurvedic technique for accomplishing this, but even if we're not acquainted with any spiritual tradition, the natural arc of life will lead us back toward the egoless consciousness that was ours in childhood. Many people in later life are able to regain something like the state of pure awareness that exists in the first few years of life. In view of this, I suspect that perhaps Wordsworth was wrong: We can regain our sense of splendor in the grass—in fact, we need never lose it at all. To the extent that we are able to maintain the unity consciousness that was once ours, the fear of separation, of isolation, that is so basic to the fear of death will melt away.

Although as young children the two brothers were inseparable, Jack and Michael became increasingly competitive as they matured. Each perceived the other as the favored child and neither ever received enough attention. Their resentment intensified as they entered college, and upon graduating and entering the business world, their competition escalated to real hostility. After years of bitter arguments, they cut off all communication and publicly derided each other's faults whenever the opportunity arose.

At the age of fifty-five, Jack developed unrelenting abdominal pain. After resisting medical care for months, he finally saw his physician, who immediately sensed the seriousness of his illness. After a series of tests, Jack was told that he was dying of untreatable pancreatic cancer. This news was the catalyst for a dramatic transformation resulting in Jack's strong desire to vent his feelings about being wounded as a child to his brother.

After almost ten years of not speaking, Jack entreated Michael to visit him. When they met, Jack's heart poured out the pain that he had been carrying, and with each remorseful tear, his anger transmuted to love. By the end of their emotional exchange, the brothers were confessing how much they had always loved each other, even though throughout their lives they had only expressed their disdain. In the melting of their egos, the unifying essence of spirit was allowed to shine.

The ego lives in fear. It fears loss of power, loss of approval, loss of money, and of course, it fears death, which is perceived as the loss of everything. Spirit, which exists beyond the needs of the ego, has no fear of death because it never dies. To the extent that we are aware of our unity with spirit, we can transcend the fear of death and experience our mortality with acceptance, and even with love.

A second component of our fear of death derives, I think, from a sense of impending powerlessness. At the last moment, after all, what if there are still a lot of things we want to do? It won't just be all the new films we'll be missing—we'll be helpless to recapture the days and nights we wasted in worry, or the hurt we inflicted on others, or the love we failed to return. We all have sins of commission and sins of omission. In short, we may be faced with our regrets.

This prospect may indeed be worthy of fear, but only if we fail to see it first as a spur to action. *Carpe diem*—"Seize the day!"—has been a theme of poetry since ancient times, and in Ayurvedic teaching it is referred to as *present-moment awareness*. Just as a blazing fire can burn a log to a fine ash, by really experiencing every day to the fullest we can eliminate regrets and residual guilt-ridden emotions from our consciousness. If we can fully process the events and relationships of our lives—really digest them—we can leave the table without hunger when the feast is finished.

The truth of this, I'm sorry to say, was made clear to me when my older sister died of cancer when I was still a teenager—

I had never been close with Jill, who had no apparent need for an annoying little brother. We kept our distance and I rarely paid her much attention throughout my teenage years. Then, while home from college on winter break, I learned that she was having trouble swallowing and was going to see a specialist. Things proceeded at a reckless pace from that point on. A biopsy showed that my twenty-one-year-old sister had a rare form of throat cancer and needed urgent hospitalization to have her voice box removed. A tracheostomy tube was placed in her, but the major surgery had to be delayed because she had contracted an upper-respiratory infection. I remember seeing the terror in her eyes when I visited her in the hospital and the tears that flowed when my parents told her I had donated blood for her. Although there seemed so much she wanted to say, she was unable to communicate verbally.

While preparing to go to the hospital the next day with my parents, I received a phone call from her surgeon saying that something tragic had happened. Because the tumor had so damaged her throat tissues, the breathing tube had eroded into her carotid artery. Despite emergency efforts to save her, she was gone.

If she had lived longer, perhaps many of the emotions that remained unresolved between us at the time of her death would have played themselves out. Perhaps she and I would have been able to express things to each other that are only dimly sensed by young people. I don't expect ever to fully recover from this experience and I know that my parents do not go a day without thinking what more they could have done for her. Almost all of us live with, "If only I had . . ." or "I should have . . ." or, "I could have . . ." and these are the big lesson opportunities that life offers. We are reminded that being human is an ephemeral, remarkable gift that must be cherished every moment we're alive.

Many years after my sister's passing, while caring for a patient as a neurology resident, I had the opportunity to try the lesson again. Although this gentleman was a dairy farmer, and I had rarely been near a cow, I was drawn to a spiritual quality I sensed in him. Although we talked very little during my busy days on the neurology ward, I felt a quiet connection with him. His condition was very serious, and I knew he was going to die. He knew it also.

One Sunday, although I was not on call, I had this strong urge to return to the hospital and spend some time with this patient. It was an unusual encounter for us. Normally he saw me in my white doctor's coat during a typically busy day, but now there was far less activity and I was in jeans and a casual shirt. Perhaps it was the removal of my professional barriers that allowed him to talk freely with me, and though he had a moderate speech impairment from the tumor in his brain, we spoke for quite a while. He talked about how much he had loved farming and getting up early in the mornings to milk the cows.

It wasn't an especially profound conversation, but it seemed meaningful and we both shed some tears. He had no regrets about his life; he had done what he'd loved for as long as he could, and if he had been offered anything in the world he would simply have chosen to do the same thing. He was alone in the hospital, but this didn't seem to trouble him particularly. He knew that his wife was at home taking care of their farm. Finally we said good-bye, and I left. He died about three hours later, and although I felt sadness, I had no regrets. He was alive when he died, as a saying goes, and his life was really over just when it ended.

This simple man reminds me that we are waves on an ocean. While we are alive, we mostly see ourselves as separate, comparing our qualities and what we have achieved to those around us. And yet, each wave is ultimately the unbounded ocean temporarily disguising itself as separate, but never losing connection to its source—which is the same source of all the other waves. Knowing that at some point our individuality will merge again with universality is a tremendous gift. The urgency it bestows upon our daily life is an opportunity to embrace the moment, living it as if it could be our last.

As I board airplanes these days, I have the thought that every person who died in an airplane crash did not believe that his or her life was about to end. Although we all know there is the possibility of our dying on any given day, we are fairly certain that it is *not* today. Throughout his stories, the sorcerer Don Juan reminds Carlos Castaneda that death is always stalking us, and this is the driving force to live a life of meaning, ever alert to the miraculous opportunities available at every moment.

Timebound and timeless, individual and universal, local and nonlocal—these are the contradictions that Ayurveda suggests can only be resolved by going beyond the realm of duality with its names and forms and becoming intimate with the silent field of spirit. When our understanding of spirit merges with our direct experience, we have wisdom—the wisdom of life—the wisdom of healing.

In my dream I am walking along the shoreline on a pristine beach. The white sand is sparkling as a brilliant sun beams its light onto the turquoise water lapping against the shore. I become entranced by the scene that is unfolding in front of me as I discover human beings silently emerging out of and returning back into the sand. I realize I am witnessing the primordial dust from which we are made and to which we all return. I recognize the endless cycle of birth, life, and death flowing in a continuous stream and I see a celestial hand compassionately performing this divine work. In the same gesture that a newborn's umbilical cord is pinched off to begin a new life, the airway of a dying man is gently closed off at the end. The wheel of life eternally turns.

Appendix A

SOURCES OF HERBAL NUTRITIONAL PRODUCTS

The Ayurvedic Institute, P.O. Box 23445, Albuquerque, NM 87192-1445. Phone (505) 291-9698.

Bazaar of India Imports, 1810 University Avenue, Berkeley, CA 94703. Phone (415) 548-4110.

Infinite Possibilities Products, P.O. Box 1088, Sudbury, MA 01776. Phone (800) 858-1808.

Nature Care Products Company, 6 Charles Park, Guilderland, NY 12084. Phone (800) 923-9338.

Nature's Herbs, 600 East Quality Drive, American Fork, UT 84003. Phone (800) 437-2257.

Planetary Formulations, P.O. Box 533, Soguel, CA 95073. Phone (408) 464-2003.

References

INTRODUCTION: TWENTY-FIRST-CENTURY HEALTH CARE

1. Reinarz, J. A., M. J. Megna, and G. T. Brown. 1979. Nosocomial infections: time for accountability. In *Infectious Diseases,* Current Topic, vol. 1, ed. D. N. Gilbert and J. P. Sanford, 219–40. New York: Grune and Stratton.

2. Phelps, C. E. 1989. Bug/Drug resistance—sometimes less is more. *Medical Care* 27:194–203.

3. Levy, S. B. 1992. *The Antibiotic Paradox: How Miracle Drugs Are Destroying the Miracle.* New York: Plenum Press.

4. Kunin, C. M., G. L. Mandel, R. G. Douglas, and J. E. Bennett. 1985. Problems in antibiotic usage. In *Principles and Practice of Infectious Disease,* 2d ed., 427–34. New York: John Wiley.

5. Editorial. 1988. Need we poison the elderly so often? *The Lancet* 2:20–22.

6. Illich, I. 1976. *Medical Nemesis: The Expropriation of Health.* New York: Pantheon Books.

7. Steel, K., P. M. Gertman., et al. 1981. Iatrogenic illness in a general medical service at a university hospital. *New England Journal of Medicine* 304:638–42.

8. Leape, L. L. 1994. Error in medicine. *Journal of American Medical Association* 272:1851–57.

9. Smith, R. 1991. Where is the wisdom? *British Medical Journal* 303:798–99.

10. Naylor, C. D. 1995. Grey zones of clinical practice: some limits to evidence-based medicine. *The Lancet* 345:840–42.

11. Four decades of achievement, 1988. In *Highlights of the Work of the World Health Organization.* Geneva, Switzerland: World Health Organization.

12. Coan, R. M., G. Wong, and P. L. Caon. 1980. The acupuncture treatment of low back pain: a randomized controlled study. *American Journal of Chinese Medicine* 8:181–89.

13. Christensen, P. A., M. Noreng, and P. E. Andersen. 1989. Electroacupuncture and postoperative pain. *British Journal of Anaesthesia* 62:258–62.

14. Helms, J. M. 1987. Acupuncture for the management of primary dysmenorrhea. *Obstetrics and Gynecology* 69:51–56.

15. Dundee, J. W., J. Yang, and C. McMillan. 1991. Non-invasive stimulation of the p-6 (Neiguan) antiemetic acupuncture point in cancer chemotherapy. *Journal of Royal Society Medicine* 84:210–12.

16. Brewington, V., M. Smith, and D. Lipton. 1994. Acupuncture as a detoxification treatment: an analysis of controlled research. *Journal of Substance Abuse Treatment* 11:289–407.

CHAPTER 1: HEALING THE HEALER

1. Nuland, S. B. 1995. *How We Die: Reflections on Life's Final Chapter.* New York: Vintage Books.

2. Simon, D. B., S. Oparil, and C. P. Kimball. 1976. The transcendental meditation program and essential hypertension. In *Scientific Research on the Transcendental Meditation Program,* collected papers, vol. 1, 268–69. West Germany: MERU Press.

CHAPTER 2: CREATING A UNIVERSE

1. Hawking, S. W. 1988. *A Brief History of Time.* Toronto: Bantam Books.

2. Bergson, H. 1983. *Creative Evolution.* Lanham, Md: University Press of America.

3. Moore, K. L., and T. V. N. Persaud. 1993. The nervous system. In *The Developing Human,* ed. K. L. Moore and T. V. N. Persaud, 385–422. Philadelphia: W. B. Saunders.

4. Stebbins, W. C. 1983. *The Acoustic Sense of Animals.* Cambridge, Mass.: Harvard University Press.

5. Green, D. G. 1994. Visual acuity, color vision and adaptation. In *Principles and Practice of Ophthalmology,* ed. D. M. Alber and F. A. Jacobiec, 332–49. Philadelphia: W. B. Saunders.

6. Masson, J., and S. McCarthy. 1995. *When Elephants Weep.* New York: Delacourt Press.

7. Moncrieff, R. W. 1970. *Odours.* London: William Heinemann Medical Books, Ltd.

CHAPTER 3: PERSONALIZING THE UNIVERSE

1. Herbert, N. 1987. How large is starlight?: a brief look at quantum reality. *Revision* 10:31–35.

2. Phillips, D. P., T. E. Ruth, and L. M. Wagner. 1993. Psychology and survival. *The Lancet* 342:1142–45.

3.   Phillips, D. P., and E. W. King. 1988. Death takes a holiday: mortality sur-
     rounding major social occasions. *The Lancet* 2:728–32.

4.   Phillips, D. P., and D. G. Smith. 1990. Postponement of death until sym-
     bolically meaningful occasions. *Journal of the American Medical Association*
     263:1947–51.

5.   Eccles, J. C. 1966. Conscious experience and memory. In *Brain and Con-
     scious Experience*, ed. J. Eccles, 414–44. New York: Springer-Verlag.

CHAPTER 4: THE ORIGINS OF HEALTH AND DISEASE

See General Ayurvedic References

CHAPTER 5: RESTFUL ALERTNESS—EAVESDROPPING ON SILENCE

1.   Cannon, W. B. 1932. *The Wisdom of the Body*. New York: Norton Press.

2.   Salk, J. 1983. *Anatomy of Reality—Merging of Intuition and Reason*. New York:
     Columbia University Press.

3.   Bagchi, B. K., and M. A. Wenger. 1957. Electro-physiological correlates of
     some yogi exercises. *Electroencephalographic and Clinical Neurophysiology.* 7
     (supplement): 132–49.

4.   Das, N. N., and H. Gastaut. 1955. Variations de l'activité électrique du
     cerveau, du coeur et des muscles sqelletiques au cours de las meditation et
     de l'extase yogique. *Electroencephalographic and Clinical Neurophysiology.* 6
     (supplement): 211–19.

5.   Onda, A. 1965. Autogenic training and Zen. In *Autogenic Training*, ed. W.
     Luthe, 251–58. New York: Grune and Stratton.

6.   Kasamatsu, A., and T. Hirai. 1966. An electroencephalographic study on
     Zen meditation (Zasen). *Folia Psychiatrica et Neurologia Japanica* 20:315–36.

7.   Anand, B. K., G. S. China, and B. Singh. 1961. Some aspects of electroen-
     cephalographic studies in yogis. *Electroencephalographic Clinical Neurophysi-
     ology* 13:452–56.

8.   Benson, H., J. W. Lehman, and M. S. Malhotra. 1982. Body temperature
     changes during the practice of tum-mo yoga. *Nature* 295:234–36.

9.   Wallace, R. K. 1970. Physiological effects of transcendental meditation. *Sci-
     ence* 167:1751–54.

10. Wallace, R. K., H. Benson, and A. F. Wilson. 1971. A wakeful hypometa-
     bolic physiologic state. *American Journal of Physiology* 221:795–99.

11. Wallace, R. K., and H. Benson. 1972. The physiology of meditation. *Scien-
     tific American* 226:84–90.

12. Seeman, W., S. Nidich, and T. Banta. 1972. A study of the influence of tran-
     scendental meditation on a measure of self-actualization. *Journal of Coun-
     seling Psychology* 19:184–87.

13. Hjelle, L. A. 1974. Transcendental meditation and psychological health.
     Perceptual and Motor Skills 39:623–28.

14. Goleman, D. J., and G. E. Schwartz. 1976. Meditation as an intervention in
     stress reactivity. *Journal of Consult Clinical Psychology* 44:456–66.

15. Kabat-Zinn, J. 1982. An outpatient program in behavioral medicine for chronic pain patients based on the practice of mindfulness meditation. *General Hospital Psychiatry* 4:33–47.

16. Funch, D. P., and E. N. Gale. 1984. Biofeedback and relaxation therapy for chronic temporomandibular joint pain: predicting successful outcome. *Journal of Consult and Clinical Psychology* 52:928–35.

17. Kabat-Zinn, J., L. Lipworth, and R. Burney. 1985. The clinical use of mindfulness meditation for the self-regulation of chronic pain. *Journal of Behavioral Medical* 8:163–90.

18. Kabat-Zinn, J., and A. Chapman-Waldrop. 1988. Compliance with an outpatient stress reduction program: rates and predictors of program completion. *Journal of Behavioral Medical* 11:333–52.

19. Eppley, K. R., and A. I. Abrams. 1989. Differential effects of relaxation techniques on trait anxiety: a meta-analysis. *Journal of Clinical Psychology* 45: 957–74.

20. Kabat-Zinn, J., A. Massion, et al. 1992. Effectiveness of a meditation-based stress reduction program in the treatment of anxiety disorders. *American Journal of Psychiatry* 149:936–43.

21. Eisenberg, D. M., T. L. Delbanco, et al. 1993. Cognitive behavioral techniques for hypertension: are they effective? *Annals of Internal Medicine* 118:964–72.

22. Domar, A. D., M. M. Seibel, and H. Benson. 1990. The mind/body program for infertility: a new behavioral treatment approach for women with infertility. *Fertility and Sterility* 53:246–49.

23. Benson, H. 1975. *The Relaxation Response.* New York: Morrow.

24. Goleman, D. 1977. *The Varieties of the Meditative Experience.* New York: Dutton.

25. Riegel, B., D. Simon, et al. Submitted for publication 1997. *Teaching Ayurvedic and Western Health Promotion Strategies to Healthy Adults.*

26. For a beautiful visual journey of the relationship between the microcasm and macrocasm of life, see *The Powers of Ten Video* by Charles and Ray Eames. 1989. Pyramid Film and Video, Santa Monica, Calif. (800) 421-2304.

CHAPTER 6: ACCESSING THE INNER PHARMACY THROUGH THE DOORS OF PERCEPTION

1. DeCaspar, A. J., and W. P. Fifer. 1980. Of human bonding: newborns prefer their mother's voice. *Science* 208:1174–76.

2. Lind, J., V. Vuorenkoshi, and O. Wasz-Hockert. 1972. The effect of cry stimulus on the temperature of the lactating breast of primipara. In *Psychosomatic Medicine in Obstetrics and Gynaecology*, 293–95. Basel, Switzerland: S. Karger.

3. Gottlieb, G. 1968. Prenatal behavior of birds. *Quarterly Review of Biology* 43:148–74.

4. Marwick, C. 1996. Leaving the concert hall for clinic: therapists now test music "charms." *Journal of The American Medical Association* 275:267–68.

5. Allen, K., and J. Blascovich. 1994. Effects of music on cardiovascular reactivity among surgeons. *Journal of American Medical Association* 272:882–84.

6. Field, T. M., S. M. Schanberg, et al. 1986. Tactile/kinesthetic stimulation effects on preterm neonates. *Pediatrics* 77:654–58.

7. Spencer-Booth, Y., and R. A. Hinde. 1967. The effects of separating rhesus monkey infants from their mothers for six days. *Journal of Child Psychology Psychiatry* 7:179–97.

8. Nerem, R. M., M. J. Levesque, and J. F. Cornhill. 1980. Social environment as a factor in diet-induced atherosclerosis. *Science* 208:1475–76.

9. Blakemore C., and G. F. Cooper. 1970. Development of the brain depends on the visual environment. *Nature* 228:477–78.

10. MacFarlane, A. 1975. Olfaction in the development of social preferences in the human neonate. In *Parent-Infant Interaction*, 103–17. Amsterdam: Ciba Foundation Symposium 33, Elsevier Publishing Company.

CHAPTER 7: HEALING BREATH AND NEUROMUSCULAR INTEGRATION FOR OPTIMAL FITNESS

General References

1. Rama, S., R. Ballentine, and A. Hymes. 1979. *Science of Breath.* Honesdale, Pa.: Himalayan Institute.

2. Douillard, J. 1995. *Body, Mind and Sport.* New York: Crown.

3. Feuerstein, G., and S. Bodian. 1993. *Living Yoga—A Comprehensive Guide for Daily Life.* New York: Jeremy Tarcher/Putnam.

4. Johari, H. 1989. *Breath, Mind and Consciousness.* Rochester, Vt.: Destiny Books.

5. Satchidananda, S. 1970. *Integral Hatha Yoga.* New York: Henry Holt.

6. Iyenger, B. K. S. 1976. *Light on Yoga.* New York: Schocken Books.

7. Desikackar, T. K. V. 1995. *The Heart of Yoga.* Rochester, Vt.: Inner Traditions International.

Yoga Videos

1. *Yoga Journal's Yoga.* 1992. Healing Arts, Venice, Calif. (800) 254-8464.

2. *Lilias Alive With Yoga.* 1990. Goldhil Media, Thousand Oaks, Calif. (805) 495-0735.

3. *Gentle Yoga.* 1994. Himalayan Institute, Honesdale, Pa. (800) 822-4547.

4. *Hatha Yoga.* 1989. Timeless Books, Spolkane, Wash. (509) 838-6652.

CHAPTER 8: FOOD AS MEDICINE

1. White, R., and E. Frank. 1994. Health effects and prevalence of vegetarianism. *Western Journal of Medicine* 160:465–71.

General References

1. Banchek, L. 1992. *Cooking for Life: Ayurvedic Recipes for Good Food and Health.* New York: Harmony Books.

2. Cousens, G. 1992. *Conscious Eating.* Patagonia, Ariz.: Vision Books.

3.   Lad, U., and V. Lad. 1994. *Ayurvedic Cookbook for Self-Healing.* Albuquerque, N.M.: Ayurvedic Press.

4.   Morningstar, A., and U. Dersai. 1991. *The Ayurvedic Cookbook.* Twin Lakes, Wisc.: Lotus Light.

5.   Murray, M. T. 1993. *The Healing Power of Foods.* Rocklin, Calif.: Prima Publishing.

6.   Bragg, G., and D. Simon. 1997. *Celebrating Nourishment.* New York: Random House.

CHAPTER 9: THE WISDOM OF HERBS

1.   Farnsworth, N. R., and D. D. Soejarto. 1985. Potential consequence of plant extinction in the United States on the current and future availability of prescription drugs. *Economic Botany* 39:231–40.

2.   Farnsworth, N. R., and R. W. Morris. 1976. Higher plants—the sleeping giant of drug development. *American Journal of Pharmacy* 147:46–52.

3.   Balandrin, M. F., J. A. Klocke, et al. 1985. Natural plant chemicals: sources of industrial and medicinal materials. *Science* 228:1154–60.

4.   Kohli, R. P., P. R. Dua, et al. 1967. Some essential effects of an essential oil of apium graveolens linn. *Indian Journal of Medical Research* 55:1099–1102.

5.   Kapoor, L. D. 1990. *Handbook of Ayurvedic Medicinal Plants.* Boca Raton, Fla.: CRC Press.

6.   Mowrey, D. B., and D. E. Clayson. 1982. Motion sickness, ginger and psychophysics. *The Lancet* 1:655–57.

7.   Gupta, L. P., S. P. Sen, and K. N. Udupa. 1976. Pharmacognostical and pharmacological studies on terminalia arjuna. *Journal of Research Indian Medicine, Yoga and Homeopathy* 11:4.

8.   Wagner, H., and H. Norr. 1992. Plant drugs with adaptogenic activity. *Winterhoff Zeitschrift fur Phytotherapie* 13:42–54.

9.   Chopra, R. N., and P. De. 1930. The action of sympathomimetic alkaloids in sida cordifolia. *Indian Journal of Medicine* 18:467.

10. Dhar, M. L., M. M. Dhar, et al. 1968. Screening of Indian plants for biological activity. *Indian Journal of Experimental Biology* 6:232.

11. Ramaswamy, A. S., S. M. Pariyswami, and N. Basu. 1970. Pharmacological studies of C. Asiatica Linn. *Journal Research of Indian Medicine* 4:160–75.

12. Chopra, R. N., S. L. Nayer, and I. C. Chopra. 1956. *Glossary of Indian Medicinal Plants.* New Delhi, India: Council of Scientific and Industrial Research.

13. Das, D., R. C. Sharma, and R. B. Arora. 1973. Antihyperlipidaemic activity of fraction a of commiphora mukul in monkeys. *Indian Journal of Pharmacology* 5:283.

14. Satyavati, G. V., M. K. Raina, and M. Sharma. 1976. *Medicinal Plants of India,* vol. 1. New Delhi, India: Indian Council on Medical Research.

15. Subahrmanyan, V., V. Sreenivasamurthy, et al. 1957. Studies on the antibacterial activity of spices. *Journal of Science Indian Research* 16 (section C):240.

16. Arora, R. B., M. Singh, and C. Kanta. 1962. Tranquilizing activity of jatamansone, a sesquiterpene from nardostachys jatamansi. *Life Science* 6:225.

17. Nath, C., G. P. Gupta, et al. 1981. Study of anti-Parkinsonian activity of seed of mucuna prurita hook. *Indian Journal of Pharmacology* 13:94.

18. Chander, R., Y. Dwivedi, et al. 1990. Evaluation of hepatoprotective activity of picroliv (from Picrorhiza kurroa) in mastomys natalensis infected with plasmodium berghei. *Indian Journal of Medical Research* 92:34–37.

19. Klein, A. D., and N. S. Penneys. 1988. Aloe vera. *Journal of American Academy Dermatology* 18:714–20.

20. Rao, A. R., S. Sukumar, et al. 1969. Study of anti-viral activity of tender leaves of Margosa tree (Melia asadirachta) on vissinia and variola virus. *Indian Journal of Medical Research* 57:495–502.

21. Grover, G. S., and J. T. Rao. 1977. Investigations on the antimicrobial efficiency of essential oils from ocimum sanctum and ocimum gratissimim. *Perfum Kosmet* 57:326.

22. Epstein, M. T., R. A. Espiner, et al. 1977. Effect of eating licorice on the renin-angiotensin aldosterone axis in normal subjects. *British Medical Journal* 1:488–90.

General References:

1. Dash, B. 1991. *Materia Medica of Ayurveda*. New Delhi, India: B. Jain Publishers.

2. Kapoor, L. D. 1990. CRC *Handbook of Ayurvedic Medicinal Plants*. Boca Raton, Fla.: CRC Press.

3. Lad, V., and D. Frawley. 1986. *The Yoga of Herbs*. Santa Fe, N.M.: Lotus Press.

4. Mabey, R. 1988. *The New Age Herbalist*. New York: Collier Books.

5. Mowrey, D. B. 1986. *The Scientific Validation of Herbal Medicine*. New Canaan, Conn.: Keats Publishing.

6. Patnaik, N. 1993. *The Garden of Life*. New York: Doubleday.

7. Ray, P., and H. N. Gupta. 1980. *Caraka Samhita*. New Delhi, India: Indian National Science Academy.

8. Tierra, M. 1988. *Planetary Herbology*. Santa Fe, N.M.: Lotus Press.

9. Tyler, V. E. 1993. *The Honest Herbal*. Binghamton, N.Y.: Pharmaceutical Products Press.

CHAPTER 10: UNDERSTANDING BIOLOGICAL RHYTHMS: THE KEYS TO BALANCE

1. Reichlin, S. 1992. Neuroendocrinology. In *William Textbook of Endocrinology*, 8th ed., ed. J. D. Wilson and D. W. Foster. 167–82. Philadelphia: W. B. Saunders.

2. Sturtevant, R. P., F. M. Sturtevant, et al. 1978. Chronopharmacokinetics of ethanol: Variation in rate of ethanolemia decay in human subjects. *International Journal of Clinical Pharmacology* 16:594–99.

3. Reinberg, A. 1992. Circadian changes in psychological effects of ethanol. *Neuropsychopharmacology* 7:149–56.

4. Mills, J. N. 1966. Human circadian rhythms. *Physiological Reviews* 46:128–71.

5. Aschoff, J. 1965. Circadian rhythms in man. *Science* 148:1427–32.

6. Scheving, L. E., J. E. Pauly, et al. 1983. Chronobiology of cell prolifera-tion—implications for cancer chemotherapy. In *Biological Rhythms and Medicine,* ed. A. Reinberg and M. H. Smolensky, 79–130. New York: Springer-Verlag.

7. Focan, C. 1995. Circadian rhythms and cancer chemotherapy. *Pharmacology and Therapeutics* 67:1–52.

8. Cavanagh, J. R. 1969. Rhythm of sexual desire in women. *Medical Aspects Human Sexuality* 3:29–39.

9. Labrecaque, G., and M. C. Vanier. 1995. Biological rhythms in pain and in the effects of opioid analgesics. *Pharmacology and Therapeutics* 68:129–47.

10. Palmer, J. D. 1976. Human rhythms. In *An Introduction to Biological Rhythms,* 173. New York: Academic Press.

11. Palmer, J. D. 1976. Introduction to biological rhythms, their properties, and clock control. In *An Introduction to Biological Rhythms,* 1–3. New York: Academic Press.

12. Hunt, N. 1992. Seasonal affective disorder. *British Journal of Hospital Medicine* 48:245–49.

13. Czeisler, C. A. 1995. The effect of light on the human circadian pace-maker. In *Circadian Clocks and Their Adjustment,* Ciba Foundation Sympo-sium 183, 254–302. Chichester, England: Wiley and Sons.

14. Kraft, M., and R. J. Martin. 1995. Chronobiology and chronotherapy in medicine. *Disease-A-Month* 41:501–75.

15. Bjarnason, G. A. 1995. Chronobiology—implications for cancer chemother-apy. *Acta Oncologica* 34:615–24.

16. Smaaland, R. S., O. D. Laerum, et al. 1991. Deoxyribonucleic acid (DNA) synthesis in human bone marrow is circadian stage dependent. *Blood* 12: 2603–11.

CHAPTER 11: DETOXIFICATION, PURIFICATION, AND REJUVENATION

General References:

1. Devaraj, T. L. 1986. *The Panchakarma Treatment of Ayurveda.* Mysore, India: Dhanvantari Oriental Publications.

2. Joshi, S. 1997. *An Introduction to Ayurveda and Panchakarma.* Santa Fe, N.M.: Lotus Press.

CHAPTER 12: RESPONSIBILITY, COMPASSION, AND FREEDOM

General References:

1. Das, R., and P. Gorman. 1985. *How Can I Help?* New York: Knopf.

2. Kornfield, J. 1993. *A Path With Heart.* New York: Bantam Books.

3. Dalai Lama. 1984. *Kindness, Clarity, and Insight.* Ed. J. Hopkins and E. Napper. Ithaca, N.Y.: Snow Lion Publications.

CHAPTER 13: PSYCHONEUROIMMUNOLOGY—MIND, BODY, AND IMMUNITY

1. Angell, M. 1985. Disease as a reflection of the psyche. *New England Journal of Medicine* 312:1570–72.

2. Renoux, G., and M. Renoux. 1992. The positive regulation of T-cells by the neocortex is likely to involve a dopamine pathway. In *Psychoneuroimmunology,* ed. H. Schmoll, U. Tewes, and N. P. Plotnikoff, 39–47. Lewiston, N.Y.: Hogrefe and Huber Publishers.

3. Nossal, G. J. V. 1993. Life, death and the immune system. *Scientific American* 269:52–62.

4. Cannon, W. B. 1932. *The Wisdom of the Body.* New York: Norton Press.

5. Selye, H. 1978. *The Stress of Life.* 2d ed. New York: McGraw-Hill.

6. Felten, S. Y., and D. L. Felten. 1991. Innervation of lymphoid tissue. In *Psychoneuroimmunology,* ed. R. Ader, D. L. Felten, and N. Cohen, 27–69. San Diego: Academic Press.

7. Besedovsky, H. O., and A. Del Rey. 1991. Physiological implications of the immune-neuro-endocrine network. In *Psychoneuroimmunology,* ed. R. Ader, D. L. Felten, and N. Cohen, 589–608. San Diego: Academic Press.

8. Ader, R. 1975. Behaviorally conditioned immunosuppression. *Psychosomatic Medicine* 37:333–42.

9. Shibata, H., R. Fujiwara, et al. 1992. Restoration of immune function by olfactory stimulation with fragrance. In *Psychoneuroimmunology,* ed. H. Schmoll, U. Tewes, and N. P. Plotnikoff, 161–71. Lewiston, N.Y.: Hogrefe and Huber Publishers.

10. Kiecolt-Glaser, J. K., R. Glaser, et al. 1986. Modulation of cellular immunity in medical students. *Journal of Behavioral Medicine* 9:5–21.

11. Kiecolt-Glaser, J. K., W. Garner, et al. 1984. Psychosocial modifiers of immunocompetence in medical students. *Psychosomatic Medicine* 46:7–14.

12. Cohen, S., and D. A. J. Tyrell. 1991. Psychological stress and susceptibility to the common cold. *New England Journal of Medicine* 325:606–12.

13. Linn, M. W., B. S. Linn, and J. Jensen. 1984. Stressful life events, deysphoric mood and immune responsiveness. *Psychological Reports* 54:219–22.

14. Kiecolt-Glaser, J. K., L. Fisher, et al. 1987. Marital quality, marital disruption and immune function. *Psychosomatic Medicine* 49:13–34.

15. Kiecolt-Glaser, J. K., J. R. Dura, et al. 1991. Spousal caregivers of dementia victims: longitudinal changes in immunity and health. *Psychosomatic Medicine* 53:345–62.

16. Helsing, K. J., M. Szklo, and G. W. Comstock. 1981. Factors associated with mortality after widowhood. *American Journal of Public Health* 71:802–9.

17. Persky, V. W., J. Kempthorne-Rawson, and R. B. Shekelle. 1987. Personality and risk of cancer: twenty-year follow-up of the Western Electric study. *Psychosomatic Medicine* 49:435–49.

18. Kiecolt-Glaser, J. K., and R. Glaser, et al. 1985. Psychosocial enhancement of immunocompetence in a geriatric population. *Health Psychology* 4:25–41.

19. Antoni, M. H. 1991. Psychosocial stressors and behavioral interventions in gay men with HIV-1 infection. *International Review of Psychiatry* 3:383–99.

20. Pennebaker, J. W., J. K. Kiecolt-Glaser, and R. Glaser. 1988. Disclosures of traumas and immune function: health implications for psychotherapy. *Journal of Consulting and Clinical Psychology* 56:239–45.

21. Cousins, N. 1979. *Anatomy of An Illness as Perceived by the Patient.* New York: W. W. Norton.

22. Fry, W. F. 1992. The physiologic effects of humor, mirth and laughter. *Journal of The American Medical Association* 267:1857–58.

23. Ziegler, J. 1995. Immune system may benefit from the ability to laugh. *Journal of National Cancer Institute* 87:342–43.

24. Spiegel, D., J. R. Bloom, et al. 1989. Effect of psychosocial treatment on survival of patients with metastatic breast cancer. *The Lancet* 2:888–91.

25. Fawzy, F., N. Cousins, et al. 1990. A structured psychiatric intervention for cancer patients. *Archives of General Psychiatry* 47:720–25.

26. Fawzy, F., N. Cousins, et al. 1990. A structured psychiatric intervention for cancer patients (phase-two): changes over time in immunological measures. *Archives of General Psychiatry* 47:729–35.

27. Salk, J. 1983. *Anatomy of Reality—Merging of Intuition and Reason.* New York: Columbia University Press.

CHAPTER 14: MIND BODY INTERACTIONS IN DIGESTIVE DISORDERS

1. Furness, J. B., and M. Costa. 1980. Types of nerves in the entire nervous system. *Neuroscience* 5:1–20.

2. Brooks, F. P. 1983. Central nervous system and the digestive tract. In *Functional Disorders of the Digestive Tract,* ed. W. Y. Chey, 21–27. New York: Raven Press.

3. Dockray, G. J., and D. H. Walsh. 1994. Regulatory Peptide Systems of the Gut. In *Gut Peptides: Biochemistry and Physiology,* ed. G. J. Dockray and D. H. Walsh, 1–9. New York: Raven Press.

4. Smith, G. P., and J. Gibbs. 1985. The satiety effect of cholecystokinin: recent program and current problems. *Annals of The New York Academy of Science* 448:417–23.

5. Stengaard-Pedersen, K., and L. I. Larsson. 1981. Localization and opiate receptor binding of enkephalin, CCK and ACTH / β-endorphin in the rat central nervous system. *Peptides* 2:3–19.

6. Dockray, G. J. 1994. Vasoactive intestinal polypeptide and related peptides. In *Gut Peptides: Biochemistry and Physiology,* ed. G. J. Dockray and D. H. Walsh, 447–72. New York: Raven Press.

7. Bienenstock, J., and A. P. Befus. 1985. The gastrointestinal tract as an immune organ. In *Gastrointestinal Immunity for the Clinician,* ed. J. B. Kirsner and R. G. Shorter, 1–22. Orlando, Fla.: Grune and Stratton.

8. Andersen, L. P., and H. Nielsen. 1993. Peptic ulcer: an infectious disease? *Annals of Medicine* 25:563–68.

9. Thompson, W. G., and K. W. Heaton. 1980. Functional bowel disorders in apparently healthy people. *Gastroenterology* 79:283–88.

10. Sandler, R. S. 1990. Epidemiology of irritable bowel syndrome in the United States. *Gastroenterology* 99:409–15.

11. Kirsner, J. B. 1983. Foreword to *Functional Disorders of the Digestive Tract*, ed. W. Y. Chey, xvii–xix. New York: Raven Press.

12. Sullivan, M. A., S. Cohen, and W. Snape. 1978. Colonic myoelectrical activity in irritable bowel syndrome. *New England Journal of Medicine* 298:878–83.

13. Mayer, E. A., and H. E. Raybould. 1990. Role of visceral afferent mechanisms in functional bowel disorders. *Gastroenterology* 99:1688–1704.

14. Phillips, S. F., N. J. Talley, and M. Camilleri. 1992. The irritable bowel syndrome. In *Motility Disorders of the Gastrointestinal Tract*, ed. S. Anuras, 299–326. New York: Raven Press.

15. Drossman, D. A., D. C. McKee, et al. 1988. Psychosocial factors in irritable bowel syndrome. *Gastroenterology* 95:701–8.

16. Klein, K. B. 1988. Controlled treatment trials in the irritable bowel syndrome: a critique. *Gastroenterology* 95:232–41.

17. Whorwell, P. J., A. Prior, and E. B. Faragher. 1984. Controlled trial of hypnotherapy in the treatment of severe, refractory irritable bowel syndrome. *The Lancet* 2:1232–34.

18. Whorwell, P. J., A. Prior, and S. M. Colgan. 1987. Hypnotherapy in severe irritable bowel syndrome: further experience. *Gut* 28:423–25.

19. Harvey, R. F., R. A. Hinton, et al. 1989. Individual and group hypnotherapy in treatment of refractory irritable bowel syndrome. *The Lancet* 1:424–25.

CHAPTER 15: MIND BODY INTERACTIONS IN DIABETES

1. Ratner, R. E. 1992. Overview of diabetes mellitus. In *Management of Diabetes Mellitus*, ed. D. Haire-Joshe, 3–20. St. Louis, Mo.: Mosby Year Book.

2. Carter Center of Emory University. 1995. Closing the gap: the problem of diabetes in the United States. *Diabetes Care* 8:391–406.

3. The Diabetic Control and Complications Trial Research Group. 1993. The effect of intensive treatment of diabetes on the development and prognosis of long-term complications in insulin-dependent diabetes mellitus. *New England Journal of Medicine* 329:977–86.

4. Brief, D. J., and J. D. Davis. 1984. Reduction of food intake and body weight by chronic intraventricular insulin infusion. *Brain Research Bulletin* 12:571–75.

5. LeRoith, D., W. Lowe, et al. 1985. Insulin Receptors in the Brain. In *Neural and Endocrine Peptides and Receptors*, ed. T. E. Moody, 289–98. New York: Plenum Press.

6. Surwit, R. S., M. N. Feinglos, et al. 1984. Behavioral manipulation of the diabetic phenotype in ob/ob mice. *Diabetes* 33:616–18.

7.   Capponi, R., M. E. Kawada, et al. 1980. Diabetes mellitus by repeated stress in rats bearing chemical diabetes. *Hormone and Metabolic Research* 12: 411–12.

8.   Surwit, R. S., J. A. McCubbin, et al. 1990. Glycemic reactivity to stress: a biologic marker for development of type 2 diabetes? *Diabetes* 39 (supplement):8A.

9.   Bhishagratna, K. K. 1981. *An English Translation of The Sushruta Samhita.* Varanasi, India: Chokhamba Sanskrit Series Office.

10.   Wilkinson, G. 1987. The influence of psychiatric, psychological and social factors on the control of insulin dependent diabetes mellitus. *Journal of Psychosomatic Research* 31:277–96.

11.   Cox, D. J., A. G. Taylor, et al. 1984. The relationship between psychological stress and insulin dependent diabetic blood glucose control: preliminary investigations. *Health Psychology* 3:63–75.

12.   Turkat, I. D. 1982. Glycosylated hemoglobin levels in anxious and non-anxious diabetic patients. *Psychosomatics* 23:1056–58.

13.   Delamater, A. M., S. M. Kurtz, et al. 1987. Stress and coping in relations to metabolic control of adolescents with type-one diabetes. *Journal of Developmental and Behavioral Pediatrics* 8:136–40.

14.   Frenzel, M. P., K. D. McCaul, et al. 1988. The relationship of stress and coping to regimen adherence and glycemic control of diabetes. *Journal of Social and Clinical Psychology* 6:77–87.

15.   Kuttner, M. J., A. M. Delamaater, and J. V. Santiago. 1990. Learned helplessness in diabetic youths. *Journal of Pediatric Psychology* 15:581–94.

16.   Marcus, M. D., and R. R. Wing. 1990. Eating disorders and diabetes. In *Neuropsychological and Behavioral Aspects of Diabetes,* ed. C. S. Holmes, 102–121. New York: Springer-Verlag.

17.   Rosenbaum, L. 1983. Biofeedback-assisted stress management for insulin-treated diabetes mellitus. *Biofeedback and Self-Regulation* 8:519–32.

18.   Lammers, C. A., B. D. Naliboff, and A. J. Straatmeyer. 1984. The effects of progressive relaxation on stress and diabetic control. *Behavioral Research Therapy* 22:641–50.

19.   McGrady, A., B. K. Bailey, and M. P. Good. 1991. Controlled study of biofeedback-assisted relaxation in type-one diabetes. *Diabetes Care* 14: 360–65.

20.   Bailey, B. K., M. Good, and A. McGrady. 1990. Clinical observations on behavioral treatment of a patient with insulin-dependent diabetes mellitus. *Biofeedback and Self-Regulation* 15:7–13.

21.   Surwit, R. S., and M. N. Feinglos. 1983. The effects of relaxation of glucose tolerance in non-insulin dependent diabetes. *Diabetes Care* 6:176–79.

22.   Lane, J. D., C. C. McCaskill, et al. 1993. Relaxation training for NIDDM. *Diabetes Care* 16:1087–94.

23.   Boardway, R. H., and A. M. Delamater, et al. 1993. Stress management training for adolescents with diabetes. *Journal of Pediatric Psychology* 18: 29–45.

24. Guthrie, D., T. Moeller, and R. Guthrie. 1983. Biofeedback and its application to the stabilization and control of diabetes mellitus. *American Journal of Clinical Biofeedback* 2:82–87.

25. Rice, B. I., and J. V. Schindler. 1992. Effect of thermal biofeedback–assisted relaxation training on blood circulation in the lower extremities of a population with diabetes. *Diabetes Care* 15:853–58.

26. Shulimson, A. D., P. F. Lawrence, and C. V. Iacono. 1986. The effect of thermal biofeedback-mediated relaxation training on healing. *Biofeedback and Self Regulation* 4:311–19.

27. Perri, M. G., A. M. Nezu, and B. J. Viegener. 1992. The effectiveness of treatment for obesity. In *Improving the Long-Term Management of Obesity*, ed. M. G. Perri, A. M. Nezu, and B. J. Viegener, 53–78. New York: John Wiley and Sons.

CHAPTER 16: MIND BODY INTERACTIONS IN HEART DISEASE

1. *1993 Heart and Stroke Facts Statistics.* 1994. Dallas: American Heart Association.

2. Preston, T. A. 1989. Assessment of coronary bypass surgery and percutaneous transluminal coronary angioplasty. *International Journal of Technical Assessment Health Care* 5:431–42.

3. Dawber, T. R., C. F. Meadors, and F. E. Moore. 1951. Epidemiological approaches to heart disease: the Framingham study. *American Journal of Public Health* 41:279–90.

4. Fielding, J. E. 1984. Smoking: health effects and control. *New England Journal of Medicine* 313:491–96, 555–61.

5. Bellin, L. J. 1988. Non-pharmacological control of blood pressure. *Clinical Experimental Pharmacology Physiological* 15:215–33.

6. Resnicow, K., J. Barone, et al. 1991. Diet and serum lipids in vegan vegetarians: a model for risk reduction. *Journal of The American Diet Association* 91:447–53.

7. Keen, H., and B. Thomas. 1988. Diabetes mellitus. In *Nutrition in the Clinical Management of Diseases*, 2d ed. J. W. T. Dickerson and H. A. Lee, 167–90. London: Edward Arnold.

8. Multiple risk factor intervention trial. 1982. *Journal of The American Medical Association* 248:1465–71.

9. Keys, A., C. Aravinis, et al. 1972. Probability of middle-aged men developing coronary heart disease in five years. *Circulation* 45:815–28.

10. Gordon, T., M. R. Garcia-Palmieri, et al. 1974. Differences in coronary heart disease in Framingham, Honolulu and Puerto Rico. *Journal of Chronic Diseases* 27:329–44.

11. Friedman, M., and R. H. Rosenman. 1959. Association of specific overt behavior patterns with blood and cardiovascular findings: blood cholesterol level, blood clotting time, incidence of arcus senilis and clinical coronary artery disease. *Journal of The American Medical Association* 169:1286–96.

12. Harvey W. 1963. De motu cordis, 1628. In *Three Hundred Years of Psychiatry*, ed. R. Hunter and D. MacAlpine, page 130. London: Oxford University Press.

13. Burns, J. W., and E. Katkin. 1993. Psychological, situational and gender predictions of cardiovascular reactivity to stress: a multivariate approach. *Journal of Behavioral Medical* 16:445–65.

14. Ellwood, P., S. Renaud, et al. 1991. Ischaemic heart disease and platelet aggregation: the caerphilly collaborative heart disease study. *Circulation* 83:38–44.

15. Schneiderman, N. 1983. Animal behavior models of coronary heart disease. In *Handbook of Psychology and Health*, vol. 3, ed. D. S. Krantz, A. Baum, and J. E. Singer, 19–56. Hillsdale, N.J.: Lawrence Erlbaum Associates.

16. Celsus, 30 A. D. Quoted in J. C. Buell and R. S. Eliot, 1979: Stress and cardiovascular disease. *Modern Concepts of Cardiovascular Disease* 4:19–24.

17. Charaka. 1981. *Charaka Samhita*, vol. 1, Chapter XXX, trans. P. V. Sharma. Varanasi, India: Chaukhambha Orientalia.

18. Rosenman, R. H., R. J. Brand, et al. 1975. Coronary heart disease in the western collaborative group study. *Journal of The American Medical Association* 233:872–77.

19. Matthews, K. A., and S. G. Haynes. 1986. Type-A behavior and coronary disease risk. *American Journal of Epidemiology* 123:923–60.

20. Ragland, D. R., and R. J. Brand. 1988. Type-A behavior and mortality from coronary heart disease. *New England Journal of Medicine* 318:65–69.

21. Shekelle, R. B., S. B. Halley, et al. 1985. The MRFIT behavior pattern study. *American Journal of Epidemiology* 122:559–70.

22. Williams, R. B., T. L. Haney, et al. 1980. Type-A behavior, hostility and coronary atherosclerosis. *Psychosomatic Medical* 42:539–49.

23. Shelkelle, R. B., M. Gale, et al. 1983. Hostility, risk of coronary heart disease and mortality. *Psychosomatic Medicine* 45:109–114.

24. Barefoot, J. C., W. G. Dahlstrom, and R. B. Williams. 1983. Hostility, CHD incidence and total mortality: a twenty-five-year follow-up study of two hundred and fifty-five physicians. *Psychosomatic Medicine* 45:59–63.

25. Barefoot, J. C., K. A. Dodge, et al. 1989. The cook-medley hostility scale: item content and ability to predict survival. *Psychosomatic Medicine* 51:46–57.

26. Dembroski, T. M., J. M. MacDougall, et al. 1989. Components of hostility as predictors of sudden death and myocardial infarction in the multiple risk factor intervention trial. *Psychosomatic Medicine* 51:514–22.

27. Smith, T. W. 1992. Hostility and health: current status of a psychosomatic hypothesis. *Health Psychology* 11:139–50.

28. Roskies, E. 1983. Modification of coronary risk behavior. In *Handbook of Psychology and Health*, vol. 3, ed. D. S. Krantz, A. Baum, J. E. Singer, 231–76. Hillsdale, N.J.: Lawrence Erlbaum Associates.

29. Allison, T. G., D. E. Williams, et al. 1995. Medical and economic costs of psychologic distress in patients with coronary artery disease. *Mayo Clinic Proceedings* 70:734–42.

30. Goodman, M., J. Quigley, et al. 1996. Hostility predicts restonosis after percutaneous transluminal coronary angioplasty. *Mayo Clinic Proceedings* 71:729–34.

31. O'Keefe, J. H., R. D. Conn, et al. 1996. The new paradigm for coronary artery disease: altering risk factors, atherosclerotic plaques, and clinical prognosis. *Mayo Clinic Proceedings* 71:957–65.

32. Berkman, L. F., and S. L. Syme. 1979. Social networks, host resistance and mortality: a nine-year follow-up study of Alameda County residents. *American Journal of Epidemiology* 109:186–204.

33. Frasure-Smith, N., and R. Prince. 1985. The ischemic heart disease life stress monitoring program: impact on mortality. *Psychosomatic Medicine* 47:431–45.

34. Williams, R., J. C. Barefoot, et al. 1992. Prognostic importance of social and economic resources among medically treated patients with angiographically documented coronary artery disease. *Journal of The American Medical Association* 276:520–24.

35. Case, R. B., A. J. Moss, et al. 1992. Living alone after myocardial infarction. *Journal of The American Medical Association* 267:515–19.

36. Medalie, J. H., and U. Goldbourt. 1976. Angina pectoris among ten thousand men. *American Journal of Medicine* 60:910–21.

37. Sales S. M., and J. House. 1971. Job dissatisfaction as a possible risk factor in coronary heart disease. *Journal of Chronic Disease* 23:861–73.

38. Kornitzer, M., F. Kittel, et al. 1982. Job stress and coronary heart disease. *Advances in Cardiology* 29:56–61.

39. Karasek, R., D. Baker, et al. 1981. Job decision latitude, job demands and cardiovascular disease: a prospective study of Swedish men. *American Journal of Public Health* 71:694–705.

40. Karasek, R., T. G. Theorell, et al. 1982. Job, psychological factors and coronary heart disease. *Advances in Cardiology* 29:62–67.

41. Rabkin, S. W., F. A. L. Mathewson, and R. B. Tate. 1980. Chronobiology of cardiac sudden death in men. *Journal of The American Medical Association* 244:1357–58.

42. Kolata, G. 1986. Heart attacks at 9:00 A.M. *Science* 233:417–18.

43. Muller, J. E., P. L. Ludmer, et al. 1987. Circadian variation in the frequency of sudden cardiac death. *Circulation* 75:131–38.

44. Arntzenius, A. C., D. Kromhout, et al. 1985. Diet, lipoproteins and the progression of coronary atherosclerosis—the Leiden intervention trial. *New England Journal of Medicine* 312:805–11.

45. Ornish, D., S. E. Brown, et al. 1990. Can lifestyle changes reverse coronary heart disease? The lifestyle heart trial. *The Lancet* 336:129–33.

46. Lappe, F. M. 1991. *Diet for a Small Planet*. New York: Ballantine Books.

47. De Lorgeril, M., S. Renaud, et al. 1994. Mediterranean alpha-linolenic acid-rich diet in secondary prevention of coronary heart disease. *The Lancet* 343:1454–59.

48. Knekt, P., A. Reunanen, et al. 1994. Antioxidant vitamin intake and coronary mortality in a longitudinal population study. *American Journal of Epidemiology* 139:1180–89.

49. Watts, G. F., B. Lewis, et al. 1992. Effects on coronary artery disease of lipid-lowering diet, or diet plus cholestyramine, in the St. Thomas' atherosclerosis regression study. *The Lancet* 339:563–69.

50. Thomas, C. B., and F. F. Eisenberg. 1957. Observations on the variability of total serum cholesterol in Johns Hopkins medical students. *Journal of Chronic Diseases* 6:1–32.

51. Thomas, C. B., and E. A. Murphy. 1958. Further studies on cholesterol levels in the Johns Hopkins medical students: the effect of stress at examinations. *Journal of Chronic Diseases* 8:661–68.

52. Nerem, R. M., M. J. Levesque, and J. F. Cornhill. 1980. Social environment as a factor in diet-induced atherosclerosis. *Science* 208:1475–76.

53. Crichton, M. 1988. *Travels.* New York: Knopf.

CHAPTER 17: MIND BODY INTERACTIONS IN CANCER

1. Boring, C. C., T. S. Squires, and T. Tong. 1993. Cancer statistics. *California Cancer Journal Clinical* 43:7–26.

2. Mettlin, C., F. Lee, et al. 1991. The American Cancer Society national prostate cancer detection project. *Cancer* 67:2949–58.

3. Miller, B. A., E. J. Feuer, and B. F. Hankey. 1993. Recent incidence trends for breast cancer in women and the relevance of early detection: an update. *California Cancer Journal Clinical* 43:27–41.

4. Scheffler, R. M., and N. L. Andrew, ed. 1989. *Cancer Care and Cost.* Ann Arbor, Mich.: Health Administration Press Perspectives.

5. Bried, E. M., and R. M. Scheffler. 1992. The financial stages of cancer in the elderly. *Oncology* 6 (supplement):153–60.

6. Cassileth, B. R., E. J. Lusk, et al. 1984. Contemporary unorthodox treatments in cancer medicine. *Annals of International Medical* 101:105–12.

7. Cassileth, B. R. 1986. Unorthodox cancer medicine. *Cancer Investigation* 4:591–98.

8. Selye, H. 1978. *The Stress of Life.* 2d ed. New York: McGraw-Hill.

9. Riley, V., and D. H. Sparkman. 1977. Housing stress. *Lab Animal* 6:16–21.

10. Riley, V., M. A. Fitsmaurice, and D. H. Spackman. 1981. Psychoneuroimmunologic factors in neoplasia: studies in animals. In *Psychoneuroimmunology,* ed. R. Ader, 31–102. New York: Academic Press.

11. Ader, R. 1975. Behaviorally conditioned immunosuppression. *Psychosomatic Medicine* 37:333–42.

12. Bovnjerg, D. H., and W. H. Redd. 1992. Anticipatory nausea and immune suppression in cancer patients receiving cycles of chemotherapy: conditioned responses. In *Psychoneuroimmunology,* ed. H. Schmoll, U. Tewes, et al., 237–50. Lewiston, N.Y.: Hogrefe and Huber Publishers.

13. Shelkelle, R. B., W. J. Raynor, et al. 1981. Psychological depression and the seventeen-year risk of cancer. *Psychosomatic Medicine* 43:117–25.

14. Kiecolt-Glaser, J. K., L. Fisher, et al. 1987. Marital quality, marital disruption and immune function. *Psychosomatic Medicine* 49:13–34.

15. Kiecolt-Glaser, J. K., S. Kennedy, et al. 1988. Marital discord and immunity in males. *Psychosomatic Medicine* 50:213–29.

16. Persky, V. W., J. Kempthorne-Rawson, and R. B. Shelkelle. 1987. Personality and risk of cancer: twenty-year follow-up of the Western Electric study. *Psychosomatic Medicine* 49:435–49.

17. Greer, S., and T. Morris. 1975. Psychological attributes of women who develop breast cancer: a controlled study. *Journal of Psychosomatic Research* 19:147–53.

18. Kneier, A. W., and L. Temoshok. 1984. Repressive coping reactions in patients with malignant melanoma as compared to cardiovascular disease patients. *Journal of Psychosomatic Research* 28:145–55.

19. Temoshok, L., B. W. Heller, et al. 1985. The relationship of psychosocial factors to prognostic indicators in cutaneous malignant melanoma. *Journal of Psychosomatic Research* 29:139–53.

20. Temoshok, L. 1987. Personality, coping style, emotion and cancer: towards an integrative model. *Cancer Survival* 6:545–67.

21. Cassileth, B., E. J. Lusk, et al. 1985. Psychosocial correlates of survival in advanced malignant disease. *New England Journal of Medicine* 312:1551–55.

22. Jamison, R. N., T. G. Burish, and K. A. Walston. 1987. Psychogenic factors in predicting survival of breast cancer patients. *Journal of Clinical Oncology* 5:768–72.

23. Holland, J. C. 1990. Behavioral and psychosocial risk factors in cancer: human studies. In *Handbook of Psychooncology*, ed. J. C. Holland and J. H. Rowland, 705–26. New York: Oxford University Press.

24. U.S. Department of Health and Human Services. 1982. *The Health Consequences of Smoking: Cancer. A Report of the Surgeon General*. USDHHS, PHS, DHHS publ. no. 82-50179. Washington, D.C.: United States Government Printing Office.

25. Higginson, J., and M. J. Sheridan. 1991. Nutrition and human cancer. In *Cancer and Nutrition*, ed. R. B. Alfin-Slater and D. Kritchvesky, 1–5. New York: Plenum Press.

26. Turjman, N., G. T. Goodman, et al. 1984. Diet, nutrition intake and metabolism in populations at high and low risk for colon cancer: metabolism of bile acids. *American Journal of Clinical Nutrition* 40 (supplement): 937–41.

27. White, R., and E. Frank. 1994. Health effects and prevalence of vegetarianism. *Western Journal of Medicine* 160:465–71.

28. Bloom, J. 1982. Social support, accommodation to stress and adjustment to breast cancer. *Social Science Medical* 16:1329–38.

29. Nealing, S., and H. Winefield. 1988. Social support and recovery after surgery for breast cancer: frequency and correlates of supportive behaviors by family, friends and surgeon. *Social Science Medical* 27:385–92.

30. Berkman, L., and S. L. Syme. 1979. Social networks, host resistance and mortality: a nine-year follow-up study of Alameda county residents. *American Journal of Epidemiology* 109:186–204.

31. Bloom, J. R., and D. Spiegel. 1984. The relationship of two dimensions of social support to the psychological well being and social functioning of women with advanced breast cancer. *Social Science Medical* 19:831–37.

32. Holland, J. C., and S. Lewis. 1993. Emotions and cancer: what do we really know. In *Mind/Body Medicine,* ed. D. Goleman, and J. Gurin, 85–110. New York: Consumer Reports Books.

33. Waxler-Morrison, N., T. G. Hislop, et al. 1991. Effects of social relationships on survival for women with breast cancer: a prospective study. *Social Science Medical* 33:177–83.

34. Fawzy, F. I., M. E. Kemeny, et al. 1990. A structured psychiatric intervention for cancer patients (phase-two): changes over time in immunologic measures. *Archives of General Psychiatry* 47:729–35.

35. Fawzy, F. I., N. W. Fawzy, et al. 1993. Malignant melanoma: effects of a structured psychiatric intervention, coping and affective state on recurrence and survival six years later. *Archives of General Psychiatry* 50:681–89.

36. Richardson, J. L., D. R. Shelton, et al. 1990. The effect of compliance with treatment on survival among patients with hematologic malignancies. *Journal of Clinical Oncology* 8:356–64.

37. Spiegel, D., J. R. Bloom, et al. 1989. Effect of psychosocial treatment on survival of patients with metastatic breast cancer. *The Lancet* 2:888–91.

38. Spiegel, D. 1993. *Living Beyond Limits.* New York: Times Books.

CHAPTER 18: MIND BODY INTERACTIONS IN REPRODUCTION AND PREGNANCY

1. Herzog A. 1992. The Neuroendocrine Basis of Infertility. In *Technology and Infertility,* ed. M. M. Seibel, J. Bernstein, et al., 213–22. New York: Springer-Verlag.

2. Domar, A. D., and M. M. Seibel. 1990. Emotional aspects of infertility. In *Infertility—A Comprehensive Text,* ed. M. M. Seibel, 23–35. Norwalk, Conn.: Appleton and Lange.

3. Seibel, M. M., and M. L. Taymor. 1982. Emotional aspects of infertility. *Fertility and Sterility* 37:137–45.

4. Burden, H. W., and I. E. Lawrence. 1977. The effect of denervation on compensatory ovarian hypertrophy. *Neuroendocrinology* 23:367–78.

5. Edwards, R. 1980. The female reproductive tract. In *Conception in the Human Female,* ed. R. Edwards, 416–524. London: Academic Press.

6. Dunkel-Schetter, C., and M. Lobel. 1991. Psychological reactions to infertility. In *Infertility—Perspectives from Stress and Coping Research,* ed. A. L. Stanton, and C. Dunkel-Schetter, 29–57. New York: Plenum Press.

7. Moghisi, K. S., and E. E. Wallach. 1983. Unexplained infertility. *Fertility and Sterility* 391:5–16.

8. McGrady, A. V. 1984. Effects of psychological stress on male reproduction: a review. *Archives of Andrology* 131:1–10.

9. Giblin, P. T., M. L. Poland, et al. 1988. Effects of stress and characteristic adaptability on semen quality in healthy men. *Fertility and Sterility* 49:127–32.

10. Palti, Z. 1969. Psychogenic male infertility. *Psychosomatic Medicine* 31:326–30.

11. Alonso-Uriarte, R., I. Sojo-Aranda, and V. Cortes-Gallegos. 1991. Role of stress in male fertility. *Archives of Invest Medical* 22:223–28.

12. Stoleru S., J. P. Teglas, et al. 1993. Psychological factors in the aetiology of infertility: a prospective cohort study. *Human Reproduction* 8:1039–46.

13. Rodriguez, B., L. Bermudez, et al. 1983. The relationship between infertility and anxiety: some preliminary findings. Presented at the Second World Congress of Behavior Therapy, Washington, D.C., December 8–11.

14. Domar, A. D., M. M. Seibel, and H. Benson. 1990. The mind/body program for infertility: a new behavioral treatment approach for women with infertility. *Fertility and Sterility* 53:246–49.

15. Domar, A. D., P. C. Zuttermeister, et al. 1992. Psychological improvement in infertile women after behavioral treatment: a replication. *Fertility and Sterility* 58:144–47.

16. Rue, J., and R. K. Burke. 1991. Participation in a support group improves pregnancy success rates in infertile couples. *American Association of Gynaecologic Laparoscopists: Twentieth Annual Meeting Abstracts,* 183. Las Vegas, Nev.: The American Association of Gynaecologic Laparoscopists.

17. Blomberg, S. 1980. Influence of maternal distress during pregnancy on fetal malformations. *Acta Psychiatrica Scandinavica* 62:315–30.

18. Seibel, M., and J. A. McCarthy. 1993. Infertility, pregnancy and the emotions. In *Mind/Body Medicine,* ed. D. Goleman, and J. Gurin, 214. New York: Consumer Reports Books.

19. Bradley, R. M., and C. M. Mistretta. 1975. Fetal sensory receptors. *Physiology Reviews* 55:352–82.

20. Langman, J. 1990. Ear. In *Medical Embryology,* 6th ed., 328–37. Baltimore: Williams and Wilkins.

21. Goodlin, R. C., and W. Schmidt. 1972. Human fetal arousal levels as indicated by heart rate recordings. *American Journal of Obstetrics Gynecology* 114:613–21.

22. Goodlin, R. C. 1979. The fetus as a person. In *Care of the Fetus,* 1–13. New York: Masson Publishing.

23. Ando, Y., and H. Hattori. 1977. Effects of noise on human placental lactogen levels in maternal plasma. *British Journal of Obstetrics Gynecology* 84:115–18.

24. Schell, L. M. 1982. The effects of chronic noise exposure on human prenatal growth. In *Human Growth and Development,* ed. J. Borms, R. Haupsie, et al., 125–29. New York: Plenum Press.

25. Gottlieb, G. 1968. Prenatal behavior of birds. *Quarterly Review of Biology* 43:148–74.

26. Vince, M. A. 1969. Embryonic communication, respiration and the synchronization of hatching. In *Bird Vocalizations,* ed. R. A. Hinde, 233–60. London: Cambridge University Press.

27. Verny, T., and J. Kelly. 1981. *The Secret Life of the Unborn Child.* New York: Dell Publishing.

28. Ibuka, M. 1991. Remarkable abilities of fetuses and newborn babies. In *Behavioral Development of Human Fetus and Neonates,* ed. N. Kobayashy and M. Ibuka, 9–10. Farmington, Conn.: S. Karger.

29. Salam, M. Z., and R. D. Adams. 1966. New horizons in the neurology of childhood. *Perspectives in Biology and Medicine.* (Spring) 384–410.

30. Natsuyama, E. 1991. In utero behavior of human embryos at the spinal-cord stage of development. In *Behavioral Development of Human Fetus and Neonates,* ed. N. Kobayashy and M. Ibuka, 11–29. Farmington, Conn.: S. Karger.

31. Liley, A. 1971. The fetus as a personality. *The Australian and New Zealand Journal of Psychiatry* 6:99–105.

32. Smyth, C. N. 1965. Exploratory methods for testing the integrity of fetus and neonate. *Journal of Obstetrics and Gynecology of the British Commonwealth* 72:920–25.

33. Kooi, K. A., R. P. Tucker, and R. E. Marshall. 1978. Spontaneous electrical activity of the normal brain. In *Fundamentals of Electroencephalography,* ed. K. A. Kooi, R. P. Tucker, and R. E. Marshall, 49–66. Hagerstown, Md.: Harper and Row.

34. Sontag, L. W. 1970. Parental determinants of postnatal behavior. In *Fetal Growth and Development,* ed. H. A. Weisman and G. R. Kerr, 265. New York: McGraw-Hill.

CHAPTER 19: MIND BODY INTERACTIONS IN WOMEN'S HEALTH—MENSTRUATION AND MENOPAUSE

1. Smith, S., and I. Schiff. 1989. The premenstrual syndrome—diagnosis and management. *Fertility and Sterility* 52:527–43.

2. Hammaarback, S., and J. E. Damber. 1989. Relationship between symptoms severity and hormone changes in women with premenstrual syndrome. *Journal of Clinical Endocrinology and Metabolism* 68:125–30.

3. Watts, J. F. F., W. R. Butt, et al. 1985. Hormonal studies in women with premenstrual tension. *British Journal of Obstetrics and Gynecology* 92:247–55.

4. Steinberg, S. 1991. The treatment of late luteal phase dysphoric disorder. *Life Science* 49:767–802.

5. Budoff, P. W. 1987. Use of prostaglandin inhibitors in the treatment of premenstrual syndrome. *Clinical Obstetrics Gynecology* 30:453–64.

6. Barr, W. 1984. Pyridoxine supplements in the premenstrual syndrome. *Practitioner* 228:425–27.

7. Kendall, K. E., and P. P. Schnurr. 1987. The effects of vitamin B-6 supplementation on premenstrual syndrome. *Obstetrics Gynecology* 70:145–49.

8. Malmgren, R., A. Collins, and C. Nilsson. 1987. Platelet serotonin uptake and effects on vitamin B-6 treatment in premenstrual tension. *Neuropsychobiology* 18:83–88.

9. Williams, M. J., R. Harris, and B. Dean. 1985. Controlled trial of pyridoxine in the premenstrual syndrome. *Journal of Internal Medicine Research* 13:174–79.

10.   Rapkin, A. J., E. Edelmuth, et al. 1987. Whole-blood serotonin in premenstrual syndrome. *Obstetrics Gynecology* 70:533–37.

11.   Veeninga, A. T., and G. H. M. Westenberg. 1990. Serotonergic function and late luteal phase dysphoric disorder. *Psychopharmacology* 102:414–16.

12.   Rickels, K., E. W. Freeman, et al. 1990. Fluoxetine in the treatment of premenstrual syndrome. *Current Therapeutic Research* 48:161–66.

13.   Sundblad C., K. Modigh, et al. 1992. Clomopramine effectively reduces premenstrual irritability and dysphoria—a placebo controlled trial. *Acta Psychiatr Scand* 85:39–47.

14.   Taylor D., N. F. Woods, et al. 1991. Perimenstrual negative affect: development and testing of an explanatory model. In *Menstruation, Health and Illness*, ed. D. L. Taylor and N. F. Woods, 103–18. New York: Hemisphere.

15.   Gallant S. J., D. A. Popiel, et al. 1992. Using daily ratings to confirm premenstrual syndrome/late luteal phase dysphoric disorder, one and two. *Psychosomatic Medicine* 54:149–81.

16.   Graham, C. A., and B. B. Sherwin. 1987. The relationship between retrospective premenstrual symptom reporting and oral contraceptive use. *Journal of Psychosomatic Research* 31:45–53.

17.   Graham, C. A., and B. B. Sherwin. 1992. A prospective treatment study of premenstrual symptoms using triphasic oral contraceptive. *Journal Psychosomatic Research* 36:257–66.

18.   Freeman, E. W., K. Rickesl, et al. 1990. Ineffectiveness of progesterone suppository treatment for premenstrual syndrome. *Journal of The American Medical Association* 264:349–53.

19.   Corney, R. H., R. Stanton, et al. 1990. Comparison of progesterone, placebo and behavioral psychotherapy in the treatment of premenstrual syndrome. *Journal of Psychosomatics Obstetrics Gynecology* 11:211–20.

20.   Rossignol, A. M., and H. Bonnlander. 1991. Prevalence and severity of the premenstrual syndrome: effects of food and beverages that are sweet or high in sugar content. *Journal of Reproductive Medicine* 36:131–36.

21.   Boyd, N. F., P. Shannon, et al. 1988. Effect of a low-fat high-carbohydrate diet on symptoms of cyclical mastopathy. *The Lancet* 1:128–32.

22.   Rossignal, A. M. 1985. Caffeine-containing beverages and premenstrual syndrome in young women. *American Journal of Public Health* 75:1335–37.

23.   Abraham, G. E., and J. T. Hargrove. 1980. Effect of vitamin B-6 on premenstrual symptomatology in women with premenstrual tension syndromes: a double-blind crossover study. *Infertility* 3:155–65.

24.   London, R. S., L. Murphy, et al. 1987. Efficacy of alpha-tocopherol in the treatment of premenstrual syndrome. *Journal of Reproductive Medicine* 32:400–404.

25.   Thys-Jacobs, S., S. Ceccarelli, et al. 1989. Calcium supplementation in premenstrual syndrome: a randomized crossover trial. *Journal of General Internal Medicine* 4:183–89.

26.   Facchinetti, F., P. Borella, et al. 1991. Oral magnesium successfully relieves premenstrual mood changes. *Obstetrics Gynecology* 78:177–81.

27. Paddison, D. L., L. H. Gise, et al. 1988. Premenstrual syndrome and sexual abuse. *American Psychiatric Association Abstracts* 35:73.

28. Chandraiah, S., J. L. Levenson, and J. B. Collins. 1991. Sexual dysfunction, social maladjustment and psychiatric disorders in women seeking treatment in a premenstrual syndrome clinic. *International Journal of Psychiatry in Medicine* 21:189–204.

29. Margolis, A. 1985. The use of cognitive restructuring intervention in the treatment of premenstrual syndrome: a controlled study. *Dissertation Abstracts International* 47:381

30. Morse, C. A., L. Dennerstein, et al. 1991. A comparison of hormone therapy, coping skills training and relaxation for the relief of premenstrual syndrome. *Journal of Behavioral Medicine* 14:469–89.

31. Goodale, I. L., A. D. Domar, and H. Benson. 1990. Alleviation of premenstrual syndrome symptoms with the relaxation response. *Obstetrics Gynecology* 75:649–55.

32. Slade, P. 1989. Psychological therapy for premenstrual emotional symptoms. *Behavioral Psychotherapy* 17:135–50.

33. Timonen, S., and B. Procopé. 1971. Premenstrual syndrome and physical exercise. *Acta Obstetrica et Gynecologica Scandinavica* 50:331–37.

34. Prior, J. C., and Y. Vigna. 1987. Conditioning exercise and premenstrual syndrome. *Journal of Reproductive Medicine* 32:423–28.

35. Lemon, D. 1991. The effects of aerobic training on women who suffer from premenstrual syndrome. *Dissertation Abstracts International* 52:563.

36. Kaufert, P. A., M. Lock, et al. 1994. Menopause as a normal physiological event or as a disease. In *Comprehensive Management of Menopause*, ed. J. Lorrain, 59–65. New York: Springer-Verlag.

37. Lock, M., P. Kaufert, and P. Gilbert. 1988. Cultural construction of the menopausal syndrome: the Japanese case. *Maturitas* 10:317–32.

38. Eiken, P., and N. Kolthoff. 1995. Compliance with long-term oral hormonal replacement therapy. *Maturitas* 22:97–103.

39. Wren, B. G., and L. Brown. 1991. Compliance with hormonal replacement therapy. *Maturitas* 13:17–21.

40. Redi, D., D. Torgerson, et al. 1996. Randomized trial of perimenopausal screening for osteroporosis risk: effect on HRT uptake and quality of life. *Journal of Bone Mineral Research,* 11(supplemental 1):S109.

41. Weiss, N. C., C. L. Ure, et al. 1980. Decreased risks of fractures of the hip and lower forearm with post-menopausal use of estrogen. *New England Journal of Medicine* 303:1195–98.

42. Writing Group for the Post Menopausal Estrogen and Progestin Intervention Trail. 1996. Effects of hormone therapy on bone mineral density. *Journal of The American Medical Association* 276:1389–96.

43. Speroff, L., J. Rowan, et al. The comparative effect on bone density, endometrium, and lipid of continuous hormones as replacement therapy. *Journal of The American Medical Association* 276:1397–1403.

44. Grodstein, F., and M. J. Stampfer. 1995. The epidemiology of coronary heart disease and estrogen replacement. *Progress Cardiovascular Disease* 38:199–210.

45. Gallagher, J. C., B. S. Hulka, et al. 1996. Why HRT Makes Sense. *Patient Care,* August 15, 166–92.

46. Reid, A. R., R. W. Ames, et al. 1993. Effect of calcium supplementation on bone loss in postmenopausal women. *New England Journal of Medicine* 328:460–64.

47. Barzel, U. S. 1996. Osteoporosis: taking a fresh look. *Hospital Practice,* May 15, 59–68.

48. Ross, P. D. 1996. Osteoporosis. *Archives of Internal Medicine* 156:1399–1411.

49. Nelson, M. E., M. A. Fiatarone, et al. 1994. Effects of high-intensity strength training on multiple risk factors for osteoporotic fractures. *Journal of The American Medical Association* 272:1909–14.

50. Adlercreutz, H., E. Hamalainen, et al. 1992. Dietary phyto-oestrogens and the menopause in Japan. *The Lancet* 339:1233.

51. Knight, D. C., and J. A. Eden. 1996. A review of the clinical effects of phytoestrogens. *Obstetrics and Gynecology* 87:897–904.

CHAPTER 20: MIND BODY INTERACTIONS IN FATIGUE AND CHRONIC PAIN

1. Cox, B., M. Blaxter, et al. 1987. *The Health and Lifestyle Survey.* London: Health Promotion Research Trust.

2. Kroenke, K., D. R. Wood, et al. 1988. Chronic fatigue in primary care. *Journal of The American Medical Association* 260:929–34.

3. Cobb, I. 1920. *A Manual of Neurasthenia (Nervous Exhaustion).* London: Balliere, Tindall and Cox.

4. Beard, G. 1881. *American Nervousness.* New York: GP Putnam's.

5. Ferrier, D. 1911. Neurasthenia and Drugs. *Practitioner* 86:11–15.

6. Rabinbaach, A. 1982. The body without fatigue: a nineteenth century utopia. In *Political Symbolism in Modern Europe: Essays in Honor of George Mosse,* ed. S. Drescher, D. Sabean, and A. Sharlin, 42–62. London: Transaction Books.

7. Browning, W. 1911. Is there such a disease as neurasthenia? A discussion and classification of the many conditions that appear to be grouped under that head. *New York State Journal of Medicine* 11:7–17.

8. Buchwald, D., J. L. Sullivan, and A. L. Komaroff. 1987. Frequency of chronic active Epstein-Barr virus infection in a general medical practice. *Journal of The American Medical Association* 257:2303–7.

9. Kim, E. 1994. A brief history of chronic fatigue syndrome. *Journal of The American Medical Association* 272:1070–71.

10. Jones, J. F., C. G. Ray, et al. 1985. Evidence for active Epstein-Barr virus infection in patients with persistent, unexplained illness: elevated anti-early antigen antibodies. *Annals of Internal Medicine* 107:1–7.

11. Straus, S. E., G. Tosato, et al. 1985. Persisting illness and fatigue in adults with evidence of Epstein-Barr virus infections. *Annals of Internal Medicine* 107:7–16.

12. Buchwald, D., and A. L. Komaroff. 1991. Review of laboratory findings for patients with chronic fatigue syndrome. *Review Infectious Diseases* 13: S12–18.

13. Klimas, N., F. Salvato, et al. 1990. Immunologic abnormalities in chronic fatigue syndrome. *Journal of Clinical Microbiology* 28:1403–10.

14. Chao, C. C., E. N. Janoff, et al. 1991. Altered cytokine release in peripheral blood mononuclear cell cultures from patients with the chronic fatigue syndrome. *Cytokine* 3:292–98.

15. Homes, G. P., J. E. Kaplan, et al. 1988. Chronic fatigue syndrome: a working case definition. *Annals of Internal Medicine* 108:387–89.

16. Komaroff, A. L., and A. Geiger. 1989. Does the Center for Disease Control working case definition of chronic fatigue identify a distinct group? *Clinical Research* 37:778A.

17. Katon, W. J., D. S. Buchwald, et al. 1990. Psychiatric illness in patients with chronic fatigue and rheumatoid arthritis. *Journal of General Internal Medicine* 6:277–85.

18. Bou-Holaigh, I., P. C. Rowe, et al. 1995. The relationships between neurally mediated hypotension and chronic fatigue syndrome. *Journal of The American Medical Association* 274:961–67.

19. Cope, H., and A. S. David. 1996. Neuroimaging in chronic fatigue syndrome. *Journal of Neurology Neurosurgery Psychiatry* 60:471–73.

20. Ware, N. C. 1988. An anthropological approach to understanding chronic fatigue syndrome. In *Chronic Fatigue Syndrome*, ed. S. E. Straus, 85–97. New York: Marcel Dekker.

21. Straus, S. E., J. K. Dale, et al. 1988. Acyclovir treatment of the chronic fatigue syndrome: lack of efficacy in a placebo-controlled trial. *New England Journal of Medicine* 319:1692–98.

22. Dismukes, S. E., J. S. Wade, et al. 1990. A randomized, double-blind trial of nystatin for the candidiasis hypersensitivity syndrome. *New England Journal of Medicine* 323:1717–23.

23. Gracious, B., and K. L. Wisner. 1991. Nortriptyline in chronic fatigue syndrome: a double-blind placebo-controlled single case study. *Biological Psychiatry* 30:405–408.

24. Goldstein, J. A. 1986. Cimetidine, ranitidine, and Epstein-Barr virus infection. *Annals of Internal Medicine* 105:139.

25. Lloyd, A., I. Hickie, et al. 1990. A double-blind placebo-controlled trial of intravenous immunoglobulin therapy in patients with chronic fatigue syndrome. *American Journal of Medicine* 89:561–68.

26. Behan, P. O., W. M. H. Behan, and D. Horrobin. 1990. Effects of high doses of essential fatty acids on the post-viral fatigue syndrome. *Acta Neurologica Scandinavica* 82:209–16.

27. Gantz, N. M. 1991. Magnesium and chronic fatigue. *The Lancet* 338:66.

28. Vercoulen, J. H., C. M. Swanink, et al. 1996. Prognosis in chronic fatigue syndrome: a prospective study on the natural course. *Journal of Neurology Neurosurgery Psychiatry* 60:489–94.

29. Sharpe, M., K. Hawton, et al. 1996. Cognitive behaviour therapy for the chronic fatigue syndrome: a randomized controlled trial. *British Medical Journal* 312:22–26.

30. Buchwald, D., J. Blair, and P. Mease. 1991. Treatment of chronic fatigue syndrome with acupuncture. *International Journal of Clinical Acupuncture* 2:231–36.

31. McCluskey, D. R., and M. S. Riley. 1992. Chronic fatigue syndrome. *Comprehensive Therapies* 18:13–16.

32. Marcus, N. J. and J. M. D. Norman. 1994. *Freedom from Chronic Pain*. New York: Simon and Schuster.

33. Kabat-Zinn, J., L. Lipworth, and R. Burney. 1985. The clinical use of mindfulness meditation for the self-regulation of chronic pain. *Journal of Behavioral Medicine* 8: 163–90

34. Kabat-Zinn, J. 1982. An outpatient program in behavioral medicine for chronic pain patients based on the practice of mindfulness meditation. *General Hospital Psychiatry* 4:33–47.

35. Nigl, A. J. 1984. *Biofeedback and Behavioral Strategies in Pain Treatment*. Jamaica, N.Y.: Spectrum Publications.

36. Orne, M. T. 1992. Non-pharmacological approaches to pain relief: hypnosis, biofeedback, placebo effect. In *Evaluation and Treatment of Chronic Pain*, 2d ed., ed. G. M. Aronoff, 430–39. Baltimore: Williams and Wilkins.

37. National Institutes of Health Technology Assessment Panel. 1996. Integration of behavioral and relaxation approaches into the treatment of chronic pain and insomnia. *Journal of The American Medical Association* 276:313–18.

38. Osler, W. 1904. *Principles and Practice of Medicine*. New York: Appleton.

39. Lewith, G. T., and D. Machine. 1983. On the evaluation of the clinical effects of acupuncture. *Pain* 16:111–27.

General Ayurvedic References

1. Adhikari, N. D. 1978. *Lessons from the Ayurveda*. Washington, Miss.: New Jaipur Press.

2. Bhishagratna, K. K. 1981. *The Sushruta Samhita*. Vols. 1, 2 and 3. Varanasi, India: Chowkhamba Sanskrit Series Office.

3. Dash, B. 1978. *Fundamentals of Ayurvedic Medicine*. Delhi, India: Bansal and Company.

4. Dash, B. 1992. *Massage Therapy in Ayurveda*. New Delhi, India: Concept Publishing.

5. Dash, B. 1991. *Materia Medica of Ayurveda*. New Delhi, India: B. Jain Publishers.

6.   Dash B., and L. Kashyap. 1980. *Basic Principles of Ayurveda.* New Delhi, India: Concept Publishing.

7.   Dash B., and M. M. Junius. 1983. *A Handbook of Ayurveda.* New Delhi, India: Concept Publishing.

8.   Devaraj, T. L. 1980. *The Panchakarma Treatment of Ayurveda.* Bangalore, India: Dhanvantari Oriental Publications.

9.   Dutt, U. C. 1993. *Materia Medica of the Hindus.* Calcutta, India: Krishnadas Sanskrit Studies.

10. Frawley, D. 1989. *Ayurvedic Healing—A Comprehensive Guide.* Salt Lake City, Utah: Passage Press.

11. Heyn, B. 1990. *Ayurveda—The Indian Art of Natural Medicine and Life Extension.* Rochester, Vt.: Healing Arts Press.

12. Joshin, S. 1996. *Ayurveda and Panchakarma.* Twin Lakes, Wis.: Lotus Press.

13. Kapoor, L. D. 1990. *Handbook of Ayurvedic Medicinal Plants.* Boca Raton, Fla.: CRC Press.

14. Lad, V. 1984. *Ayurveda—The Science of Self-Healing.* Santa Fe, N.M.: Lotus Press.

15. Lee, R. D. 1986. *Ayurveda and Modern Medicine.* Bombay, India: Bharatiya Vidya Bhavan.

16. Lonsdorf, N., V. Butler, and M. Brown. 1993. *A Woman's Best Medicine.* New York: Putnam.

17. Murthy, N. A., and D. P. Pandey. 1982. *Ayurvedic Cure for Common Diseases.* New Delhi, India: Orient Paperbacks.

18. Patnaik, N. 1993. *The Garden of Life.* New York: Doubleday .

19. Priyadaranjan, R., and H. N. Gupta. 1965. *Caraka Samhita—A Scientific Synopsis.* New Delhi, India: Indian National Science Academy.

20. Ranade, S. 1993. *Natural Healing Through Ayurveda.* Salt Lake City, Utah: Passage Press.

21. Rhyner, H. H. 1994. *Ayurveda—The Gentle Health System.* New York: Sterling Publishing.

22. Ros, F. 1994. *The Lost Secrets of Ayurvedic Acupuncture.* Twin Lakes, Wisc.: Lotus Press.

23. Sachs, M. 1994. *Ayurvedic Beauty Care.* Twin Lakes, Wisc.: Lotus Press.

24. Sharma, P. 1983. *Caraka-Samhita.* Vols. 1 and 2. Delhi, India: Chaukhamba Orientalia.

25. Srikantamurthy, K. R. 1993. *Clinical Methods in Ayurveda.* Varanasi, India: Chaukhambha Orientalia.

26. Svoboda, R. E. 1992. *Ayurveda—Life, Health and Longevity.* London: Arkana Penguin Books.

27. Svoboda, R. E. 1988. *Prakruti: Your Ayurvedic Constitution.* Albuquerque, N.M.: Geocom Limited.

28. Tiwari, M. 1995. *Ayurveda—Secrets of Healing.* Twin Lakes, Wisc.: Lotus Press.

Index

About the Author

Dr. David Simon has had a lifelong interest in healing. In his undergraduate college years, he majored in anthropology, where his primary focus was on the role of the healer in non-Western cultures. He became intrigued by the *shaman,* or medicine man, whose purpose was to help those with emotional or physical suffering reestablish health through the integration of body, mind, and spirit. As scientific information on altered states of consciousness and meditation emerged, he became engrossed in understanding the interaction between the mind and brain.

After graduating medical school from the University of Chicago, David received training in internal medicine and neurology, while continuing to explore his interest in holistic and consciousness-based medicine. Upon completion of his residency and fellowship, Dr. Simon opened a neurology practice in San Diego with a focus on neurophysiology and brain injury. In addition to his role as medical director for the neurological and neurorehabilitation services at Sharp Cabrillo Hospital, Dr. Simon served two years as chief of the medical staff.

Dr. Simon's association with Dr. Deepak Chopra began in 1986 when he participated in an Ayurvedic training program sponsored by the American Association of Ayurvedic Medicine, of which

Dr. Chopra was president. Their relationship developed over the years, leading to a shared vision of creating a program to bring the principles of mind body medicine into the health-care mainstream.

In 1993, they opened their program in San Diego, dedicated to providing health providers and the community with the information and practical approaches of mind body medicine. Since launching this project, Dr. Simon has given numerous presentations to health-care providers, the general public, and the media. He has been instrumental in developing courses with Dr. Chopra, including "Training in Mind Body Medicine for Health Professionals," "The Magic of Healing," "The Seduction of Spirit," "Magical Beginnings, Enchanted Lives," and "Return to Wholeness."

Dr. Simon serves as medical director of The Chopra Center for Well Being in La Jolla, California, overseeing the patient care, research, development, and educational components of the program.

For more information on health-enhancing programs at The Chopra Center for Well Being, and to contact Dr. David Simon, please call 1-888-424-6772.